CANADIAN RED CROSS

Emergency Care

The Canadian Red Cross Society ("CRCS") has made reasonable efforts to ensure the contents of this publication are accurate and reflect the latest in available scientific research on the topic as of the date published. The information contained in this publication may change as new scientific research becomes available. Certain techniques described in this publication are designed for use in lifesaving situations. However, the CRCS cannot guarantee that the use of such techniques will prevent personal injury or loss of life.

The information contained in Chapter 11: Pharmacology, is based on information gathered from a variety of third party sources, such as members of the National Committee on Emergency Medical Care, the National Medical Advisory Committee, and Compendium of Pharmaceuticals and Specialties. The CRCS has made reasonable efforts to ensure that the content of Chapter 11, including drug names and profiles and routes of drug administration, is accurate and conforms to the standards accepted at the time of publication and is provided as information only. However, constant changes in information resulting from continuing research and clinical experience, reasonable differences in opinions among authorities, unique aspects of individual clinical situations, and the possibility of human error in preparing Chapter 11 require that the reader exercise individual judgment when making a clinical decision and, if necessary, consult and compare information from other sources. The CRCS shall not be held liable for any damage arising out of human error or possible omission or inaccuracy of the information contained in Chapter 11.

All the content in Chapter 11 is provided for informational purposes only; it is meant to be used in the context of the CRCS training course on the subject, and it is not to be relied upon for any other purpose. It is the responsibility of the Emergency Medical Responder authorized to provide medical assistance to ascertain the status of each drug, to check the product information provided by the manufacturer of each drug for any changes, and to obtain from the relevant sources or authorities the approved instructions for the administration of drugs. The CRCS does not accept responsibility or liability of any kind whatsoever for the application or use of the information contained in Chapter 11 by any individual in the course of a medical emergency or otherwise.

This publication is available in English and French.

The terms "he" and "she" have been used throughout *Emergency Care* to ensure representation of both genders and to correspond to any photos within a particular section.

Glossary terms are in blue.

Illustrations by Scott Mooney and Jackie Wald
Composition by Tinge Design Studio Inc.

Printed in Canada by:
The StayWell Health Company Ltd.
2 Quebec Street, Suite 107, Guelph, ON N1H 2T3
A part of Krames StayWell Strategic Partnerships Division
780 Township Line Road, Yardley, PA 19067-4200 USA

ISBN: 978-1-58480-560-1

Contents

Acknowledgements

Over the past 65 years, the Canadian Red Cross First Aid Programs have grown and flourished. Each time a program is revised, its foundation is built on the great work completed in the previous revisions. In 1997, the original version of the *First Responder* manual was developed and produced through a joint effort of the American Red Cross and Mosby-Year book Inc. In 2005, the Canadian Red Cross developed an *Emergency Medical Responder Supplement* for the *First Responder* manual, which created the first Canadian Red Cross Emergency Medical Responder Program. The Canadian Red Cross would like to recognize everyone who worked on developing these programs in the past; their hard work and dedication set the foundations for revising and updating these First Responder and Emergency Medical Responder programs.

We would like to thank the American Red Cross for permission to use content from its *Emergency Medical Response* (copyright © 2011 by The American National Red Cross).

There was excellent market research that guided the project's direction and vision. We would like to thank our Training Partners, Instructor Trainers, and Instructors who participated in the market research. Their input and guidance helped shape the look of our programs and products.

This incredible project required the hard work and dedication of the many teams who put in countless hours to contribute to its success. Canadian Red Cross extends its thanks to each team and its members.

The Canadian Red Cross National Medical Advisory Committee (NMAC) reviewed the content of the program and thanks go to Andrew MacPherson, MD, CCFP-EM, and Brendan J. Hughes, MD, CCFP.

The Volunteer Technical Committee members were responsible for developing the technical content and direction that laid the foundation for the program: Nolan Baggett (Newfoundland), Frédérick Beauchamp (Quebec), Jason Brinson (Ontario), Rob Briscoe (British Columbia), Marc R. Côté (Quebec), Ian Fitzpatrick (British Columbia), Lyle Karasiuk (Saskatchewan), Roger Mayo (Ontario), Paul Myroon (Alberta), and Caroline Sparks (Yukon).

The following organizations reviewed the *Emergency Care* text and endorsed the program and we thank them for their valuable contributions: Karen Roche, Canadian Association of Fire Chiefs (CAFC); the Canadian Athletic Therapists Association (CATA); the Canadian Ski Patrol; Philip Groff, PhD, and Jayne Morrish, MA, Parachute; the Paramedic Chiefs of Canada; and Agnes Makowski, MScPT, Sport Physiotherapy Canada (SPC).

The Canadian Association of Fire Chiefs (CAFC) supports the important work of First Responders across Canada and was pleased to review *Emergency Care*.

The Canadian Athletic Therapists Association (CATA) was pleased to review Chapter 13: Musculoskeletal Injuries of *Emergency Care*.

The Canadian Ski Patrol recognizes the importance of First Responder training and was pleased to review *Emergency Care*.

Parachute was pleased to review *Emergency Care* and supports the work of our partners at the Canadian Red Cross.

The Paramedic Chiefs of Canada is pleased to support the important work of the Canadian Red Cross in developing this text.

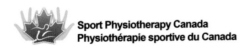

Sport Physiotherapy Canada (SPC) recognizes the unique value of the Canadian Red Cross First Responder program and is proud to support *Emergency Care*.

The Red Cross

In June 1859, Henry Dunant saw an unforgettable scene: 40,000 dead and wounded soldiers left on the field after the Battle of Solferino in Italy. Dunant organized local villagers into first aid teams to help as many of the wounded as possible, saving thousands of lives.

To prevent this horror from happening again, he decided to create a neutral organization to care for wounded soldiers and prisoners—an organization that would be respected and protected by both sides in any conflict. The result was the Red Cross.

Dunant spent the rest of his life trying to reduce the suffering caused by war. He lobbied governments, organized Red Cross Societies in different countries, and spoke to the public. Today, the symbol chosen for the Red Cross is recognized around the world: a red cross on a white background.

In 1901, Dunant won the first Nobel Peace Prize. By founding the International Red Cross and Red Crescent Movement, he has saved the lives of millions of people over the years.

On May 19, 1909, Parliament passed the Canadian Red Cross Society Act, which established the Canadian Red Cross to serve Canadians as an auxiliary to government and the public authority, in accordance with the Geneva Conventions. (Prior to 1909, the Red Cross operated in Canada as a branch of the British Red Cross.) As a result, for more than a century, Canadians have had their own national Red Cross Society dedicated to improving the situations of the most vulnerable people in Canada and around the world.

NOTE:

In December 2005, the International Red Cross and Red Crescent Movement welcomed the decision to create an additional emblem alongside the red cross and red crescent, the red crystal.

The Red Cross—The Fundamental Principles

There are Red Cross or Red Crescent Societies in more than 190 countries around the world. In every country, our programs and activities are guided by seven Fundamental Principles. The Tanzanian Red Cross has created a short, simple version of these principles:

Humanity: We serve people, but not systems.

Impartiality: We care for the victims and the aggressors alike.

Neutrality: We take initiatives, but never take sides.

Independence: We bow to needs, but not rulers.

Voluntary Service: We work around the clock, but never for personal gain.

Unity: We have many talents, but a single idea.

Universality: We respect nations, but our work knows no bounds.

Essentially, we provide help to people in need, whatever their race, political beliefs, religion, social status, or culture.

Henry Dunant

Who We Are—The Canadian Red Cross

Our Mission

The Canadian Red Cross's mission is to improve the lives of vulnerable people by mobilizing the power of humanity in Canada and around the world.

Our Vision

The Canadian Red Cross is the leading humanitarian organization through which people voluntarily demonstrate their caring for others in need.

Our Values

Our actions and decisions are based on:

- Humanitarian values
- Respect, dignity, and care for one another within and outside the Canadian Red Cross
- Integrity, accountability, effectiveness, and transparency

Our Volunteers

Volunteers are the heart of the Canadian Red Cross. More than 25,000 Red Cross volunteers give their time and energy to help others every day. If you are looking for opportunities to give back to your community, meet new people, have new experiences, learn new skills, or develop your professional skills training, volunteering for the Canadian Red Cross is the right choice for you.

How We Help

Disaster Management

The Canadian Red Cross helps people affected by emergencies and disasters. We work with governments and with other humanitarian organizations to meet people's basic needs. We provide food, clothing, shelter, first aid, and emotional support. When families have been separated by disasters, we help bring them back together.

International Operations

The Canadian Red Cross works in other countries to help people who have been affected by wars and natural disasters. We bring urgently needed supplies, reunite families, and help rebuild communities. Each year, we send about 100 professional relief workers on overseas missions.

First Aid Programs

Canadian Red Cross First Aid Programs have been training Canadians in first aid for the past 65 years. Our courses give people the knowledge and skills to deal with emergency situations and prevent injuries from happening.

Swimming and Water Safety Program

Since 1946, more than 32 million Canadians have learned how to swim and safely enjoy water activities with the Canadian Red Cross. Our Red Cross Swim programs are unique because they consider each swimmer's individual needs and offer participants of all abilities and ages (preschool, kids, teens, and adults) opportunities to learn swimming and water-safety skills. Teens and adults can also enjoy aquatic sports and enroll in lifeguarding courses.

RespectED: Violence and Abuse Prevention

Since 1984, in communities across the country, the Canadian Red Cross has been helping to break the cycle of hurt. RespectED: Violence and Abuse Prevention programs promote healthier relationships and safer communities through education and partnerships.

Homecare Services

The Canadian Red Cross provides in-home community services to help individuals in Ontario and Atlantic Canada live as independently as possible. These services enhance people's well-being and dignity, whether they are frail or elderly, children at risk, people with disabilities, or palliative patients.

Health Equipment Loan Programs (HELP)

For more than 50 years, the Canadian Red Cross has been offering Health Equipment Loan Programs (HELP) that allow Canadians throughout much of the country to borrow basic health and mobility devices, such as wheelchairs or walkers. More than 200,000 Canadians use this service each year, lessening the burden on families already coping with injury or illness.

Part *1*

Preparing to Respond

1
The Responder

2
The Emergency Scene

3
Preventing Disease Transmission

The Responder

You are called to the scene at a bathroom in a mall. A man has slipped and fallen on the bathroom floor. The man is breathing but unresponsive. He was found by other mall patrons, who are now upset and concerned. You have been summoned to help. What do you do?

INTRODUCTION

As a responder, you are a key part of the emergency medical services (EMS) system. You provide a link between the first actions of bystanders and more advanced medical care. A responder is a person, paid or volunteer, who is often summoned to provide initial care in an emergency. As the first trained professional on the scene, your actions are often critical. They may determine whether a seriously ill or injured person survives.

According to the Paramedic Association of Canada (PAC), "first responders" may be included within the emergency medical responder (EMR) level, although in many settings, first responders do not transport patients.

According to PAC, the EMR "has successfully completed a recognized training program in emergency patient care and transportation." As part of the foundation of the Canadian emergency systems, EMRs are often linked with volunteer emergency services organizations in rural and remote areas and in some communities may be the sole provider of emergency services.

Responders across the country have different roles to perform, including primary and secondary surveys, the provision of safe and prudent care, effective oral and written communication, and the transport of a patient to the most appropriate healthcare facility. Responders must also learn to recognize the signs of high levels of stress in themselves and their co-workers.

By taking this course, you will gain the knowledge, skills, and confidence to give appropriate care when you are called to help someone who has become injured or suddenly ill. You will learn how to assess a patient's condition and how to recognize and care for life-threatening emergencies. You will also learn how to minimize a patient's discomfort and prevent further complications until you can obtain more advanced medical care as well as the importance of managing critical incident stress.

Components of an EMS System

The EMS system is a network of community resources and medical personnel that provides emergency care to patients with injury or sudden illness. When people at an emergency scene recognize an emergency and take action, they activate this system. The care provided by more highly trained professionals continues until a patient receives the level of care he needs. An effective EMS system includes the following components:

- Communications
- Transportation
- Facilities
- Medical control
- Trauma systems
- Public information and education
- Human resources, training, and continuing education
- Resource management
- Regulation and policy
- Evaluation

EMS systems throughout Canada vary by region and, in many cases, by city. In 2001, PAC, with the support of Human Resources Development Canada and the Canadian Medical Association, established the National Occupational Competency Profiles (NOCPs) to promote national consistency in paramedic training and practice.

Since 1988, PAC (originally The Canadian Society of Ambulance Personnel) has been the national association for paramedics. Its mandate includes:

- Promotion of paramedic self-regulation
- Promotion of a national examination
- Promotion of a national registry for paramedics
- Advocacy for paramedics to be included in the *Canada Health Act*
- Support for paramedic research through the Canadian Emergency Health Services Research Consortium
- Stewardship of the National Occupational Competency Profile for paramedics

Over the past several years, national paramedic stakeholder groups have arisen that share several aspects of PAC's mandate.

In 2002, the Emergency Medical Service Chiefs of Canada (EMSCC) was incorporated as a national forum for information gathering, policy development, and coordinated action by the leadership of Canada's EMS systems. This group works under an operating mission, "To advance and align EMS leadership in Canada."[1]

Canadian Organization of Paramedic Regulators

In 2008, paramedic regulators from across Canada began working together informally "to discuss ways to ensure compliance with the new labour mobility requirements of the Agreement on Internal Trade (AIT) that came in to effect on April 1, 2009." These regulators agreed on a statement of intent that identified a strategy to enable them to achieve AIT compliance in the short term. When it was formed, the Canadian Organization of Paramedic Regulators (COPR) received letters of support from all provincial jurisdictions, and these authorities provide the funding for COPR.

The regulators' initial success with meeting the AIT labour mobility requirements resulted in recognizing that a national organization would benefit a number of initiatives including, but not limited to, labour mobility.

In early 2010, regulators established COPR as a formal organization. "In addition, federal government and provincial labour mobility coordinators recognized the group's innovation and willingness to adapt practices to succeed with labour mobility."

This support—coupled with the group's desire to build upon the initial successes—led them to successfully apply for federal government funding to further their labour mobility work. Also, COPR submitted a set of bylaws to the federal government as part of the process for incorporation.[2]

The Society for Prehospital Educators in Canada (SPEC; rebranded in 2006 from the former Canadian Society of Prehospital Care Educators) is a national group of paramedic educators that "has demonstrated a keen desire to represent paramedic education on a national basis."[3]

The concept of labour mobility is the freedom of workers to practice their occupation wherever opportunities exist.[4] In 2008, with the help of Human Resources and Skills Development Canada, several provincial regulators established a national body of paramedic regulators, whose purpose is "to address national standards within the context of labour mobility. In 2009, the

Canadian Organization of Paramedic Regulators was established."[5]

Today, "for the first time in the field of paramedicine, there is a national perspective representing education, regulation, operations, and professional practice."[6]

Levels of Training for Providers

An EMS system may utilize emergency care providers with many different levels of training. PAC has developed four levels of pre-hospital EMS training: emergency medical responder, primary care paramedic (PCP), advanced care paramedic (ACP), and critical care paramedic (CCP). By meeting minimum competency profiles, EMS systems can attain consistency throughout the country, which will allow for portability and achieving an appropriate standard of professional care.

Medical Control

Certification as a first responder or emergency medical responder is not a licence to perform all the skills in the *Emergency Care* text. These should only be performed if you have been delegated these acts by a physician. Physicians provide medical direction in EMS systems, through a process called medical control. This process allows a physician to direct the care given to patients by pre-hospital care professionals. Usually, a medical director, who assumes responsibility for the care given, does this monitoring.

The medical director also oversees training and the development of protocols (standardized procedures to be followed when providing care to people with illness or injury). Since it is impossible for the medical director to be present at every incident outside the hospital, he can still direct care through standing orders. Standing orders allow responders to provide certain types of care or treatments without consulting the physician. This type of medical control is called indirect or off-line medical control and it includes education, protocol review, and quality improvement of emergency care professionals. Other procedures not covered by standing orders require the responder to speak directly with the physician. This contact can be made via cellphone, radio, or telephone. This kind of medical control is called direct or on-line medical control.

COMPONENTS OF AN EMERGENCY RESPONSE

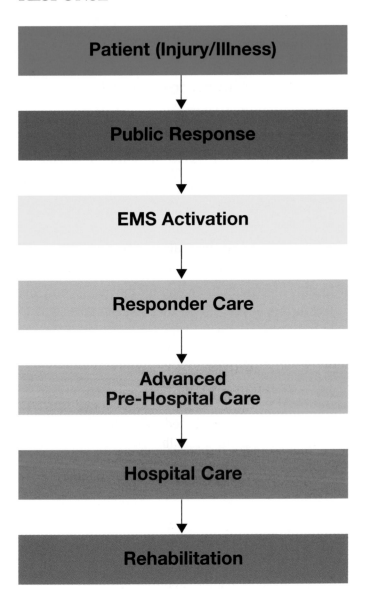

| Patient (Injury/Illness) |
| Public Response |
| EMS Activation |
| Responder Care |
| Advanced Pre-Hospital Care |
| Hospital Care |
| Rehabilitation |

THE EMERGENCY RESPONSE SUPPORTING THE EMS SYSTEM

The survival of a patient depends on all people performing their roles correctly and promptly to make the EMS system work. People must recognize emergencies and quickly get help by activating the system. They must learn what actions to take in the first critical minutes. They must also learn to prevent emergencies and prepare for them. They need to support the EMS system in their community.

When they are summoned, professionals must respond sensitively, quickly, and effectively to emergencies. They must keep their training current and stay abreast of new issues in emergency response. When each component of the system works effectively, this enhances the patient's chances for a full recovery.

So what happens if one of these components breaks down? Since the patient's life may depend on each or all of these components, a break can cause serious consequences.

For instance, if a person does not recognize a life-threatening emergency, such as the early signals of a heart attack, and does not quickly call EMS personnel, the patient may not live. Poor information given to the EMS dispatcher may delay advanced medical care. Improper care of the patient before more advanced medical care is obtained can result in the patient's condition worsening, possibly leading to permanent disability or death.

In a serious injury or illness, survival and recovery are not a matter of chance. Survival results from a carefully orchestrated continuum of events in which all participants fulfill their roles. The EMS system can make the difference between life and death or a partial or full recovery. You as a responder play a critical role in this system.

THE RESPONDER

Responders, unlike lay people, are more likely to respond to the scene of a medical emergency and to provide emergency medical care to a patient while on duty. They should have ready access to supplies and equipment for providing care until more advanced medical care is obtained. More advanced medical care refers to someone with a higher level of training, who takes over the care of the patient.

Some occupations, such as law enforcement and firefighting, require personnel to respond to and assist at the scene of an emergency. These personnel are dispatched through an emergency number, such as 9-1-1 or the local EMS number, and often share common communication networks. When a person dials 9-1-1 or the local EMS number, he will contact police, fire, or ambulance personnel. These are typically considered public safety personnel. However, responders do not necessarily work in public safety agencies. People in many other occupations are called to help in the event of an injury or sudden illness, for example:

- Athletic therapists
- Disaster team members
- Emergency management personnel
- First aid station attendants
- Industrial safety personnel
- Ski patrol members
- Workplace first aid attendants

As a responder, you have a duty to quickly and safely respond to the scene of an emergency. Your duty is also to assess the patient's condition and provide necessary care, act as the patient's advocate, make sure that any necessary additional help has been summoned, assist other medical personnel at the scene, and document your actions.

Personal Characteristics

As an emergency care provider who deals with the public, you must be willing to take on responsibilities beyond giving care. These responsibilities require you to demonstrate certain characteristics that include:

- *Maintaining a caring and professional attitude.*

  Patients are sometimes difficult to work with. Be compassionate; try to understand their concerns and fears. Realize that any anger a patient may show is often the result of fear. Someone who helps at the emergency may also be afraid. Try to be reassuring. Even though a bystander may not have done everything perfectly, be sure to thank him for taking action. Recognition and praise help affirm people's willingness to act. Also, be careful about what you say. Do not give distressing news about the emergency to the patient or his family or friends.

- *Controlling your fears.*

  Try not to reveal your anxieties to the patient or bystanders. The presence of blood, vomit, unpleasant odours, or torn or burned skin is disturbing to most people. You may need to compose yourself before

acting. If you must, turn away for a moment and take a few deep breaths before providing care.

- *Presenting a clean and professional appearance.*

  This helps ease a patient's fears and inspires confidence.

- *Keeping your skills and knowledge up to date.*

  Involve yourself in continuing education, professional reading, and refresher training.

- *Staying fit with daily exercise and a healthy diet.*

  Job stresses can adversely affect your health. Exercise and diet can help you manage physical, mental, and emotional stress.

- *Maintaining a safe and healthy lifestyle.*

  As a responder, it is important to maintain a safe and healthy lifestyle both on and off the job. Identify the risk factors in your life so that you can take steps to reduce them.

Responsibilities

Since you will often be the first trained professional to arrive in many emergencies, your primary responsibilities centre on safety and early emergency care. Your six major responsibilities are to:

1. *Ensure safety for yourself and any bystanders.*

   Your first responsibility is to not make the situation worse by getting hurt yourself or letting bystanders get hurt. By making sure the scene is safe as you approach it, you can avoid unnecessary injuries.

2. *Gain access to the patient.*

   Carefully approach the patient unless the scene is too dangerous to handle without help. Electrical hazards, unsafe structures, and other dangers may make it difficult to reach the patient. Recognize when a rescue requires specially trained emergency personnel and know how to activate this response.

3. *Determine any threats to the patient's life.*

   Check first for immediate life-threatening conditions and care for any you find. Next, look for other conditions that could eventually threaten the patient's life or health if not cared for.

4. *Obtain more advanced medical care as needed.*

   After you quickly assess the patient, notify more advanced medical personnel of the situation if someone has not already done so. Transport the patient if it is necessary and you are trained and able to do so.

5. *Provide needed care for the patient.*

   Remain with the patient and provide whatever care you can until more advanced personnel take over.

6. *Assist more advanced medical personnel.*

   Transfer your information about the patient and the emergency to more advanced personnel. Tell them what happened, how you found the patient, any problems you found, and any care you gave. Assist them as needed and help with care for any other patients. When possible, try to anticipate the needs of those giving care.

In addition to these major responsibilities, you have secondary responsibilities that include:

- Controlling or directing bystanders or asking them for help.

- Taking additional steps, if necessary, to protect bystanders from dangers such as traffic or fire.

- Recording what you saw, heard, and did at the scene.

- Reassuring the patient's family or friends.

Interpersonal Communication

Medical emergencies can be frightening to people. When speaking to the patient and family, be sure to speak slowly and clearly. Use language they can understand. Avoid technical terms that will confuse and possibly frighten them.

When speaking to people, get down to their level, if possible, to avoid appearing threatening. Make eye contact. Use body language that shows you are open and interested in what people have to say. One way to put people at ease is to address them by name, whenever possible. Note, however, that if the person is an older adult, you should not call him by his first name unless invited to do so.

Listen carefully to what the patient tells you. Observe the patient when he talks. Provide reassurance if someone appears reluctant to speak about a topic. Tell him that any information he may have about the problem is important, even if it is upsetting to talk about.

Listen to what bystanders tell you. They may have seen or heard something that will help you in determining how you will treat the patient. Many times, people will want to stay with the patient or watch to see what is going on. Be firm but reasonable with bystanders. Ask them to move away for the safety and comfort of everyone. Consider allowing a parent of a child or an immediate family member to stay, although this is not always possible. If there are hostile bystanders, ensure your safety, and the safety of the patient, and call for help from the appropriate source, if required.

You can also learn a lot about physical problems just by observing the patient while he talks. If someone can only speak a few words before needing to take a breath, for example, he may be having a breathing emergency. Be observant. If someone is holding his stomach or clutching his chest—and may do so without being aware of it—this might give you information. Someone who winces with pain should be questioned about the pain.

From the patient's perspective, nothing is more annoying than not being listened to. Consider the last time you had to repeat information to someone several times; it is not a pleasant experience. Listening lets a patient know that you believe he is important. If you ask someone a question, listen for the answer. Make notes, if necessary, so you do not forget what the patient said. If you forget too often, the patient may stop answering your questions altogether.

Remember that everyone deserves equal care. One patient should be treated with the same respect and dignity afforded to any other. If you are called to care for someone who does not speak a language you understand, call for someone who can translate. A family member or neighbour, for example, may be able to speak both your language and that of the patient.

Watch the patient's body language, whether he speaks your language or another. Nonverbal clues can help you determine what is wrong. Be sensitive to cultural differences; in some cultures or religions, it may be inappropriate to make eye contact or for someone of a different gender to help the patient. Respect this and do what you can to help.

PAC lists several competencies for paramedics under the area of practising effective oral communication skills. Some of these can be summarized as follows:

To use appropriate language for a specific situation, you must be able to:

- Identify basic communication needs.
- Describe common communication barriers.
- Describe methods of meeting basic communication needs.
- Adapt communication techniques effectively.
- Use appropriate terminology.
- Integrate medical and non-medical terminology.[7]

CRITICAL INCIDENT STRESS MANAGEMENT

Researchers have recognized for years that individuals who provide emergency care can experience high levels of stress. Incidents involving multiple patients, rescues, children, failed resuscitation attempts, and death or serious injury to co-workers tend to cause more stress than most other incidents. Critical incident stress can cause a number of signs and symptoms, some of which may appear as long as weeks after the incident. They include:

- Confusion
- Lowered attention span
- Poor concentration
- Denial
- Guilt
- Depression
- Anger
- Change in interactions with others
- Increased or decreased eating
- Uncharacteristic, excessive humour or silence
- Unusual behaviour

NOTE:

Stress management techniques should also be used for children and adolescents.

From the time you begin to establish a rapport with someone, you become involved in the person's pain and stress. You share to some degree the thoughts and emotions of the person.

As a result, the emotional impact of a situation may be too great for you to handle alone. For this reason, you may need counselling to deal with the stress.

Counselling is not just for those incidents involving death or major disasters. Any incident is a potential source of emotional crisis for you. Even though the outcome of such an incident would be completely different from one involving death, the emotions and stress factors would all still be present.

Some people think that participating in counselling is an admission of weakness—quite the contrary. Counselling should be, and in many areas is, a routine part of any overwhelming incident, such as an airline disaster. Counselling can help in any situation, regardless of how minor you may think the event was. The most important thing you can do to minimize the effects of any emergency is to express your feelings and thoughts after the incident. Check with your local agency to see what resources are available to you.

NOTE:

Critical incident stress can affect anyone involved in an emergency.

LEGAL AND ETHICAL ISSUES

Many people are concerned about lawsuits. Lawsuits against those who give care at the scene of an emergency are highly unusual and rarely successful. By being aware of some basic legal principles, you may be able to avoid the possibility of legal action in the future.

The following sections address, in general terms, the legal principles that concern emergency care. Because laws vary between provinces, territories, and possibly regions, your instructor may need to update you on the laws that apply to you or tell you where you can find such information.

Duty to Act

Most responders, either by case law, statute, or job description, have a duty to act at the scene of an emergency. This duty applies to public safety officers, government employees, licensed and certified professionals, and paraprofessionals while on duty. For instance, members of a volunteer fire department have a duty to act based on their agreement to participate in the fire department. An athletic therapist has a duty to give care to an injured athlete. Failure to adhere to these agreements could result in legal action.[8]

If your actions do not meet the standards set for you, you may be successfully sued if your actions harm someone.

Scope of Practice

A responder's scope of practice is defined as the range of duties and skills he is allowed and expected to perform when necessary to his level of training and using reasonable care and skill. The responder is governed by legal, ethical, and medical standards. Be aware that when you practise a medical act, you may be doing so as an extension of your medical director. These standards establish the scope and the limits of care the responder provides. Since practices may differ by region, responders must be aware of the variations existing for their level of training and licencing in their region.

Ethical Responsibilities

As a responder, you have an ethical obligation to carry out your duties and responsibilities in a professional manner. This includes showing compassion when dealing with a patient's physical and mental needs and communicating sensitively and willingly at all times. You should never become satisfied with meeting minimum training requirements but rather strive to develop your professional skills to surpass the standards for your region. Doing so includes not only practising and mastering the skills taught in the course, but also seeking further training and information through workshops, continuing medical education, conferences, and supplemental or advanced educational programs.

In addition, be honest in reporting your actions and the events that occurred at a scene or when responding to an emergency. You have not only an ethical responsibility but also a legal one to document events accurately. Make it a personal goal to be a person whom others trust and can depend on to give accurate reports and provide effective care. You should address your responsibilities to the patient at each and every emergency. You must also periodically conduct a self-review of performance to help improve any weaknesses, including skills such as providing care to the patient, communication with him, and documentation.

Consent

An individual has a basic right to decide what can and cannot be done with his body. Therefore, to provide care for a patient, you must first obtain that person's consent. Usually, the person needs to tell you clearly that you have permission to provide care.

To obtain consent, you must:

1. Identify yourself to the person.

2. State your level of training.

3. Explain what you think may be wrong.

4. Explain what you plan to do.

After you have provided this information, the person can decide whether to grant his informed (or actual) consent. A person can withdraw consent for care at any time.

There is no specific age at which one is old enough to give or reject first aid treatment. In general, the person to receive the treatment must be mature enough to understand the circumstances he is in, the nature of the treatment to be provided, and the consequences of refusal.

A person who is unconscious, confused, or seriously ill or injured may not be able to grant informed consent. In these cases, the law assumes that the person would grant consent for care if he were able to do so. This is termed implied consent. Implied consent also applies to minors who obviously need emergency assistance when a parent or guardian is not present.

Consent: Special Situations

Unless an illness or injury is life-threatening, a parent or guardian must be present and give consent for minors before care can be given. If you encounter a parent or guardian who refuses to let you provide care, try to explain the consequences if care is not given to the ill or injured child. Use terms that the parent or guardian will understand. A law enforcement officer can help obtain the necessary legal authority to provide care. Do not argue with the parent or guardian as doing so can create a potentially unsafe scene. If the person is an adult whom you know or learn is under a legal guardian's care, you must also get the guardian's consent to give care. In certain situations, a person's cultural or religious beliefs may prevent that person from receiving care or being cared for by strangers or members of the opposite sex. In such a situation, you should respect the person's wishes and obtain other trained personnel to deal with the situation.

Competence

Competence refers to the person's ability to understand the responder's questions and to understand the implications of decisions. Responders must obtain permission from competent people before providing any care. Before receiving consent or refusal of care, the responder should determine if the person is competent. A person may not be competent to make rational decisions if he is intoxicated or on drugs, has a serious injury that might affect his judgment, or has a mental illness or disability. In such cases, call additional or appropriate personnel to evaluate the person. A law enforcement officer may need to be present to obtain the necessary legal authority so that care can be provided by the responder or advanced medical personnel.

Advance Directives and Do Not Resuscitate (DNR) Orders

Advance directives and do not resuscitate (DNR) orders are documented instructions from a person or his substitute decision maker and may be signed by a medical authority that protect a person's right to refuse efforts to resuscitate him in the case of cardiac arrest. Advance directives and DNR orders may differ by province, territory, or region. You must be aware of your relevant legislation and protocols relative to these orders. In some provinces/territories, a "No CPR" bracelet has been introduced to assist in identifying those wishes.

Negligence

Negligence is the failure to follow a reasonable standard of care, thereby causing injury or damage to another. A person could be negligent either by acting wrongly or failing to act at all.

The following scenario is an example of a case in which negligence may be suspected: A responder is called to the scene at a construction site, where a construction worker fell from a scaffolding several flights above. When the responder arrives, the worker is lying on the ground, moaning in pain, with both his hands holding his lower back.

The arriving responder notes the severity of the incident but fails to consider that the worker may have a spinal injury. The responder attempts to get the injured worker to stand up and move away from the construction area, even though there is no immediate threat of danger. This movement causes him to experience severe pain, and he suddenly loses feeling in his legs. In this case, the responder may be negligent because he failed to follow a reasonable standard of care.

Four components must be present for a lawsuit charging negligence to be successful:

1. Duty of care
2. Breach of duty
3. Cause of harm due to what someone did or failed to do
4. Damage caused

As a responder, you have a duty to respond in a professional manner, obeying traffic laws and protocols that govern your action. If you fail to act within this duty, then you commit a breach of duty. Sometimes your actions can cause improper care to be rendered, which can result in further harming a patient.

Laws That Protect Responders

Most provinces and territories have enacted laws that protect people providing emergency care. These laws,

A 16-year-old boy is the star defenceman for his hockey team. During a game, one of his teammates accidentally smacks him on the side of the head with his stick, sending him falling to the ice. He loses consciousness for 30 seconds, and when he wakes up, he is confused and disoriented. The coach assesses him despite his protesting that he's feeling fine and is keen to get back to the game. After a few minutes, the coach and parents agree that he can go back and play. What is your responsibility in this case?

which differ across Canada, are often called "Good Samaritan laws" and will generally protect you from legal liability as a responder as long as you act in good faith, are not negligent and act with reasonable care and skill, and act within the scope of your training. In times when you have a duty to respond, these laws may not be applicable.

Refusal of Care

Some people, even those who desperately need care, may refuse the care you offer. Even though the person may be seriously injured, you should honour his refusal of care. Try to convince the person of the need for care but do not argue. Allow other trained personnel to evaluate the situation. If possible, to make it clear that you did not abandon the person, have a witness hear the person's refusal and document it. Many EMS systems have a "Refusal of Care" form that you can use in these situations.

Before allowing a person to refuse care:

- Ensure that the person is competent and can make a rational decision.

- Try to persuade the person to accept care; repeat your offer to help at least once.

- Advise the person of the risks associated with refusing care.

- Consult the medical director (if required).

These factors should all be documented, and, as always, follow local protocol.

Abandonment

Just as you must have consent from a person before beginning care, you must also continue to give care once you have begun. Once you have started emergency care, you are legally obligated to continue that care until a person with equal or higher training relieves you. Usually, your obligation for care ends when more advanced medical personnel take over. If you stop your care before that point, you can be legally responsible for the abandonment of a patient in need.

Confidentiality

While providing care, you may learn things about the patient that are generally considered private and confidential. Information such as previous medical problems, physical problems, and medications being taken is personal to the individual. Respect his privacy by maintaining confidentiality, including any documentation you may create. Television and newspaper reporters may ask you questions. Lawyers may also approach you at the scene. Never discuss the patient or the care you gave with anyone except law enforcement personnel with a direct interest in the patient or other personnel caring for the individual. Once transfer of care has taken place, your responsibilities for data gathering terminate, unless asked to act further. Any information gathered to that point must be documented.

Communication

There are several aspects to the responder's role. You must be able to determine the person's major complaint, obtain a medical history, and properly reassure and comfort the patient. But just as important are tasks such as updating incoming EMS units on the person's status, requesting help from dispatch, asking the medical director for advice, and providing a hand-off report to any advanced medical care personnel who take over care. Both the former and latter types of tasks take skill; the latter depend on your skills as a good communicator.

Some of your communications with other EMS personnel will be on the radio or phone; others will be in person. In these situations, it is important for you to be accurate and speak slowly and clearly. Clear communication is critical to be able to provide accurate, complete information. Ineffective communication could result in harm to the patient in your care.

Radio Communication

Radios operate on specific frequencies that are regulated and licensed by Industry Canada's Spectrum Management and Telecommunications. Unauthorized people do not have access to these frequencies, so they cannot disrupt emergency radio traffic.

A radio system is made up of several components, usually including the following (Figure 1–1):

- *A base station:* The base system is the stationary radio located in a dispatch centre, station, or hospital.

- *Mobile radios:* These radios are mounted inside vehicles.

- *Portable radios:* These are hand-held radios that may be carried on your belt or in your pocket.

- *Repeaters:* Repeaters are devices that receive a low-power radio transmission and rebroadcast it with increased power.

- *Cellphones:* In common use by the public, cellphones are useful where radio coverage is unavailable to contact the medical director or the dispatcher.

During an emergency call, you will need to keep the dispatcher aware of your activities, assuming that your EMS system has a dispatch centre and radios. The specific times to report your activities are when you:

- Are en route to a call

- Arrive at the scene of a call

- Require additional assistance or specialized personnel

- Return to service and are available for the next call

You will also use the radio to update incoming EMS units or to speak with the medical director.

It's important to become familiar with the use of a radio so that you don't have to learn how to use it during an emergency situation, when you'll be feeling anxious. Remember to speak slowly and clearly. When you are

Figure 1–1 There are several components of a radio system.

ready to speak, push the "push to talk" button and then wait one second before you begin to speak. Hold the microphone approximately 5 to 7 cm (2 to 3 in.) away from your mouth. Keep your transmission brief; others may be waiting to use the frequency. Listen before you transmit so that you don't disrupt another conversation.

Assume that anything you say over the radio can be heard by others. People with scanners can hear what you say, for example. So never say anything personal or confidential, such as a patient's name. Of course, the public nature of radio transmission also means you should always keep your language and tone of voice professional.

Communicating with the Medical Director

While you are on the scene, you may need to consult with a physician, who can help you and the patient in your care. Whenever you have questions about someone's condition that cannot be resolved by protocols, consult with the medical director.

Called medical control, it is a process whereby a physician directs care given by pre-hospital care providers (through standing orders). The physician oversees training and development of protocols, which are standardized procedures to be followed when providing care. Standing orders allow certain types of care or treatment to be undertaken without speaking to the physician; this is called indirect, or off-line, medical control. If something is not covered by standing orders, the responder must speak directly with the physician; this is called direct, or on-line, medical control.

Since the physician may be far from the emergency scene, it is up to you to present the information clearly and concisely. Prepare yourself ahead of the call so that you're ready to provide the following information in your report:

- Your unit identifier and the fact that you are a responder
- The patient's age, sex, and chief complaint
- A brief, pertinent history of the events leading to the injury or illness
- Results of the patient's physical exam, including vital signs
- The care provided to the patient and her response to that care
- The reason you are calling

If the physician gives you orders, repeat the orders back to verify them. Be sure that all orders and advice given to you by the physician are clear. If you have any questions, ask the physician for clarification.

NOTE:

This information is what you would relay to any other healthcare provider when giving a verbal report.

Documentation

Documenting your care is as important as the care itself. Your record will help healthcare professionals assess and continue care for the patient. Because a patient's condition may change before he arrives at the hospital, a record of the condition immediately after the emergency will provide useful information for healthcare providers. They can compare the current condition with what you recorded earlier.

Your record is a legal document and is important if legal action occurs. Should you be called to court for any reason, your record will support what you saw, heard, and did at the scene of the emergency. It is

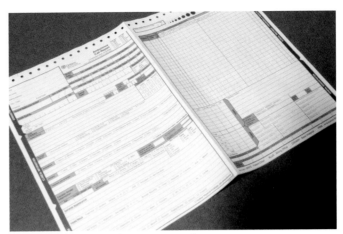

Figure 1–2 Printed care report form.

important to write the record as soon as possible after the emergency, while all the facts are fresh in your memory. Many systems have electronic forms for responders to use while others use printed forms (Figure 1–2).

Reasons for Documentation

- Medical—To document care you provided
- Legal—To defend against lawsuits, as well as possible evidence in court proceedings (e.g., if an act of violence was involved)
- Administration—To transfer information about the individual from one person to another
- Research—To improve your EMS system

PAC lists several competencies for paramedics under the area of professional responsibilities. Some of these pertain to written reports and can be summarized as follows:

- Record organized, accurate, and relevant patient information.
  - Organize patient information for the purposes of a written report.
  - Communicate accurate, organized, and relevant documentation.[9]
- Include all pertinent and required information on reports and medical records.
  - Organize information for documentation.
  - Apply principles of correct documentation.

- ■ Acknowledge the importance of appropriate documentation.
- ■ Demonstrate proper documentation.[10]

Elements of Good Documentation

- Completeness and accuracy (see Appendix A: Common Abbreviations for Documentation)
- Legibility
- Timeliness
- Absence of alterations

Documentation should include the following:

- Administrative information: names of responders, unit number, call number, and address to which the responders were sent
- Patient's information: name, age, sex, birth date, address, and any care given prior to the responder's arrival
- Vital signs
- Chief complaint
- History (SAMPLE and OPQRST) and assessment findings (see Chapter 5 for information on SAMPLE and OPQRST)
- Care given

Local protocols often dictate what specifics are to be included in a report, as well as in what format the information is to be documented.

There are some situations when other documentation, or variance in the usual documentation, may be required, such as in the care of injury to responders, multiple casualty incidents, infectious disease exposure, and other such reasons.

It may be necessary to provide a verbal report of information about the patient to another healthcare provider. To do this, report the facts. Tell the other person what you found and what you have done up to that point.

Medical Terminology

For healthcare providers to be able to accurately communicate about patients, it is important to have a common language, and part of this common language is a basic understanding of medical terminology. One of

TABLE 1–1: COMMON COMBINING FORMS

Combining Form	What Does It Mean?
Cardi/o-	Heart, cardiac
Neur/o-	Nerve, neural
Oro-	Mouth
Arteri/o-	Artery, arterial
Hem/o-	Blood
Therm/o-	Heat
Vas/o-	Duct, vessel, vascular

the key elements to understanding medical terminology is the ability to break down the terms into their parts.

Medical terms are often made up of a combining form (a root word plus a combining vowel; Table 1–1) that contains the core meaning of the term along with a suffix (a word ending) and/or prefix (a word beginning) that qualifies the combining form (Table 1–2). For example, the medical term endotracheal is made up of the combining form *trache*, which means "trachea"; the prefix *endo*, which means "within"; and the suffix *al*, which means "pertaining to." By understanding the parts of the word, we understand the term endotracheal to mean "pertaining to something within the trachea." This term might be used with the word *tube* to describe a type of tube used within the trachea. The easiest way to learn medical combining forms, their prefixes, and their suffixes is to memorize them. A few of the more common suffixes are *-emic* (pertaining to the blood), *-emia* (condition of the blood), and *-a* or *-ia* (condition).

SUMMARY

The survival and recovery of a severely ill or injured patient depend on all parts of the EMS system working together efficiently. Early response by the public, rapid EMS response, responder care, advanced pre-hospital care, hospital care, and extended care are the components for survival. The responder, the first trained person to arrive on the emergency scene, takes over

TABLE 1–2: COMMON PREFIXES

Combining Form	What Does It Mean?
A-	Without, no
Hyper-	Excessive, above, over, beyond
Hypo-	Less than normal, under
Tachy-	Fast, swift, rapid, accelerated
Brady-	Slow, dull

care of the patient from any member of the public present.

After arriving on the scene, the responder must make sure the scene is safe and then reach the patient, give care for any life-threatening conditions, and obtain more advanced medical care, if needed. The responder should give more advanced medical personnel any assistance they need.

In your role as a responder, you are guided by certain legal parameters, such as the duty to act, and professional standards of care. Part of this professionalism includes effective documentation, which is important for maintaining the standard of care for a patient and provides legal protection for you and the organization you represent. If you are a responder who falls under medical direction, you must follow protocols and standing orders within your scope of practice. In addition, there are legal and ethical requirements you must carry out, such as determining competence, obtaining consent, and adhering to advance directives when providing care. Since legal and medical standards and licensure can vary by region, it is important that you become knowledgeable about the standards in your area and the variations that exist for your level of training.

The ability to communicate clearly and accurately is one of the most critical skills for a responder. As a responder, you must be able to effectively update incoming EMS units on the status of the patient in your care, request help from dispatch, ask the medical director for advice, and provide a hand-off report to the more advanced personnel who take over care. It's also important to learn how to use radio equipment competently.

Regardless of your profession, when you are called to help a person with an injury or sudden illness, you assume the role of an emergency care provider. When an emergency occurs, the patients in your care, as well as assisting bystanders, will expect you to know what to do. Be prepared to think and act accordingly. What to do, however, often involves more than giving emergency care. Chapter 2 provides an overview of the responder's role in assessing and managing emergency scenes.

It is important to recognize the powerful impact critical incident stress can have on you and to learn to recognize the signs. You must address your own emotional needs in addition to those of the patients and families you are helping. The ability to cope with job-related stress and to realize that, in some situations, you may be overcome by emotion are necessary skills. Self-help involves sharing your feelings with others. It is only by caring for your own well-being that you can help others.

As you survey the scene, you think about everything at once: How seriously is the man injured? What do I need to do first to make it easier to help the man? How do I get the information I need in the quickest way so that I can get to work? What are my responsibilities as a responder?

Emergency Care

Chapter *2*

The Emergency Scene

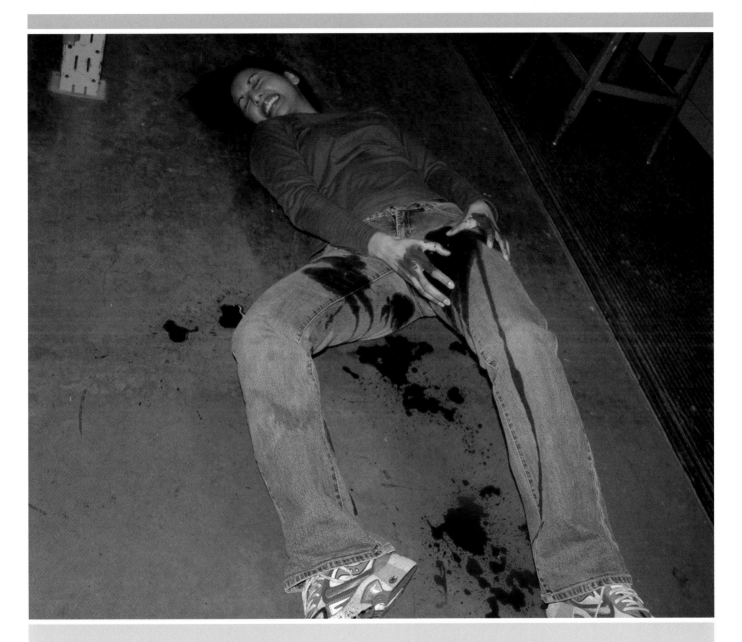

You are called to a factory and find a woman bleeding profusely from a deep wound in her upper thigh. She is in obvious pain and appears to be losing consciousness. Her breathing is rapid and her skin looks paler than normal. The factory is filled with loud machines, and you find it hard to communicate with anyone due to the noise. There are no witnesses to the incident. What do you do?

INTRODUCTION

As a responder, you have a duty to respond to an emergency when summoned. Although you should immediately proceed to the scene of an emergency when notified, you must do so safely. When you arrive, carefully evaluate the entire scene. Emergency scenes are often dangerous. Never enter a dangerous emergency scene unless you have been trained to do so and have the necessary equipment. Follow your established operating procedures, including when and how to access the EMS system.

This chapter describes the responsibilities for preparing for an emergency response and for identifying and managing initial dangers at an emergency scene.

PREPARING FOR THE EMERGENCY RESPONSE

Equipment and Personnel

The emergency response begins with the preparation of the vehicle/equipment and personnel before an emergency occurs. The first aid kit, or trauma kit, for the responder should be a standard part of your equipment for performing your duties. It should be checked on a regular schedule to ensure that it is well stocked at all times. You should be familiar with the location of all equipment within the kit. Emergency equipment must always be clean and in good working condition. Dressings, bandages, and other supplies kept in kits should be restocked as soon as possible after use. Automated external defibrillators (AEDs) must be properly maintained as per manufacturers' guidelines, making sure batteries are charged. Oxygen cylinders should be kept full. The quantity of specific items should be determined by individual need, local protocol, or legislation.

Plan of Action

To respond most efficiently to certain emergencies, you need a plan of action. A plan of this type is prepared in advance and rehearsed with personnel. Emergency plans should be established based on anticipated needs and available resources. All personnel should become familiar with these plans. For example, many businesses and industrial sites have emergency plans

Figure 2–1 Posted evacuation routes may be part of an emergency plan.

that identify trained personnel, locations of supplies and equipment, a communication network, and evacuation routes (Figure 2–1).

Many fire departments and EMS systems plan responses for large facilities requiring special resources, such as sports stadiums, public buildings, and facilities with hazardous materials. These are generally referred to as emergency response plans. A plan for evacuating a stadium crowded with fans, for example, could save thousands of lives in an emergency. Developing the plan involves inspecting the site, noting potential dangers, and identifying the type of equipment and personnel that will probably be needed. Once developed, plans must be rehearsed, evaluated, and modified periodically.

Learn about the real or potential dangers in your area and familiarize yourself with existing emergency response plans. Evaluate your role and the available local resources. Know the resources in your community for handling special situations, such as a hazardous materials spill, that require specially trained personnel and special equipment.

Communications

Emergency response depends on a reliable and efficient communication system. Make sure you are always able to contact more advanced medical personnel and other special resources. This means having a backup communication system in place. Check communications equipment often to make sure it is working.

Be sure you know how to contact the special resources in your area. Some responders may use communication networks outside 9-1-1 or the local EMS number system. Become familiar with your communication networks and develop an alternative plan in case regular communications fail. Some types of communication devices are Family Radio Service (FRS), pagers, computers, two-way radios, cellphones, satellite phones, and CB radios. For more information on communications, see Chapter 1.

Training

An important part of being prepared for emergencies is keeping your training current. Continue to practise the skills you use less often. Pursue activities that will help you perform your job better, including reading appropriate articles and publications and participating in workshops, emergency response exercises, and seminars.

RESPONDING TO THE EMERGENCY SCENE

Mental and Emotional Aspects

Just as it is important to keep equipment ready for emergencies, it is also important for you to be prepared psychologically. You can never predict how the next emergency may affect you. Certain injuries, smells, sights, and sounds can make you feel weak, nauseated, or faint the first time you encounter them. The sight of blood or gaping wounds, cries of pain, the threat of danger, or other factors may so distress well-intentioned responders that they become barriers to prompt action.

You may never get used to some sights and sounds. With experience and by being prepared, however, you can learn to cope with your feelings. To calm yourself, take a deep breath and look away for a moment. Stay relaxed. Remind yourself that the person needs you and you need to be in full control of yourself to give the required care. If you feel nauseated, step back, take several deep breaths, mentally review your task, and then proceed. The person's life may depend on you.

Recognizing your emotions and the emotions of others will help you manage the situation in a more understanding and responsive way.

Notification and Transportation

If you are in a police department, fire department, or rescue squad, for example, you may be notified to go to an emergency by telephone, pager, or radio. Lifeguards, ski patrollers, and athletic therapists may already be near or at the scene when an emergency occurs. If you are at a distance from the scene, you will probably need to use a vehicle to get there. Laws and established procedures govern the use of emergency vehicles and their warning equipment, such as lights and sirens. You must remember that emergency vehicles do not have an absolute right-of-way.

Never drive a private vehicle as if it were an emergency vehicle. Even if you have lights and sirens, people do not always see you, hear you, or yield the right-of-way. People hurrying to an emergency or a hospital sometimes cause vehicle collisions because they fail to drive safely.

MANAGING DANGERS AT THE EMERGENCY SCENE

Some emergency scenes are immediately dangerous. Others may become dangerous while you are providing care. Sometimes the dangers are obvious, such as fire or hostile patients or bystanders. Other dangers may be less obvious, such as the presence of a hazardous material or unstable structures. Table 2–1 lists a number of hazards you may find at an emergency scene.

Primary Responsibilities of the Responder
1. Ensure safety for yourself and any bystanders.
2. Gain access to the patient.
3. Determine any threats to the patient's life.
4. Obtain more advanced medical care, as needed.
5. Provide needed care for the patient.
6. Assist advanced medical personnel, as needed.

Personal Safety

Of the six primary responsibilities of the responder, safety should always be foremost. You cannot overlook the importance of ensuring your own safety. Often it requires only simple tasks to make an emergency scene safe. Approach all emergency scenes cautiously until you can size up the situation. If you arrive at the scene by vehicle, park a safe distance away. If the scene appears safe, continue to evaluate the situation as you approach.

Pay particular attention to the:

• Location of the emergency

• Extent of the emergency

• Apparent scene dangers

• Apparent number of patients

• Behaviour of the patient(s) and bystanders

If at any time the scene appears unsafe, retreat to a safe distance. Notify additional personnel and wait for their arrival. Never enter a dangerous scene unless you have the training and equipment to do so safely. Well-meaning responders have been injured or killed because they forgot to look for scene hazards. If your training has not prepared you for a specific emergency, such as a fire or an incident involving hazardous materials, notify appropriately trained personnel.

When arriving on an emergency scene, always follow these four guidelines to ensure your personal safety and that of anyone else at the scene:

1. Take time to evaluate the scene. This will enable you to recognize existing and potential dangers.

2. Wear appropriate personal protective equipment (PPE).

3. Perform only the skills you are trained to do. Know what resources are available to help.

4. Get the help you need. If you have not already done so, notify additional personnel. Be able to describe the scene and the type of additional help required.

TABLE 2–1: POTENTIAL HAZARDS AT AN EMERGENCY SCENE

• Pets (or other animals)	• Debris	• Weather
• Weapons	• Confined spaces	• Ice
• Low lighting	• Pathogens	• Terrain
• Furniture scattered about	• People	• Hazardous materials
• Blocked or cluttered exits	• Unstable/unsafe structures	• Downed electrical lines
• Loud noise	• Fire	• Low-oxygen
• Traffic	• Water	• Sharp glass or metal

Safety of Others

You have a responsibility for the safety of others at the scene, as well as for your personal safety. Discourage bystanders, family members, or unprepared responders from entering an area that appears unsafe. You can use these well-intentioned individuals to help you keep unauthorized people away from unsafe areas and to summon more appropriate help. Some dangers may require you to take special measures, such as placing physical barriers to prevent onlookers from getting too close. Other situations may require you to act quickly to free someone who is trapped or move a patient in immediate danger to safety.

Ideally, you should move patients only after you have assessed and properly cared for them. If, however, immediate dangers threaten their life, you must decide whether to move them. If the situation is dangerous and you cannot move them, retreat to safety yourself. If you can move them, do so quickly and safely.

Situations that may require an emergency move include:

- The presence of dangerous or hazardous materials or situations

- Moving a patient with more minor injuries to reach someone who may have a life-threatening condition

- Moving a patient to provide appropriate care

Chapter 21 provides more detailed information about how to move patients safely.

Specific Emergency Situations

Certain emergency scenes present a special set of problems. These situations include crime scenes, scenes with hazards, and scenes with multiple patients.

Since every emergency scene has potential dangers, always expect the unexpected. Never attempt a rescue for which you are not properly trained and equipped. Always wear appropriate protective gear, such as gloves and goggles. Be aware that at any time even a seemingly safe emergency scene can turn dangerous. Always take the necessary precautions when you suspect or identify certain dangers. Several of the following situations are also discussed in Chapters 21 and 22.

Crime Scene

If you arrive at the scene of a crime or potential suicide, do not try to reach any person until you are sure the scene is safe. A person who has been shot, stabbed, or beaten may have severe injuries, but until the scene is safe, there is nothing you can do to provide care. For the scene to be safe, law enforcement personnel must have made it secure. Police usually gather evidence at a crime scene, so do not touch anything except what you must in order to give care. Use one path of entrance and exit. Your duty is to the patient; provide necessary care and then vacate the crime scene area. Once you enter a crime scene to give care, make sure that police are aware of your presence and actions. Document what you did, moved, and touched.

As a responder, when you arrive at a scene where criminal activity is suspected, take the following steps:

- Notify law enforcement personnel if they are not already at the scene.

- Take precautions not to remove or disturb anything at the scene unless it is absolutely necessary in order to perform critical patient care.

- Document any situations in which you need to disturb the scene in the interest of patient care.

- In situations where sexual assault is suspected or alleged by the patient, notify law enforcement personnel and discourage the patient from washing, showering, or changing clothing.

- When removing clothing following gunshot wounds, stabbings, or other assaults, if at all possible do not cut clothing through or near the bullet or stab wound holes.

- Allow bloody clothing to dry.

- Avoid allowing blood or debris to contaminate another area or clothing.

- Do not roll clothes up in a ball.

- Never put wet or bloody clothes in plastic bags.

- Handle clothing as little and as carefully as possible, as powder flakes from gunshot wounds may be present and handling may decrease the value of powder-deposit examination.

- Consider bagging the patient's hands if the situation permits.

- Minimize the introduction of foreign objects into a crime scene. Communicate with law enforcement concerning any items you left behind (such as medical supplies) and if you disturbed anything (such as moving furniture to access a patient).

- Yield to the primary investigative agency on the scene.

If you happen to be on the scene when an unarmed person threatens suicide, try to reassure and calm the person. Make sure that appropriate personnel have been notified. You cannot physically restrain a suicidal person without medical or legal authorization. Listen to her and try to keep her talking until help arrives. Try to be understanding. Many suicide attempts are a call for help. Do not dare the person to act or trivialize her feelings. Unless your personal safety is threatened, never leave a suicidal person alone.

Drug Labs

Drug labs are places where people illegally manufacture drugs. Clues such as the possession of chemical glassware, or unusual chemicals, by someone not working in the chemical field may indicate the presence of a drug lab.

Specific dangers in illegal drug lab situations are:

- Booby traps

- Electrical hazards

- Fire and explosion hazards

- Air quality, due to moulds or chemical reactions

- Biohazards

- General existence of large volumes of potentially hazardous materials

Wait until trained personnel arrive; this is an unsafe environment.

Traffic

Traffic is often the most common danger you and other emergency personnel will encounter when responding to a motor vehicle collision. If you drive to the collision scene, always try to park where your vehicle will not block other traffic, such as an emergency vehicle that needs to reach the scene. The only time you should park in a roadway or block traffic is to:

- Protect a patient.

- Protect any responders, including yourself.

- Warn oncoming traffic if the situation is not clearly visible.

Others can help you put reflectors, flares, or lights along the road. These items should be placed well back of the scene to enable oncoming motorists to stop or slow down in time.

Emergency personnel have been injured or killed by traffic at emergency scenes. If you are not a law enforcement officer and dangerous traffic makes the scene unsafe, wait for more help to arrive before giving care.

Fire

Any fire can be dangerous. Make sure that the local fire department has been summoned. Only firefighters, who are highly trained and use equipment that protects them against fire and smoke, should approach a fire. Do not let others approach. Gather information to help the responding fire and EMS units. Give this information to emergency personnel when they arrive. If you are not trained to fight fires or lack the necessary equipment, follow these basic guidelines:

- Stay away from a burning vehicle.

- Never enter a burning or smoke-filled building.

- If you are in a building that is on fire, always check doors before opening them. If a door is hot to the touch, do not open it.

- Since smoke and fumes rise, stay close to the floor and put a moist cloth over your mouth and nose.

- Never use an elevator in a building that may be burning.

Electricity

Downed electrical lines also present a major hazard to responders. Always look for downed wires at a scene and always treat them as dangerous. If you find downed wires, follow these guidelines:

Figure 2–2 Hazardous material placard.

- Move any crowd back from the danger zone. The safe area should be established at a point twice the length of the span of the wire.

- Never attempt to move downed wires.

- Notify the fire department and power company immediately. Always assume that the wires are energized.

- If downed wires contact a vehicle, do not touch the vehicle and do not let others touch it. Tell anyone in the vehicle to stay still and stay inside the vehicle. Never attempt to remove people from a vehicle with downed wires across it, no matter how seriously injured they may seem.

- Do not touch any metal fence, metal structure, or body of water in contact with a downed wire. Wait for the power company to shut off the power source.

Water and Ice

Water and ice can also be serious hazards. To help a conscious person in the water, reach out to her with a branch, a pole, or even your hand, being careful not to be pulled into the water. When the person grasps the object, pull her to safety.

If you cannot reach the person, try to throw her something nearby that floats. If you have a rope available, attach a floatable object, such as a lifejacket, plastic jug, ice chest, or empty gas can, to one end. Never enter a body of water to rescue someone unless you have been trained in water rescue and then enter only as a last resort.

Fast-moving water is extremely dangerous and often occurs with floods, hurricanes, and low-head dams. Ice is also treacherous. It can break under your weight, and the cold water beneath can quickly overcome even the best swimmers. Never enter fast-moving water or venture out on ice unless you are trained in this type of rescue. Such rescues require careful planning and proper equipment. Wait until trained personnel arrive.

Hazardous Materials

Hazardous materials are common and are a special risk for responding personnel. When you approach an emergency scene, look for clues that indicate the presence of hazardous materials. These include:

- Signs (placards) on vehicles, storage facilities, or railroad cars identifying the presence of hazardous materials

- Clouds of vapour

- Spilled liquids or solids

- Unusual odours

- Leaking containers, bottles, or gas cylinders

- Chemical transport tanks or containers

Those who transport or store hazardous materials in specific quantities are required to post placards identifying the specific hazardous material, by name or by number, and its dangers (Figure 2–2). This information is available from various reference materials. If you do not see a placard but suspect that a hazardous material is present, try to get information before you approach the scene.

Unsafe Structures

Buildings and other structures, such as mines, wells, and unreinforced trenches, can become unsafe because of fire, explosions, natural disasters, deterioration, or other causes. An unsafe building or structure is one in which:

- The air may contain debris or hazardous gases

- There is a possibility of being trapped or injured by collapsed walls, weakened floors, and other debris

Try to establish the exact or probable location of anyone in the structure. Gather as much information as you can, call for appropriate help, and wait for the arrival of properly trained and equipped personnel.

Wreckage

The wreckage of automobiles, aircraft, or machinery may contain hazards such as sharp pieces of metal or glass, fuel, and moving parts. The wreckage may be unstable. Do not try to rescue someone from wreckage unless you have the proper equipment and training. Rescue is made only after the wreckage has been stabilized. Gather as much information as you can and be sure that advanced medical personnel have been called.

Natural Disasters

Natural disasters include tornadoes, hurricanes, earthquakes, forest fires, ice storms, and floods (Figure 2–3). Rescue efforts after a natural disaster are usually coordinated by local resources until they become overwhelmed. Then the rescue efforts are coordinated by government agencies. Typically, you would report to the person or people in charge at the scene and then work with the disaster response team and follow the rescue plan.

Natural disasters pose more risks than you might be aware of. A large number of injuries and deaths result

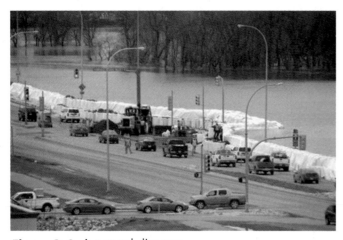

Figure 2–3 A natural disaster.

from electricity, hazardous materials, rising water, and other dangers as opposed to the disaster itself. When responding to a natural disaster, be sure to carefully survey the scene, avoid obvious hazards, and use caution when operating rescue equipment. Never use gasoline-powered equipment, such as chainsaws, generators, and pumps, in confined spaces.

Multiple Patients

Scenes that involve more than one patient are referred to as multiple casualty incidents. Such scenes make your task more complex since you must determine who needs immediate care and who can wait for more help to arrive. To make these decisions, you use a process called triage that helps you prioritize the care you give to the patients involved.

A large multiple casualty incident, such as a plane or train crash or natural disaster, may overwhelm the capabilities of the local EMS system. To effectively handle any emergency involving multiple patients, EMS uses an incident command system (ICS). An ICS establishes a chain of command at the scene that permits one person to direct all the agencies that are helping. For example, when police, fire, and ambulance personnel are called to a major urban fire, the fire chief takes charge and all other resources report to her. These resources may include police evacuating nearby buildings, firefighters fighting the blaze, and ambulance personnel providing emergency care and transportation for patients. In this way, all available resources will be used effectively and efficiently.

Hostile Situations

Environmental factors, such as hazardous materials, electricity, and unsafe structures, are not the only dangers you may encounter. You may sometimes encounter a hostile ill or injured person or family member. Any unusual or hostile behaviour may be a result of the emergency. A person's rage or hostility may be caused by the injury or illness or by fear. Many ill or injured people are afraid of losing control and may show this as anger. Hostile behaviour may also result from the use of alcohol or other drugs, lack of oxygen, or an underlying medical condition.

If a person needing care is hostile toward you, try to explain calmly who you are and that you are there to help. Remember that you cannot give care without the person's consent. If the person accepts your offer to help, keep talking to her as you assess her condition. When she realizes that you are not a threat, the hostility usually goes away.

If the person refuses your care or threatens you, withdraw from the scene. Never try to restrain, argue with, or force your care on a person. If she does not let you provide care, wait for additional help. Sometimes a close friend or a family member will be able to reassure a hostile person and convince her to accept your care.

Family members or friends who are angry or hysterical, however, can make your job more difficult. Sometimes they may not allow you to provide care. At other times, they may try to move the patient before you have stabilized her. A terrified parent may cling to a child and refuse to let you help. When family members act this way, they often feel confused, guilty, and frightened. Be understanding and explain the care you are giving. By remaining calm and professional, you will help calm them. Hostile crowds are a threat that can develop when you least expect it. If you decide the crowd at a scene is hostile, wait at a safe distance until law enforcement and other trained personnel arrive. Approach the scene only when police officers declare it safe and ask you to help. Never approach a hostile crowd unless you are trained in crowd management and supported by other trained personnel.

Hostage Situations

If you encounter a hostage situation, your first priority is to not become a hostage yourself. Assess the scene from a safe distance and call for law enforcement personnel. A police officer trained in hostage negotiations should take charge.

Try to get any information from bystanders that may help law enforcement personnel. Ask about the number of hostages, any weapons seen, and other possible hazards. Report any information to the first law enforcement official on the scene. Remain at a safe distance until law enforcement personnel summon you.

SUMMARY

Emergency scenes by their nature can be dangerous, so never approach a scene until you are sure it is safe. Your personal safety is always your first concern. Potential hazards at emergency scenes include traffic, fire, electricity, water, ice, and unsafe structures. Other dangers include ill or injured people or family members who are violent or hostile or hostile crowds.

If you have any doubt about the safety of a scene or if you are not trained and equipped to handle the situation, stay back. Be sure that appropriate help has been called and wait for properly trained and equipped personnel.

Once you are sure the scene is safe, you will be expected to provide care to ill and injured people. Information on how the human body normally functions, which you will learn in Chapter 4, will help you assess a person's condition and provide the appropriate emergency care.

You are treating a wound that is spurting blood uncontrollably. There is a crowd of workers gathered around trying to see what is going on. There is blood and blood-soaked dressings all over the floor. What do you do?

Chapter *3*

Preventing Disease Transmission

A woman has collapsed in her office. As the first trained person on the scene, you find her bleeding from the mouth. Vomit and blood are around her. She is not breathing. What do you do?

INTRODUCTION

It is not unusual to be faced with a situation in which you are concerned about disease transmission. You may encounter such concerns during everyday tasks you carry out within your job or other activities. It is important to understand how infections occur, how they are passed from one person to another, and what you can do to protect yourself and others from disease.

The types of diseases that can be contracted from other people, objects, animals, or insects are referred to as infectious diseases. Some of these infectious diseases can be transmitted more easily than others. In this chapter, you will learn how to recognize situations with the potential for disease transmission and how to protect yourself and others from contracting disease.

HOW INFECTIONS OCCUR

Disease-Causing Pathogens

The disease process begins when a pathogen gets into the body. When pathogens enter the body, they can sometimes overpower the body's defence systems and cause illness. This illness is an infection. Most infectious diseases are caused by one of the six types of pathogens identified in Table 3–1. The most common pathogens are bacteria and viruses.

Bacteria are everywhere. They do not depend on other organisms for life and can live outside the human body. Most bacteria do not infect humans. Those that do may cause serious illness. Meningitis, scarlet fever, and tetanus are examples of disease caused by bacteria.

TABLE 3–1: DISEASE-CAUSING PATHOGENS

Pathogen	Definition	Condition They Cause
Viruses	A disease-causing agent that requires another organism in order to live and reproduce	Hepatitis, measles, mumps, chicken pox, meningitis, rubella, influenza, warts, colds, herpes, shingles, human immunodeficiency virus (HIV) infection including acquired immune deficiency syndrome (AIDS), genital warts
Bacteria	Single-celled micro-organism that may cause infection	Tetanus, meningitis, scarlet fever, strep throat, tuberculosis, gonorrhea, syphilis, chlamydia, toxic shock syndrome, legionnaires' disease, diphtheria, food poisoning
Fungi	A single-celled or multicellular organism	Athlete's foot and ringworm
Protozoa	A single-celled organism that can only divide within a host organism	Malaria and dysentery
Rickettsia	A group of micro-organisms (like viruses) that require other living cells for growth but (like bacteria) use oxygen, have metabolic enzymes and cell walls, and are susceptible to antibiotics	Typhus, Rocky Mountain spotted fever
Parasitic worms	A worm classified as a parasite, which is a disease-causing organism that lives on or in a human or other animal and derives its nourishment from its host	Abdominal pain, anemia, lymphatic vessel blockage, lowered antibody response, respiratory and circulatory complications

The body has difficulty fighting infections caused by bacteria. Doctors may prescribe medications called antibiotics that either kill the bacteria or weaken them enough for the body to get rid of them.

Unlike bacteria, viruses depend on other organisms to live and reproduce. Viruses cause many diseases, including the common cold. Once they become established within the body, they are difficult to eliminate because very few medications are effective against them. Antibiotics do not kill or weaken viruses. The body's immune system is the main defence against them.

The Body's Natural Defences

The body has a series of natural defences that prevent germs from entering. The body depends on intact skin and mucous membranes in the mouth, nose, and eyes to keep germs out. When the skin is damaged, germs can enter through openings, such as cuts or sores. Mucous membranes in the mouth, nose, and eyes also work to protect the body from intruding germs, often by trapping them and forcing them out through a cough or sneeze. However, mucous membranes are less effective than skin at keeping blood-borne pathogens out of the body. If these barriers fail and a germ enters the body, the body's immune system begins working to fight the disease.

The immune system's basic tools are antibodies and white blood cells. Special white blood cells travel around the body and identify invading pathogens. Once they detect a pathogen, white blood cells gather around it and release antibodies that fight infection.

These antibodies attack the pathogens and weaken or destroy them. Antibodies can usually rid the body of pathogens. However, once inside the body, some pathogens can thrive and, under ideal conditions, multiply and overwhelm the immune system.

This combination of preventing pathogens from entering the body and destroying them once they enter is necessary for good health (homeostasis). Sometimes, however, the body cannot fight off infection. When this occurs, an invading pathogen can become established in the body, causing infection, which may range from mild to serious and brief (acute) to long-lasting (chronic). Fever and exhaustion often signal that the

body is fighting off an infection. Other common signals include headache, nausea, and vomiting.

There are three different types of human immunity: innate, adaptive, and passive.

1. **Innate immunity** is the type of protection with which we are born. The term "innate immunity" also refers to the natural barriers our bodies have, such as the skin and mucous membranes in the nose, throat, and gastrointestinal tract, which prevent most diseases from entering our bodies.

2. **Adaptive immunity** develops throughout our lives as we are exposed to diseases or are immunized against them.

3. **Passive immunity** is immunity we gain from external sources, such as from a mother's breast milk to a baby.

How Diseases Are Transmitted

You need to understand these four conditions to understand how infections occur. Think of these conditions as the pieces of a puzzle. All the pieces have to be in place for the picture to be complete (Figure 3–1). If any one of these conditions is missing, an infection cannot occur:

1. A pathogen is present.

2. There is enough of the pathogen to cause disease.

3. A person is susceptible to the pathogen.

4. There is a route of entry.

Pathogens enter the body in four ways (Table 3–2):

1. *Direct contact*

   Direct contact transmission (Figure 3–2) occurs when a person touches body fluids from an infected person.

2. *Indirect contact*

   Indirect contact transmission (Figure 3–3) occurs when a person touches objects that have touched the blood or another body fluid, such as saliva and vomit, of an infected person. These include soiled dressings, equipment, and work surfaces with which an infected person comes in contact. Sharp objects present a particular risk. If sharp objects

Figure 3–1 For an infection to occur, all four conditions must be present.

have contacted the blood or body fluids of an infected person and are handled carelessly, they can pierce the skin and transmit infection.

3. *Airborne*

   Airborne transmission (Figure 3–4) occurs when a person breathes in droplets that become airborne when an infected person coughs or sneezes. Exposure to these droplets is generally too brief for transmission to take place; however, it may if a person is coughing heavily.

4. *Vector-borne*

   Vector-borne transmission (Figure 3–5) occurs when an animal, such as a dog or raccoon, or an insect, such as a tick, transmits a pathogen into the body through a bite. A bite from an infected human is also a vector-borne transmission. The carrier is a vector and passes the infection to another animal or person. Rabies and Lyme disease are transmitted this way.

Figure 3–2 Direct contact transmission.

Figure 3–3 Indirect contact transmission.

TABLE 3–2: HOW DISEASES ARE TRANSMITTED

Mode of Transmission	Example of Disease	Definition	Route of Entry	Signs and Symptoms
Direct contact	Herpes	Family of viruses; infection with one of the human herpes viruses, especially herpes simplex types 1 and 2	Broken skin, mucous membranes	Lesions, general ill feeling, sore throat
Airborne, direct, and indirect contact	Meningitis	Inflammation of the membranes that envelop the central nervous system (meninges), usually due to a bacterial infection but sometimes from viral, protozoan, or other causes	Food and water, mucus	Respiratory illness, sore throat, nausea, vomiting
Airborne, direct, and indirect contact	Tuberculosis	A highly contagious infection caused by the bacterium *Mycobacterium tuberculosis*	Mucus, broken skin	Weight loss, night sweats, occasional fever, general ill feeling
Direct and indirect contact	Hepatitis	Inflammation of the liver from any cause; most often viral due to infection with one of the hepatitis viruses (A, B, C, D, and E) or another virus	Blood, saliva, semen, feces, food, water, other products	Flu-like, jaundice
Direct and indirect contact	HIV/AIDS	Disease due to infection with the HIV virus	Blood, semen, vaginal fluid	Fever, night sweats, weight loss, chronic diarrhea, severe fatigue, shortness of breath, swollen lymph nodes, lesions

Figure 3–4 Airborne transmission.

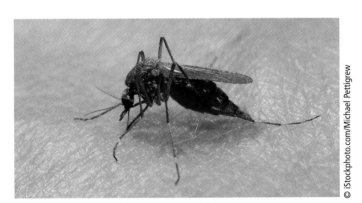

Figure 3–5 Vector-borne transmission.

Diseases That Cause Concern

Hepatitis A, B, C, D, and E

Hepatitis is a type of liver disease. Hepatitis A is caused by the hepatitis A virus (HAV). This disease is spread primarily through food or water that has been contaminated by stool from an infected person.

HAV is transmissible by:

- Eating food prepared by someone with HAV who did not wash his hands after using the bathroom

- Engaging in certain sexual activities, such as oral-anal contact with someone who has HAV

- Changing a diaper and then not washing hands

- Drinking water that has been contaminated with HAV

HAV causes inflammation and swelling of the liver. The person may feel ill, with flu-like symptoms, or may experience no symptoms at all. Symptoms of HAV usually disappear after several weeks. This disease rarely causes permanent damage or chronic illness.

HAV can be prevented with the hepatitis A vaccine, which is a series of two injections administered at least six months apart. The most effective prevention, though, is healthy habits. Always wash your hands thoroughly before preparing food, after using the toilet, and after changing a diaper. International travellers should be careful about drinking tap water.

Hepatitis B is a liver infection caused by the hepatitis B virus (HBV). Hepatitis B may be severe or even fatal, and it can be in the body for up to six months before symptoms appear. These may include flu-like symptoms, such as fever, fatigue, abdominal pain, loss of appetite, nausea, vomiting, and joint pain, as well as dark urine and clay-coloured bowel movements. Later-stage symptoms include jaundice, which causes a yellowing of the skin and eyes.

Medications are available to treat chronic hepatitis B infection, but they do not work for everyone. The most effective means of prevention is the hepatitis B vaccine. This vaccine, given in a series of three doses, provides immunity to the disease. Scientific data show that hepatitis B vaccines are safe for adults, children, and babies. There is no confirmed evidence indicating that the hepatitis B vaccine causes chronic illnesses.

The hepatitis B vaccination series should be made available to all employees who may have occupational exposure after they have completed appropriate training and within 10 working days of their initial assignment. However, employees may decide not to have the vaccination. If an employee decides not to be vaccinated, the person must sign a form affirming this decision. However, if an employee who initially declines hepatitis B vaccination decides to accept the vaccination at a later date, the employer must make the hepatitis B vaccination available at that time, so long as the standard still covers the employee.

Hepatitis C is a liver disease caused by the hepatitis C virus (HCV). In Canada, an estimated 242,500 people are infected with hepatitis C.[11] Its symptoms are similar to those of hepatitis B infection, including fever, fatigue, abdominal pain, loss of appetite, nausea, vomiting, dark urine, clay-coloured stool, joint pain, and jaundice. There is no vaccine against hepatitis C and no treatment available to prevent infection after exposure. For these reasons, hepatitis C is more serious than hepatitis B. Hepatitis C is the leading cause of liver transplants.

Hepatitis D is a serious liver disease caused by the hepatitis D virus (HDV) and relies on HBV to replicate. It is uncommon in Canada.[12] It is transmitted through contact with infectious blood, similar to how HBV is spread. There is no vaccine for hepatitis D.

Hepatitis E is caused by the hepatitis E virus (HEV). It is commonly transmitted via the fecal-oral route and is associated with ingestion of drinking water contaminated with fecal material in countries with poor sanitation. It occurs primarily in adults. The potential for HEV transmission from contaminated food is still under investigation, and there is no evidence of transmission by percutaneous (through the skin) or sexual exposures. There is currently no hepatitis E vaccination or treatment.[13]

HIV/AIDS

HIV is the virus that causes AIDS. HIV attacks white blood cells and destroys the body's ability to fight infection. This weakens the body's immune system. Infections that strike people with weakened immune systems are called opportunistic infections. Some opportunistic infections that occur in people with AIDS include severe pneumonia, tuberculosis (TB), Kaposi's sarcoma, and other unusual cancers.

People infected with HIV may not feel or appear sick. A blood test, however, can detect the HIV antibody. When an infected person has a significant drop in a certain type of white blood cell or shows signs of having certain infections or cancers, the person may be diagnosed as having AIDS. These infections can cause fever, fatigue, diarrhea, skin rashes, night sweats, loss of appetite, swollen lymph glands, and significant weight loss. In the advanced stages, AIDS is a very serious condition. People with AIDS eventually develop life-threatening infections from which they can die. Currently, there is no vaccine against HIV.

Tuberculosis

Tuberculosis (TB) is an infection caused by a bacterium called *Mycobacterium tuberculosis*. The bacteria usually attack the lungs, but they may also damage other parts of the body, such as the brain, kidneys, or spine. TB is spread through the air when an infected person coughs, sneezes, or talks. Anyone exposed to TB should be tested. People with a weakened immune system are more likely to get TB.

Symptoms of TB in the lungs may include:

• A bad cough lasting three weeks or longer

• A pain in the chest

• Weight loss

• Loss of appetite

• Coughing up blood or bloody sputum (phlegm from inside the lungs)

• Weakness and/or fatigue

• Fever and chills

• Night sweats

TB must be treated with appropriate medication or it can lead to death. It can usually be cured with several medications over a long period of time. People with latent (asymptomatic) TB can take medicine to prevent development of active TB.

Multidrug-Resistant Tuberculosis

Multidrug-resistant tuberculosis (MDR TB) is TB that is resistant to at least two of the most effective anti-TB drugs, isoniazid and rifampin. These drugs are the ones most widely used to treat TB. MDR TB is more likely to occur in people who:

• Do not take their TB medicine regularly or who do not take all of the prescribed medication

• Get active TB after having taken medication to treat it in the past

• Come from areas of the world where MDR TB is prevalent

• Spend time with someone known to have MDR TB

Meningitis

Meningitis is a contagious meningococcal infection that attacks the meninges, the protective coverings that surround the brain and spinal cord. Several different bacteria can cause meningitis, but a virus can also cause it. The bacteria are transmitted from person to person through droplets. Close and prolonged contact (e.g., kissing, sneezing, or coughing on someone) and living in close quarters or dormitories (e.g., military or student housing) facilitate the spread of the disease. Meningitis can infect anyone but is more commonly found in those who have compromised immune systems and have trouble fighting infections.

The most common symptoms are stiff neck, high fever, sensitivity to light, confusion, headache, nausea, sleepiness, and vomiting. Bacterial meningitis is a serious infection; even when diagnosed early and properly treated, 5 to 10% of people die, typically within 24 to 48 hours of the onset of symptoms. Bacterial meningitis may result in brain damage, hearing loss, or learning disability in 10 to 20% of people. Viral meningitis is less severe and usually resolves without specific treatment.

Bacterial meningitis is potentially fatal and is a medical emergency. Admission to a hospital or health centre is necessary. There are vaccines available to prevent meningitis and antibiotics with which to treat it.

Community-Associated MRSA

Methicillin-resistant Staphylococcus aureus (MRSA) is a bacterium. As one of the staph bacteria, like other kinds of bacteria, it frequently lives on the skin and in the nose without causing any health problems. It only becomes a problem when it is a source of infection. These bacteria can be spread from one person to another through casual contact or contaminated objects. Infections with MRSA are more difficult to treat than ordinary staph infections because they are resistant to many types of antibiotics, the medications used to treat bacterial infections. Infections can occur in wounds, burns, and sites where tubes have been inserted into the body.

When MRSA occurs in groups of people who have not been recently hospitalized or have not had a medical procedure, this type of MRSA is referred to as community-associated MRSA (CA-MRSA). For example, it can occur among young people who have cuts or wounds and who are in close contact with one another, such as members of a sports team.

Severe Acute Respiratory Syndrome (SARS)

Severe acute respiratory syndrome (SARS) is a viral respiratory illness caused by the SARS-associated Coronavirus (SARS-CoV). It was first reported in Asia in February 2003. Over the following months, it spread to more than two dozen countries in North America, South America, Europe, and Asia before the outbreak was contained.

SARS usually begins with a high fever (temperature greater than 38°C/100.4°F). Those infected may also experience headache, an overall feeling of discomfort, and body aches. They may have mild respiratory symptoms at the outset. About 10 to 20% of those infected have diarrhea. After two to seven days, SARS patients may develop a dry cough, and most develop pneumonia.

SARS spreads predominantly by close, person-to-person contact. The virus that causes SARS is thought to be transmitted most easily by respiratory droplets produced when an infected person coughs or sneezes

and the droplets are deposited on the mucous membranes of the mouth, nose, or eyes of people nearby. It can also spread when a person touches a surface or an object contaminated with infectious droplets and then touches the mouth, nose, or eyes.

Influenza

Seasonal influenza is a respiratory illness caused by both human influenza A and human influenza B viruses, which can be transmitted from person to person. Most people have some immunity to influenza, and there is a vaccine available.

Seasonal influenza usually has a sudden onset, with symptoms of fever (usually high), headache, extreme tiredness, dry cough, sore throat, runny or stuffy nose, and muscle aches. Abdominal symptoms such as nausea, vomiting, and diarrhea may also be present, but these symptoms occur more often in children than in adults.

Influenza is transmitted from person to person via large virus-laden droplets from coughing or sneezing. These large droplets settle on the mucosal surfaces of the upper respiratory tracts of susceptible people who are within one metre (three feet) of infected people. Transmission can also occur through direct contact or indirect contact with respiratory secretions—for example, when touching surfaces contaminated with influenza virus and then touching the mouth, nose, or eyes.

Pandemic influenza (or pandemic flu) is a virulent human influenza A virus. The term "pandemic" refers to an epidemic occurring over a wide geographic area that affects a large number of people. Pandemic flu can cause a global outbreak, or pandemic, of serious illness in humans. Because there is little natural immunity, the disease spreads easily from person to person.

Although we do not know for sure when the next pandemic influenza will strike or that it would present in the same way as seasonal influenza, it is helpful to be aware of the symptoms of seasonal influenza in order to plan for a pandemic flu. The best defence is to take steps to prevent disease transmission, such as frequent handwashing.

Immunization

Most people receive immunization as babies against common childhood diseases such as measles and mumps. Immunization is the introduction of a substance that contains specific weakened or killed pathogens into the body. The body's immune system then builds resistance to a specific infection.

You should also be immunized against several other diseases. The following immunizations are recommended:

- DPT (diphtheria, pertussis, tetanus)
- Polio
- Hepatitis B
- MMR (measles, mumps, rubella)
- Influenza
- Chicken pox

You might not have been immunized against some of the childhood diseases. If you are not sure about which immunizations you have received or may need to update, contact your doctor or local community health nurse.

PROTECTING YOURSELF FROM DISEASE TRANSMISSION

Precautions

Sometimes we might like to vary the level of protection we use based on what a person looks like, the circumstances surrounding the incident, or where he is at the time of the incident. However, the world is not that simple. Often you will not know the health status of the people you work with or care for. The one time you stop being careful may be the very time that you

Figure 3–6 There are many ways to protect yourself from disease transmission.

TABLE 3–3: RECOMMENDED PERSONAL PROTECTIVE EQUIPMENT FOR PRE-HOSPITAL SETTINGS[14]

Task or Activity	Disposable Gloves	Gown	Mask	Protective Eyewear
Bleeding control with spurting blood	Yes	Yes	Yes	Yes
Bleeding control with minimal bleeding	Yes	No	No	No
Childbirth	Yes	Yes	Yes, if splash is likely	Yes, if splash is likely
Helping with an intravenous (IV) line	Yes	No	No	No
Oral/nasal suctioning, manually clearing airway	Yes	No	Yes	Yes, if splash is likely
Handling and cleaning contaminated equipment and clothing if body fluids are present	Yes	No, unless soiling is likely	No, unless cleaning after transporting a patient with transmissible respiratory illness	No, unless gross amounts of bodily fluid are present
Transporting or caring for a patient with signs of transmissible respiratory illness	Yes	No	Yes	Yes

become infected. Each time you prepare to provide care, you must follow basic precautions, which include the following:

- PPE (Figure 3–6)
- Personal hygiene
- Engineering and work practice controls
- Equipment cleaning and disinfecting

PPE should be used to prevent skin and mucous membrane exposure when contact with blood or other body fluids is anticipated (Table 3–3). PPE keeps you from direct contact with infected materials and includes disposable gloves, gowns, masks and shields, protective eyewear, mouthpieces, and resuscitation devices. To minimize your risk of contracting or transmitting an infectious disease, follow these universal precautions:

Personal Protective Equipment (PPE)

- Handle all blood and other body fluids as if infectious.

- Handle all patients in a way that minimizes exposure to blood and other body fluids.

- Wear disposable (single-use) gloves when it is possible you will contact blood or body fluids. This may happen directly through contact with a patient or indirectly through contact with soiled clothing or other personal articles.

- Remove gloves by turning them inside out, beginning at the wrist and peeling them off. When removing the second glove, do not touch the soiled surfaces with your bare hand. Hook the inside of the second glove at the wrist and

Figure 3–7, a-c Glove removal.

peel the glove off (Figure 3–7, a-c). Always wash your hands with soap and water after removing gloves.

- Discard gloves that are peeling, discoloured, torn, or punctured.

- Do not clean or reuse disposable gloves.

- Avoid handling items such as pens, combs, or radios, yours or another person's, when wearing soiled gloves.

- Change gloves for each patient you contact.

- Use protective coverings, such as a mask, eyewear, and a gown, whenever you are likely to contact blood or other body fluids that may splash.

- Cover any cuts, scrapes, or skin irritations you may have with protective clothing or bandages.

- Use breathing devices, such as resuscitation masks with one-way valves. These should be readily available in settings where the need for resuscitation can be anticipated.

Putting On and Removing PPE

When putting on and removing PPE, follow a specific order to avoid indirect contact with pathogens. To put on the appropriate PPE (see Table 3–3), follow this order:

1. Wash hands.
2. Put on gown.
3. Put on mask.
4. Put on protective eyewear.
5. Put on disposable gloves.

When removing PPE, follow this order:

1. Remove disposable gloves.
2. Remove gown.
3. Wash hands.
4. Remove protective eyewear.
5. Remove mask.
6. Wash hands.

Personal Hygiene

Personal hygiene habits, such as frequent handwashing (Figure 3–8, a-f), are as important in preventing infection as any equipment you might use. These habits and practices can prevent any materials that might have gone through the protective equipment from staying in contact with your body.

Engineering and Work Practice Controls

Engineering controls are controls that isolate or remove the hazard from the workplace. These include puncture-resistant containers for sharp equipment and mechanical needle recapping devices. To ensure that they work well, engineering controls should be examined and maintained or replaced on a regular basis.

Work practice controls reduce the likelihood of exposure by changing the way a task is carried out. The protection provided by work practice controls is based on the way people behave rather than on a physical device.

Engineering controls and work practice controls are established to ensure good industrial hygiene. Following

Figure 3–8, a-f Thoroughly, and properly, washing your hands helps protect you against disease transmission.

certain guidelines for engineering controls and work practice controls can greatly cut down your risk of contracting or transmitting an infectious disease.

- Ensure that all response kits are fully stocked with several pairs of disposable gloves, pocket masks or face shields, and antibacterial hand cleanser.

- Ensure that response kits are readily available and easily accessible to everyone.

- Maintain all PPE in good working order. Immediately dispose of any PPE that is peeling, discoloured, torn, or punctured.

- Check and restock response kits on a regular basis.

- Use dressings and tissues to minimize direct contact with blood, other body fluids, and wounds. If possible, have the patient wash the wound first and assist you with, for example, holding a dressing in place or applying pressure if necessary.

- Avoid needle-stick injuries by not trying to bend or recap any needles.

- If a procedure requires the recapping of a needle, use mechanical devices or one-handed techniques to recap. Never recap contaminated needles.

- Place sharp items (e.g., needles, scalpel blades) in puncture-resistant, leak-proof, labelled containers.

- Perform all procedures in a way that cuts down on splashing, spraying, splattering, and producing droplets of blood or other potentially infectious materials.

- Remove soiled protective clothing as soon as possible.

- Avoid eating, drinking, smoking, applying cosmetics or lip balm, handling contact lenses, and touching your mouth, nose, or eyes in work areas where exposure to infectious materials may occur.

- Handle all soiled equipment, supplies, or other materials with great care until they are properly cleaned and disinfected. Place all contaminated disposable items in labelled containers. Place all soiled clothing in properly marked plastic bags for disposal or washing.

- Wash your hands thoroughly with soap and water immediately after providing care. Use a utility or restroom sink, not one in a food preparation area.

- If something occurs that creates disposable waste or soiled laundry, the materials should be stored in appropriate containers until they are disposed of or laundered. The containers must have warning labels or signs, such as "biohazard," to eliminate or minimize exposure to individuals. In addition, training should be provided to ensure that everyone understands and avoids the hazard.

Equipment Cleaning and Disinfecting

- Clean and disinfect equipment and work surfaces possibly soiled by blood or other body fluids to prevent infections.

- For cleaning equipment and surfaces, gloves should be worn.

- Surfaces such as floors, woodwork, vehicle seats, and countertops must be cleaned with soap and water first, using disposable towels, and then disinfected. To disinfect equipment soiled with blood or body fluids, wash thoroughly with a solution of common household chlorine bleach and water. Each EMS system may have protocols and solution ratios for various decontamination techniques. Many decontaminating solutions are available. Follow the directions on the label.

- Wash and dry protective clothing and work uniforms according to the manufacturer's instructions. Scrub soiled boots, leather shoes, and other leather goods, such as belts, with soap, a brush, and hot water.

- Work areas should be kept in a clean and sanitary condition based on a written schedule for cleaning and decontamination. The schedule should be based on the location in the facility, the type of surface to be cleaned, the type of soil present, and the tasks or procedures being done.

Spill Management

In addition, there should be a plan in place to deal with any spill that might occur. The plan should include a system to report a spill and the action taken to resolve the spill. It should also include a list of people responsible for containment, instructions for cleanup, and the final disposition of the spill. The first step in dealing with a spill is containment. Spill containment units designed for hazardous materials are available for purchase. However, any absorbent material, such as paper towels, can be used if the material is disposed of properly.

The steps for spill management are as follows:

- Wear gloves and other appropriate PPE when cleaning spills.

- Clean up spills immediately or as soon as possible after the spill occurs.

- If the spill is mixed with sharp objects, such as broken glass and needles, do not pick these up with your hands. Use tongs, a broom and a dust pan, or two pieces of cardboard.

- Dispose of the absorbent material used to collect the spill in a labelled biohazard container.

- Flood the area with disinfectant solution and allow it to stand for at least 20 minutes.

- Use paper towels to absorb the solution and put the towels in the biohazard container.

Following these precautions will usually remove at least one of the four conditions necessary for disease transmission. Remember, if only one condition is missing, infection will not occur.

The Exposure Control Plan

Preventing infectious disease transmission begins with preparation and planning. An exposure control plan is an important step in removing or reducing exposure to blood and other possibly infectious materials. The exposure control plan is a system to protect people in a given environment from infection and should be placed where it can easily be used. The plan should be updated each year or more often if changes in exposure occur.

An exposure control plan should contain the following elements:

- Exposure determination

- Identification of who will receive training, PPE, and vaccination

- Procedures for evaluating details of an exposure incident

Exposure determination is one of the key elements of an exposure control plan. It includes identifying and making a written record of tasks in which exposure to blood or other body fluids can occur.

The following Health Canada recommendations for healthcare providers can be applied to individuals at risk in any environment:

- There should be initial orientation and continuing education on modes of transmission and prevention of infections and the need for routine use of PPE for all people.

- Equipment and supplies necessary to minimize the risk of infection with pathogens should be provided.

- Adherence to recommended protective measures should be monitored. When monitoring reveals a failure to follow recommended precautions, counselling, education, or retraining should be provided.

- Health Canada also recommends that particular vaccinations, such as hepatitis B, be offered to all susceptible healthcare providers, particularly those who work in high-risk areas.

- The exposure control plan should include reporting procedures for any first aid incidents. The procedures must ensure that incidents are reported before the end of the shift in which they occur.

- Reports of first aid incidents should include the names of all responders involved and the details of the incident. The report should also include the date and time of the incident and if an exposure incident has occurred.

- Exposure reports should be included on lists of first aid incidents.

- Responders should be trained in reporting procedure specifics.

IF AN EXPOSURE OCCURS

If you suspect you have been exposed to an infectious disease, wash any area of contact as quickly as possible and write down what happened. Exposures usually involve contact with potentially infectious blood or other fluids through a needle stick, broken or scraped skin, or the mucous membranes of the eyes, nose, or mouth. Inhaling potentially infected airborne droplets also may be an exposure. Most organizations have protocols (standardized procedures) for reporting infectious disease exposure. Be aware of provincial/territorial Occupational Health and Safety guidelines and Workers' Compensation guidelines.

The procedures should include the following elements:

- Be easy to access and user-friendly

- Ensure confidentiality

- Instill confidence in the exposed worker

- List events covered by the procedure

- List immediate actions to be taken by the exposed individual to reduce the chances of infection

- Provide direction on when or how quickly the individual should report the exposure incident

- Provide direction on where and to whom the individual should report the exposure incident

- Indicate which forms the individual should complete

- Provide directions for investigating the incident

- List information required from healthcare providers

- Indicate medical follow-up, including post-exposure vaccination

If you think you have been exposed to an infectious disease, you should report the exposure immediately. A test may be done to see if the infection was present. Even before a disease is confirmed, you should receive medical evaluation, counselling, and post-exposure care. Your medical personnel or supervisor is responsible for notifying any other personnel who might have been exposed. If your system does not have a designated physician or nurse at a local hospital for follow-up care, see your personal physician.

SUMMARY

Although the body's natural defence system defends well against disease, pathogens can still enter the body and sometimes cause infection. These pathogens can be transmitted in four ways:

1. By direct contact with an infected person
2. By indirect contact with a soiled object
3. By inhaling air exhaled by an infected person
4. By vector-borne contact, through a bite from an infected animal, insect, or even a person

Infectious diseases that you should be aware of include hepatitis, herpes, meningitis, tuberculosis, SARS, influenza, community-associated MRSA, and HIV infections. You should know how the diseases are transmitted and take appropriate measures to protect yourself from them. Remember that all four conditions of infection must be present for a disease to be transmitted:

1. A pathogen is present
2. There is enough of the pathogen to cause disease
3. A person is susceptible to the pathogen
4. There is an entry route

One of the best defences against disease and infection is to wash your hands frequently. It has been determined that individuals face a significant risk as a result of exposure to blood and other potentially infectious materials because they may contain blood-borne pathogens. This hazard can be reduced or removed using a combination of engineering and work practice controls, personal protective clothing and equipment, training, medical surveillance, vaccinations, signs and labels, and other provisions.

Organizations have responsibilities that include:

• Identifying positions or tasks potentially at risk

• Developing an annual training system for all at-risk individuals

• Offering the opportunity for individuals to get counselling and medical care, such as hepatitis vaccinations, at no cost

• Using work practices, such as following universal and other precautions to minimize the possibility of infection

• Using engineering controls, such as puncture-resistant containers for sharp objects, to minimize the possibility of infection

• Creating a system for easy identification of soiled material and its disposal

• Creating an exposure control plan to minimize the possibility of exposure

• Establishing clear procedures to follow for reporting an exposure

• Creating a system of record keeping that includes updates in protocols and exposure control plans, training, medical records, and follow-up

Following these guidelines, especially the precautions, greatly decreases your risk of contracting or transmitting an infectious disease. If you suspect you have been exposed to such a disease, always document it and notify appropriate personnel. Seek medical help and participate in any follow-up procedures.

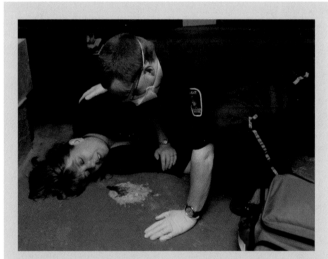

You approach the woman lying on the floor in her office. You see that her nose is bloody and blood is coming out of her mouth. The man who found her is visibly upset and asks you if you're going to be able to save her life. What do you do?

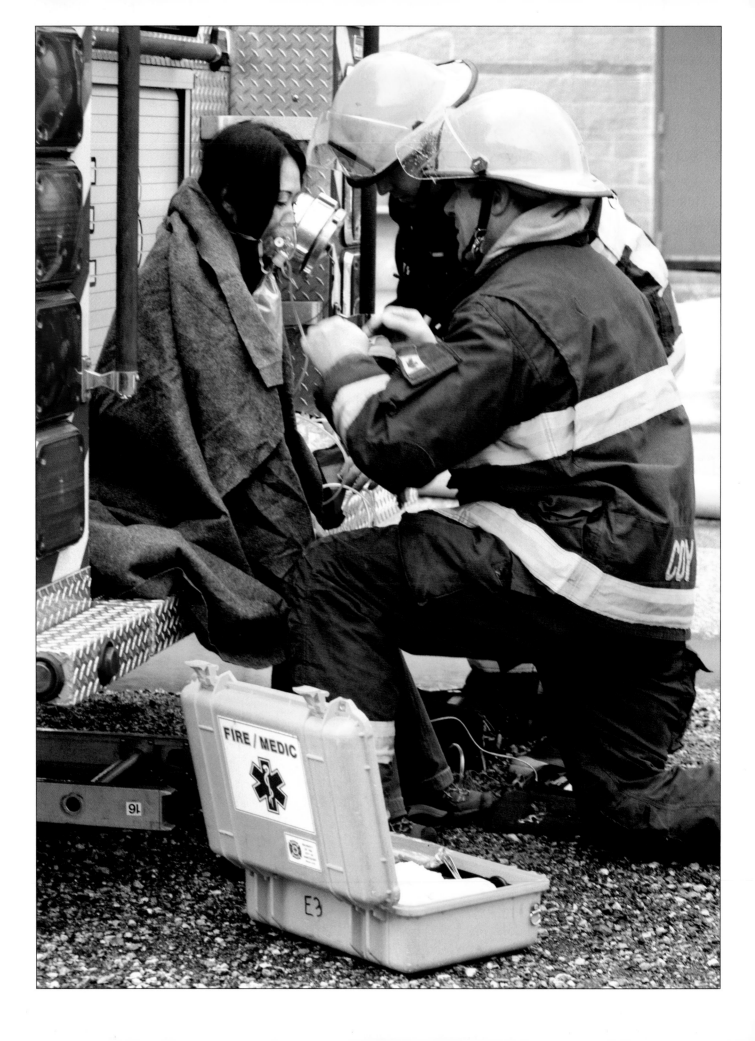

Part 2

Establishing Priorities of Care

4
Anatomy and Physiology

5
Assessment

6
Respiratory Emergencies

7
Airway and Ventilation

8
Circulatory Emergencies

9
Bleeding

10
Shock

11
Pharmacology

Chapter 4

Anatomy and Physiology

You are the responder at the scene of a motor vehicle collision involving a car with two occupants and a van driven by a woman with small children in car seats. At first glance, three people appear to be injured. The first person, a woman, was driving one of the cars, and she is going in and out of consciousness. You suspect her injuries may have crushed some of her ribs. The second person, a passenger in the same car, has injuries on the right side of his body. The third person, the driver of the van, appears to have chest and abdominal injuries, but she is conscious and you can speak to her. She is distraught because her children are in the back of the van and she is concerned about them. How would you describe the injuries and the body systems involved?

INTRODUCTION

As a responder, you need a basic understanding of normal human structure and function. Knowing the body's structures and how they work will help you more easily recognize and understand illnesses and injuries. Body systems do not function independently. Each system depends on other systems to function properly. When your body is healthy, your body systems are working well together. But an injury or illness in one body part or system will often cause problems in others. Knowing the location and function of the major organs and structures within each body system will help you to more accurately assess a patient's condition and provide the best care.

To remember the location of body structures, it helps to learn to visualize the structures that lie beneath the skin. The structures you can see or feel are reference points for locating the internal structures you cannot see or feel. For example, to locate the pulse on either side of the neck, you can use the Adam's apple on the front of the neck as a reference point. Using reference points will help you describe the location of injuries and other problems you may find. This chapter provides you with an overview of important reference points, terminology, and the functions of eight body systems.

ANATOMICAL TERMS

You do not need to be an expert in human body structure and function to provide effective care. Neither should you need a medical dictionary to effectively describe an injury. By knowing a few key structures, their functions, and locations, you can recognize a serious illness or injury and accurately communicate with other emergency care personnel about a patient's condition.

To use terms that refer to the body, you must first understand "anatomical position." All medical terms that refer to the body are based on the position shown in Figure 4–1, a-c.

The simplest anatomical terms are based on an imaginary line running down the middle of the body from the head to the ground, dividing it into two mirror-image right and left halves. This line is called the midline. In medical terms, right and left always refer to the patient in question's right and left, not the responder's.

Other terms related to the midline include lateral and medial. Anything away from the midline is called lateral. Anything toward the midline is called medial.

Another reference line can be drawn through the side of the body, dividing it into front and back halves. Anything toward the front of the body is called anterior (ventral); anything toward the back is called posterior (dorsal).

Other terms that refer to direction can also be useful. When comparing any two structures, such as two body parts, any part toward the patient's head is described as superior (cephalic). Any part toward the patient's feet is described as inferior (caudal).

Two other terms are generally used when referring to the arms and legs. These terms are proximal and distal. To understand these terms, you must think of the chest, abdomen, and pelvis as those areas that make up the trunk of the body. The arms and legs are the attachments to the trunk. Points on the body closer to the trunk are described as proximal. Points away from the trunk are described as distal.

Figure 4–2 shows other basic terms used for body regions and their specific parts. These are all standard terms used by people who provide emergency care. Some terms will be familiar, whereas others may be new to you. Study these terms and learn to use them correctly when describing body parts.

Special anatomical terms are used for the abdomen, the part of the trunk below the ribs and above the pelvis. By drawing two imaginary lines, one from the breastbone down through the navel to the lowest point in the pelvis and another line horizontally through the navel, you divide the abdomen into four areas called quadrants (Figure 4–3). These terms are important when describing injuries to the abdomen because different organs may be injured depending on the quadrant involved.

Of all these terms, it is most important to correctly use left and right, lateral and medial, and the basic terms that refer to body parts. Even though you may not use the other terms, you should know what they mean. You may need to understand what other emergency care personnel are saying when they use these terms to refer to injuries.

a

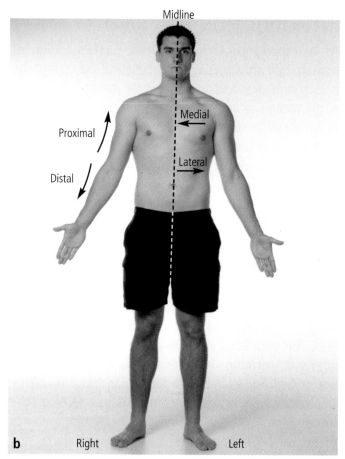

Midline

Proximal

Distal

Medial

Lateral

b   Right   Left

Superior
(Cephalic)

Anterior
(Ventral)

Posterior
(Dorsal)

Inferior
(Caudal)

c

Figure 4–1, a-c a, The anatomical position; **b**, Medical use of the terms *right* and *left* refers to the patient's right and left. *Medial* refers to anything toward the midline; *lateral* refers to anything away from the midline. *Proximal* and *distal* are usually used to refer to extremities; and **c**, *Anterior* refers to the front of the body; *posterior* refers to the back of the body; *superior* refers to anything toward the head; *inferior* refers to anything toward the feet.

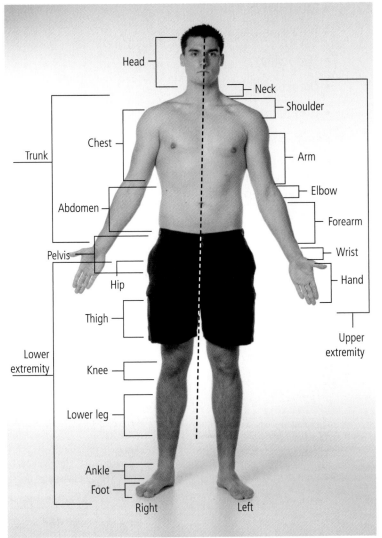

Figure 4–2 It is important to refer correctly to the parts of the body.

BODY CAVITIES

A body cavity is a hollow place in the body that contains organs such as the heart, lungs, and liver. The five major cavities, illustrated in Figure 4–4, are the:

1. Cranial cavity, located in the head, which is protected by the skull.

2. Spinal cavity, extending from the bottom of the skull to the lower back, protected by the bones of the spine.

3. Thoracic cavity, also called chest cavity, which is located in the trunk between the diaphragm and the neck. The thoracic cavity is protected by the rib cage and the upper portion of the spine.

4. Abdominal cavity, located in the trunk between the diaphragm and the pelvis.

5. Pelvic cavity, located in the pelvis, which is the lowest part of the trunk. It is protected by the pelvic bones and the lower portion of the spine.

Knowing the general location of major organs in each cavity will help you assess a patient's injury or illness. The major organs and their functions are more fully described in the next section of this chapter.

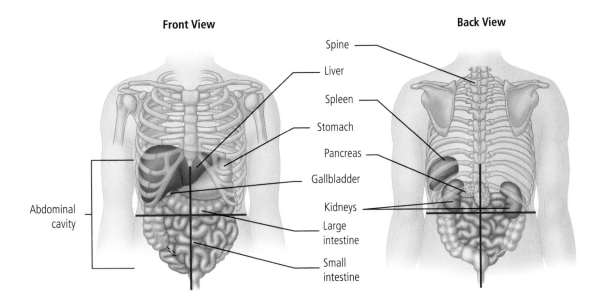

Figure 4–3 The abdominal quadrants.

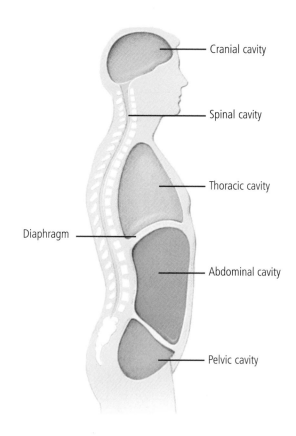

Figure 4–4 The five major cavities of the body.

BODY SYSTEMS

The human body is a miraculous machine. It performs many complex functions, each of which helps us live. Vital organs are organs whose functions are essential for life, such as the brain, heart, and lungs.

A body system is a group of organs and other structures that are especially adapted to perform specific body functions (Table 4–1). They work together to carry out a function needed for life. For example, the heart, blood, and blood vessels make up the circulatory system. The circulatory system keeps all parts of the body supplied with oxygen-rich blood.

For the body to work properly, all of the following systems must work well together:

- Respiratory
- Circulatory
- Nervous
- Musculoskeletal
- Integumentary
- Endocrine
- Digestive
- Genitourinary

When one or more of the body systems does not perform its function properly, this is referred to as pathophysiology, which is the study of abnormal changes in mechanical, physical, and biochemical functions caused by injury or illness.

The Cell

The cell is the basic unit of life (Figure 4–5). Energy, DNA, and enzymes are examples of what is created within a human cell. From cells, tissues are formed, which then form organs. Organs are grouped together to form body systems.

Figure 4–5 The basic human cell.

TABLE 4–1: BODY SYSTEMS

Systems	Major Structures	Primary Functions	How the System Works With Other Body Systems
Respiratory system	Airway and lungs	Supplies the body with oxygen through breathing	Works with the circulatory system to provide oxygen to cells; is under the control of the nervous system
Circulatory system	Heart, blood, and blood vessels	Transports nutrients and oxygen to body cells and removes waste products	Works with the respiratory system to provide oxygen to cells; works in conjunction with the urinary and digestive systems to remove waste products; helps give skin colour; is under the control of the nervous system
Nervous system	Brain, spinal cord, and nerves	One of two primary regulatory systems in the body; transmits messages to and from the brain	Regulates all body systems through a network of nerves
Musculo-skeletal system	Bones, ligaments, muscles, and tendons	Provides the body's framework; protects internal organs and other underlying structures; allows movement; produces heat; manufactures blood components	Provides protection to organs and structures of other body systems; muscle action is controlled by the nervous system
Integumentary system	Skin, hair, and nails	An important part of the body's communication network; helps prevent infection and dehydration; assists with temperature regulation; aids in production of certain vitamins	Helps protect the body from disease-producing organisms; together with the circulatory system, helps regulate body temperature under control of the nervous system; communicates sensation to the brain by way of the nerves
Endocrine system	Glands	Secretes hormones and other substances into blood and onto skin	Together with the nervous system, coordinates the activities of other systems
Digestive system	Mouth, esophagus, stomach, intestines	Breaks down food into a usable form to supply the rest of the body with energy	Works with the circulatory system to transport nutrients to the body
Genitourinary system	Uterus and genitalia	Performs the processes of reproduction	
	Kidneys, bladder	Removes wastes from the circulatory system and regulates water balance	

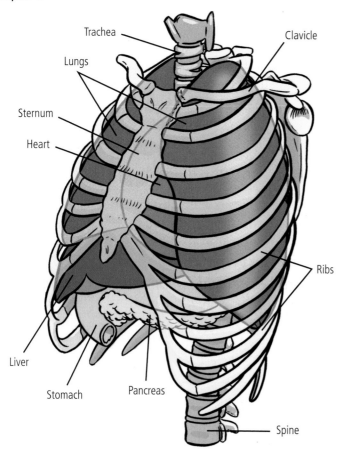

Figure 4–6 The rib cage surrounds and protects several vital organs.

Respiratory System

The body must have a constant supply of oxygen to stay alive. The respiratory system supplies the body with oxygen through breathing. When you inhale, air fills the lungs, and the oxygen in the air is transferred to the blood. The blood carries oxygen to all cells of the body. This same system removes carbon dioxide. Carbon dioxide is transferred from the blood to the lungs. When you exhale, air is forced from the lungs, expelling carbon dioxide and other waste gases. This breathing process is called respiration.

The chest is the upper part of the trunk. It is formed by 12 pairs of ribs, 10 of which attach to the sternum in front and the spine in back. The other two pairs attach only to the spine in the back and are sometimes called "floating" ribs. The rib cage is the cage of bones formed by the 12 pairs of ribs, the sternum, and the spine. It protects vital organs, such as the heart, major blood vessels,

and the lungs (Figure 4–6). Also in the chest are the esophagus, the trachea, and the muscles of respiration.

The respiratory system includes the airway and lungs. The airway, the passage through which air travels to the lungs, begins at the nose and mouth. The nose and mouth form the upper airway. Air passes through the nose and mouth and through the pharynx (the throat), larynx (the voice box), and trachea (the windpipe) on its way to the lungs (Figure 4–7). The lungs are a pair of organs in the chest that provide the mechanism for taking in oxygen and removing carbon dioxide during breathing. Behind the trachea is the esophagus. The esophagus carries food and liquids from the mouth to the stomach. A small flap of tissue, the epiglottis, covers the trachea when you swallow to keep food and liquids out of the lungs.

Air reaches the lungs through two tubes called bronchi. The bronchi branch into increasingly smaller tubes.

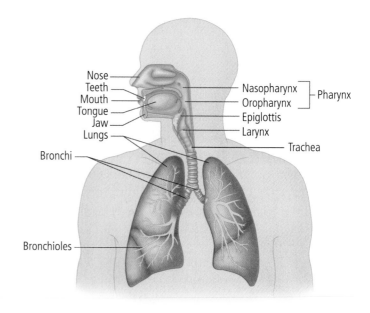

Figure 4–7 The respiratory system includes the pharynx, larynx, and trachea.

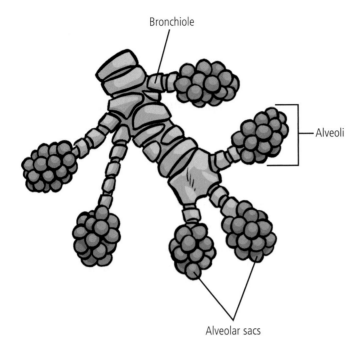

Figure 4–8 The bronchi branch into smaller tubes and end in air sacs called alveoli.

These eventually end in millions of tiny air sacs called alveoli (Figure 4–8). Oxygen and carbon dioxide pass into and out of the blood through the thin cell walls of the alveoli and tiny blood vessels called capillaries.

Air enters the lungs when you inhale and leaves the lungs when you exhale. When you inhale, the chest muscles and the diaphragm contract. This expands the chest and draws air into the lungs. When you exhale, the chest muscles and diaphragm relax, allowing air to exit from the lungs (Figure 4–9, a-b). This ongoing breathing process is involuntary and is controlled by the brain.

THE BREATHING PROCESS

Air enters the respiratory system through the nose and mouth and passes through the pharynx. The pharynx divides into two passageways: one for food, the esophagus, and one for air, the trachea. The epiglottis protects the opening of the trachea when a person swallows so that food and liquid do not enter the lungs.

The body requires a constant supply of oxygen for survival. The supply required depends on the needs of the body, which are affected by variables such as

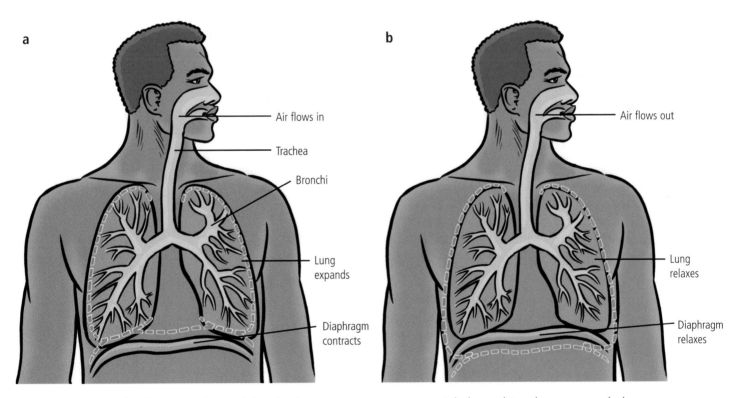

Figure 4–9, a-b The chest muscles and the diaphragm, a, contract as you inhale; and b, relax as you exhale.

activity level. A body fighting off an illness, even the common cold, uses more energy and oxygen than a body in its healthy state. With illness, the body must carry out all regular functions and also fight the illness. Some tissues, such as brain tissue, are very sensitive to oxygen starvation. Without oxygen, brain cells begin to die in as few as four to six minutes (Figure 4–10). Other vital organs will also be affected unless oxygen supplies are restored.

The brain is the control centre for breathing. It adjusts the rate and depth of breaths according to the oxygen and carbon dioxide levels in the body. Breathing requires the respiratory, circulatory, nervous, and musculoskeletal systems to work together. Injuries or illnesses that affect any of these systems may cause breathing emergencies. For example, in the event of severe bleeding, where there has been a loss of blood, the body will compensate by increasing the blood flow to the tissue and therefore increasing the respiratory rate.

Respiratory emergencies can be caused by the following:

- Choking
- Illness, such as pneumonia
- Respiratory conditions, such as emphysema and asthma
- Electrocution
- Shock
- Drowning
- Heart attack or heart disease

- Injury to the chest or lungs
- Allergic reactions, such as to food or insect stings
- Drugs
- Poisoning, such as inhaling or ingesting toxic substances

Circulatory System

The circulatory system works with the respiratory system to carry oxygen to every body cell. It also carries other nutrients throughout the body and removes waste.

The circulatory system includes the heart, blood, and blood vessels. Figure 4–11 shows this system.

The heart is a muscular organ behind the sternum, or breastbone. The heart pumps blood throughout the body through veins and arteries. Arteries are large blood vessels that carry oxygen-rich blood from the heart to the rest of the body. The arteries subdivide into smaller blood vessels and ultimately become tiny capillaries. The capillaries transport blood to all the cells of the body and nourish them with oxygen.

After the oxygen in the blood is transferred to the cells, veins carry the oxygen-poor blood back to the heart. The heart pumps this oxygen-poor blood to the lungs to pick up more oxygen before pumping it to other parts of the body. This cycle is called the circulatory cycle. The cross-section of the heart in Figure 4–12 shows how blood moves through the heart to complete the circulatory cycle.

0 minute: Breathing stops. Heart will soon stop beating. Clinical death.

4–6 minutes: Brain damage possible.

6–10 minutes: Brain damage likely.

10+ minutes: Irreversible brain damage certain. Biological death.

Figure 4–10 In clinical death the heart and breathing stops. Clinical death can lead to biological death, which is the irreversible death of brain cells.

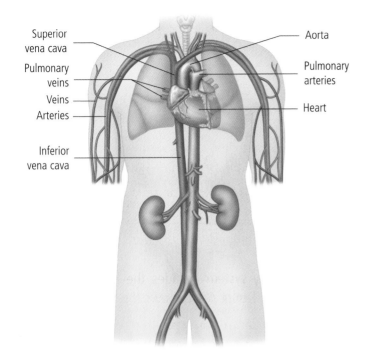

Figure 4–11 The circulatory system.

Labels:
- Superior vena cava
- Pulmonary veins
- Veins
- Arteries
- Inferior vena cava
- Aorta
- Pulmonary arteries
- Heart

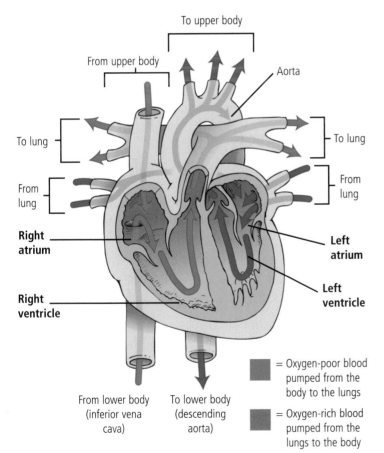

Labels:
- To upper body
- From upper body
- Aorta
- To lung
- From lung
- To lung
- From lung
- Right atrium
- Left atrium
- Right ventricle
- Left ventricle
- From lower body (inferior vena cava)
- To lower body (descending aorta)
- ■ = Oxygen-poor blood pumped from the body to the lungs
- ■ = Oxygen-rich blood pumped from the lungs to the body

Figure 4–12 The heart is a pump made up of four chambers. Various one-way valves keep the blood moving in the proper direction in order to complete the circulatory cycle.

DID YOU KNOW?

An elephant's heart beats 25 times a minute and weighs 15 kilograms (40 pounds). A man's heart beats about 70 times a minute and weighs about 1/3 kilogram (one pound). A mouse's heart beats about 700 times a minute and weighs approximately 1/2 gram (0.0175 ounce).

In a month, blood will have taken its journey around the human body 43,000 times. Blood vessels form a branching network of about 100,000 kilometres (62,000 miles), almost three times the distance around the earth.

The pumping action of the heart is called a contraction. Contractions are controlled by the heart's electrical system, which makes the heart beat regularly. You can feel the heart's contractions in the arteries that are close to the skin, for instance, at the neck or the wrist. The beat you feel with each contraction is called the pulse. The heart must beat regularly to deliver oxygen to body cells to keep the body functioning properly.

The Heart's Electrical System

To better understand both the limitations of CPR and how defibrillators work, it is helpful to understand how the heart's electrical system functions. The electrical system determines the pumping action of the heart. Under normal conditions, specialized cells of the heart initiate and carry on electrical activity. The normal point of origin of the electrical impulse is the sinoatrial (SA) node, which is situated in the upper part of the heart's right atrium.

The electrical impulse moves to the atrioventricular (AV) node, which is situated between the two atria and ventricles, and through conduction pathways within the heart muscle. From the AV node, the electrical signal is sent to the ventricles through other pathways.

These electrical impulses are the stimuli that cause the heart muscle to contract and pump the blood out of its chambers and throughout the body (Figure 4–13).

Cardiac monitors are used to read the electrical impulses in the heart to produce an electrocardiogram (ECG), which is a reading of the conduction of the electrical

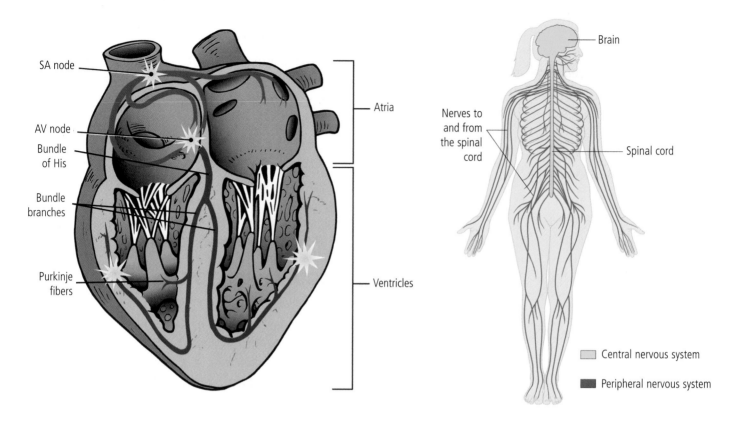

Figure 4–13 Conduction system of the heart.

Figure 4–15 The nervous system.

current through the pathways of the heart. The normal conduction of electrical impulses without any disturbances is called normal sinus rhythm (NSR) (Figure 4–14).

In NSR, the impulse is initiated in the SA node and transmitted to the atria. The stimulus from the electrical impulse causes the atria to contract and expel the blood to the ventricles. Meanwhile, the electrical current continues to travel through the atria and the AV node to the ventricles. When the ventricles receive the impulse, they contract to expel the blood throughout the body's blood vessels. This process normally takes place 60 to 100 times per minute.

Figure 4–14 Normal sinus rhythm.

Nervous System

The nervous system is the most complex and delicate of all body systems. The brain, the centre of the nervous system, is the master organ of the body. It regulates all body functions, including the respiratory and circulatory systems. The primary functions of the brain can be divided into three categories: the sensory functions, the motor functions, and the integrated functions of consciousness, memory, emotions, and use of language.

The brain transmits and receives information through a network of nerves. Figure 4–15 shows the nervous system. The spinal cord, a large bundle of nerves, extends from the brain through a canal in the spine, or backbone. Nerves extend from the brain and spinal cord to every part of the body.

Nerves transmit information as electrical impulses from one area of the body to another. Some nerves conduct impulses from the body to the brain, allowing you to see, hear, smell, taste, and feel. These are the sensory functions. Other nerves conduct impulses from the brain to the muscles to control motor functions, or movement.

Illness or injury to the brain may change a person's level of consciousness (LOC) and/or alter memory, emotions, and the ability to use language.

Nerve cells, unlike other body cells, cannot regenerate or grow back. Once brain cells die or are damaged, they are not replaced. Nerve cells may die from disease or injury. When a particular part of the brain is diseased or injured, a person may lose the body functions controlled by that area of the brain forever. For example, if the part of the brain that regulates breathing is damaged, the person may stop breathing.

The integrated functions of the brain are more complex. One of the functions of the brain, particularly the brain stem, is consciousness. When your brain stem is fully functioning and oxygenated, you are conscious. Decreased oxygen supply results in a decreased level of consciousness; at this point, you may be roused by tactile or painful stimuli. The level of consciousness may degrade to a point of unconsciousness where there is no response to any stimuli.

The spine is a strong, flexible column that supports the head and the trunk and encases and protects the spinal cord. The spinal column, which extends from the base of the skull to the tip of the tailbone, consists of small bones with circular openings, called vertebrae. The vertebrae are separated from each other by cushions of cartilage called discs (Figure 4–16, a). This cartilage, an elastic tissue, acts as a shock absorber when a person is walking, running, or jumping. The spinal cord, a bundle of nerves extending from the base of the skull to the lower back, runs through the hollow part of the vertebrae. Nerve branches extend to various parts of the body through openings on the sides of the vertebrae.

The spine is divided into five regions: the cervical or neck region, the thoracic or mid-back region, the lumbar or lower back region, the sacrum, and the

coccyx, the small triangular bone at the lower end of the spinal column (Figure 4–16, b). Injuries to the spinal column include fractures and dislocations of the vertebrae, sprained ligaments, and compression or displacement of the discs between the vertebrae.

MUSCULOSKELETAL SYSTEM

The musculoskeletal system is made up of muscles, bones that form the skeleton, and connective tissues such as tendons and ligaments. Together, these structures support the body, protect internal organs, allow movement, store minerals, produce blood cells, and produce heat. Bones and muscles connect to form various body segments.

Muscles

The body has more than 600 muscles. Most are skeletal muscles, which attach to the bones. Skeletal muscles account for most of your lean body weight (body weight without excess fat).

Muscles are able to shorten (contract) and lengthen (relax). All body movements result from skeletal muscles contracting and relaxing. Figure 4–17 shows the major muscles of the body. Skeletal muscle actions are under your conscious control. Because you control the movement, skeletal muscles are also called voluntary muscles. Skeletal muscles protect underlying structures such as bones, nerves, and blood vessels.

Most skeletal muscles are anchored to bone at each end by strong, cord-like tissues called tendons. Tendons are tissues that attach muscles to bones. Muscles and their adjoining tendons extend across joints. When the brain sends a command to move, electrical impulses travel through the spinal cord and nerve pathways to the individual muscles and stimulate the muscle fibres

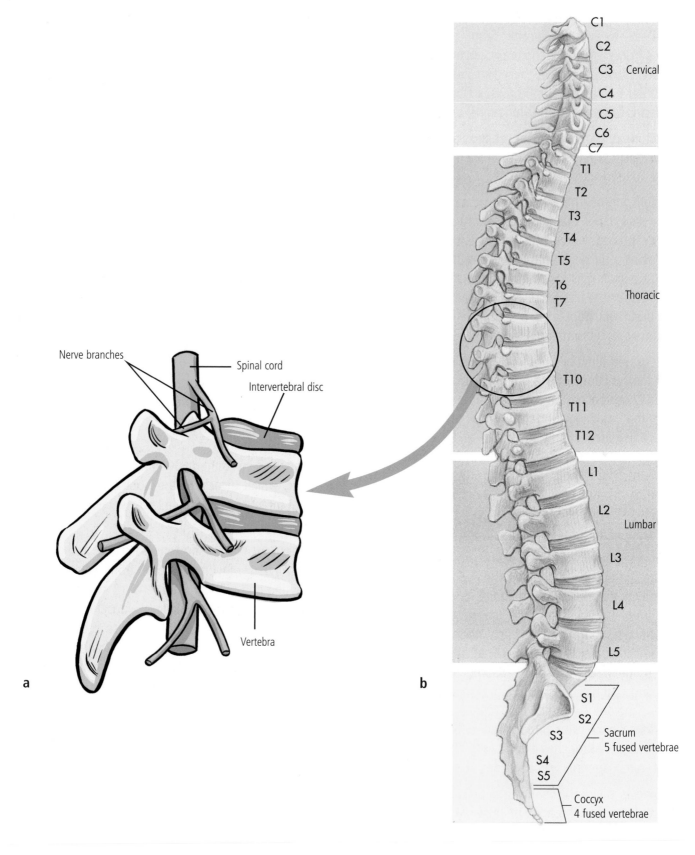

Figure 14–16, a-b a, Vertebrae are separated by pads of cartilage called invertebral discs; **b**, the spine is divided into 5 regions.

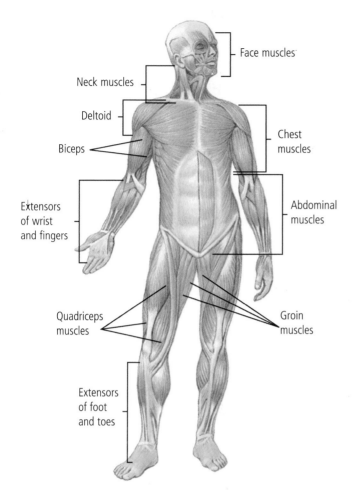

Figure 4–17 Major muscles of the body.

to move. When a muscle contracts, the muscle fibres shorten, pulling the ends of the muscle closer together. The muscles pull the bones, causing motion at the joint the muscle crosses.

Motion is usually caused by a group of muscles close together pulling at the same time. Muscle groups work together to produce movement (Figure 4–18). For instance, the hamstring muscles are a group of muscles at the back of the thigh. When the hamstrings contract, the leg bends at the knee. The quadriceps are a group of muscles at the front of the thigh. When the quadriceps muscles contract, the leg straightens at the knee. Generally, when one group of muscles contracts another group of muscles on the opposite side of the body part relaxes (Figure 4–19). Even simple tasks, such as bending to pick up an object from the floor, involve a complex series of movements in which different

Figure 4–18 Muscles work together to produce movement.

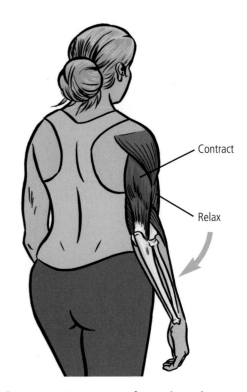

Contract

Relax

Contract

Relax

Figure 4–19 Movement occurs when one group of muscles contracts and an opposing group of muscles relaxes.

muscle groups contract and relax. Working muscles also produce heat.

Muscles protect underlying structures, such as bones, nerves, and blood vessels. Muscle action is controlled by the nervous system. Nerves carry information from the muscles to the brain. The brain takes in this information and directs the muscles through the nerves (Figure 4–20).

Muscle actions can be voluntary or involuntary. Involuntary muscles, such as the heart and diaphragm, are automatically controlled by the brain. You don't have to think about them to make them work. Voluntary muscles, such as leg and arm muscles, are most often under your conscious control. You are aware of telling them to move.

Injuries to the nervous system, brain, spinal cord, or peripheral nerves can affect muscle control. A complete loss of muscle control is called paralysis. Injuries to the nerves can also affect sensation, the ability to feel. When an isolated injury to a muscle or nerve occurs, the adjacent muscles can sometimes assume some of the function of the injured muscle (Figure 4–21).

DID YOU KNOW?
When we smile, we use 17 of our 30 facial muscles.

Figure 4–20 The brain controls muscle movement.

Figure 4–21 Adjacent muscles can often assume the function of an injured muscle.

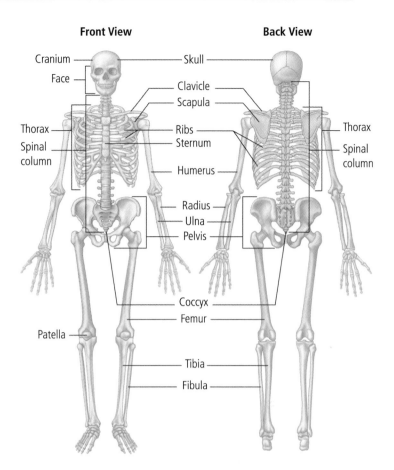

Figure 4–22 The skeleton.

Skeleton

The skeleton in an adult is formed of over 200 bones of various sizes and shapes (Figure 4–22). These bones shape the skeleton, giving each body part a unique form. For example, the head is defined by the bones that form the skull, and the chest is defined by the bones that form the rib cage. Prominent bones, bones that can be seen or felt beneath the skin, provide landmarks for locating body parts.

The skeleton protects vital organs and other soft tissues. The skull protects the brain (Figure 4–23, a). The ribs attach to the spine and breastbone, forming a protective shell for vital organs such as the heart and lungs (Figure 4–23, b), as well as the liver, kidneys, and pancreas. The spinal cord is protected by the canal formed by vertebrae, the bones that form the spinal column (Figure 4–23, c). Two or more bones come together to form joints. Ligaments, fibrous bands that hold bones together at joints, give the skeleton stability and, with the muscles, help maintain posture.

Bones

Bones are hard, dense tissues. Their strong, rigid structure helps them withstand stresses that cause injuries. The shape of bones depends on what the bones do and the stresses on them. For instance, the surfaces of bones at the joints are smooth (Figure 4–24). Although similar to the bones of the arm, the bones of the leg are much larger and stronger because they carry the body's weight.

In addition to supporting and protecting the body, bones aid movement. The bones of the arms and legs work like a system of levers and pulleys to position the hands and

Figure 4–23, a-c a, The immovable bones of the skull protect the brain; **b,** the rib cage protects the heart and lungs; and, **c,** the vertebrae protect the spinal cord.

Figure 4–24 Bone surfaces at the joints are smooth.

Femur

Patella

Tibia

Fibula

feet so they can function. Bones of the wrist, hand, and fingers are progressively smaller to allow for fine movements such as writing. The small bones of the feet enable you to walk smoothly, and together they work as shock absorbers when you walk, run, or jump. Bones also store minerals and produce certain blood cells.

Bones are classified as long, short, flat, or irregular. Long bones are longer than they are wide. These include the bones of the upper arm (humerus), the forearm (radius and ulna), the thigh (femur), and the lower leg (tibia and fibula). Short bones are about as wide as they are long. Short bones include the small bones of the hand (metacarpals) and feet (metatarsals). Flat bones have a relatively thin, flat shape. Flat bones include the breastbone (sternum), the ribs, the shoulder blades (scapula), and some of the bones that form the skull. Bones that do not fit into one of these three categories are called irregular bones. Irregular bones include the vertebrae and the bones of the face. Bones are weakest at the points where they change shape, and fractures usually occur at these points.

Bones have a rich supply of blood and nerves. Some bones store and manufacture red blood cells and supply them to the circulating blood. Bone injuries are usually very painful and can bleed excessively. The bleeding can become life-threatening if not properly cared for. Bones heal by forming new bone cells. Bone is the only body tissue that can regenerate in this way.

Bones weaken with age. Bones in young children are more flexible than in adults, so they are less likely to break. An older adult's less dense, more brittle bones are more likely to give way, even under everyday stresses. For example, an older adult may even break the strongest bone in the body, the femur, if enough stress is created on the bone when pivoting with all the body weight on one leg. When bones become gradually, progressively weaker and less dense it is called osteoporosis.

DID YOU KNOW?

A baby is born with approximately 300 bones. Why do adults have fewer bones? Some bones that are separate at birth, such as the skull, fuse together as a person grows.

Joints

A joint is a structure formed by the ends of two or more bones coming together at one place. Figure 4–25 shows a typical joint. Most joints allow motion. However, the bone ends at some joints are fused together, which restricts motion. Fused bones, such as the bones of the skull, form solid structures that protect their contents (Figure 4–26).

Joints are held together by tough, fibrous connective tissues called ligaments. Ligaments resist joint movement. Joints surrounded by ligaments have restricted movement; joints that have few ligaments move more freely. For instance, the shoulder joint, with few ligaments, allows greater motion than the hip joint, although their structure is similar. Joint motion also depends on the bone structure. Joints that move more freely have less natural support and are therefore more prone to injury. However, there is a normal range of movement for each joint. When a joint is forced beyond its normal range, ligaments stretch and tear. Stretched and torn ligaments permit too much motion, making

Figure 4–25 A typical joint consists of at least two bones that are held together by ligaments.

Figure 4–26 Fused bones, such as those of the skull, form solid structures that protect their contents.

the joint unstable. Unstable joints can be disabling, particularly when they are weight bearing, such as the knee or ankle. Unstable joints are also prone to reinjury and often develop osteoarthritis, an inflammatory condition of the joints, in later years.

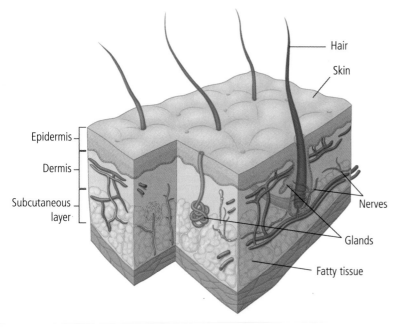

Figure 4–27 The integumentary system.

Integumentary System

The integumentary system consists of the skin, hair, and nails (Figure 4–27). Most important among these is the skin because it protects the body. The skin is the largest single organ, and without it, the human body could not function. It helps keep fluids in and prevents infection by keeping out disease-producing micro-organisms, or germs. The skin is made of tough, elastic fibres that stretch without easily tearing, protecting it from injury. The skin also helps make vitamin D and stores minerals.

The outer surface of the skin consists of dead cells that are continually rubbed away and replaced by new cells. The skin contains the hair roots, oil glands, and sweat glands. Oil glands help keep the skin soft, supple, and waterproof. Sweat glands and pores help regulate body temperature by releasing sweat. The nervous system monitors blood temperature and causes you to sweat if blood temperature rises even slightly. Although you may not see or feel it, sweat is released to the skin's surface.

Blood supplies the skin with nutrients and helps provide its colour. When blood vessels dilate (become wider), the blood circulates close to the skin's surface. This makes some people's skin appear flushed and red and makes the skin feel warm. The reddening may not appear with darker skin. When blood vessels constrict (become narrower), not much blood is close to the skin's surface, causing the skin to look pale and feel cool.

Nerves in the skin also absorb information about the environment. Nerves make the skin very sensitive to sensations, such as touch, pain, and temperature. Therefore, the skin is also an important part of the body's communication network.

The skin has two layers. The outer layer of skin, the epidermis, provides a barrier to bacteria and other organisms that can cause infection. The deeper layer, called the dermis, contains the important structures of the nerves, sweat and oil glands, and blood vessels. Because the skin is well supplied with blood vessels and nerves, most soft tissue injuries are likely to bleed and be painful.

The body's soft tissues include the structures of the integumentary system above as well as muscles that, together, protect the underlying body structures (Figure 4–28).

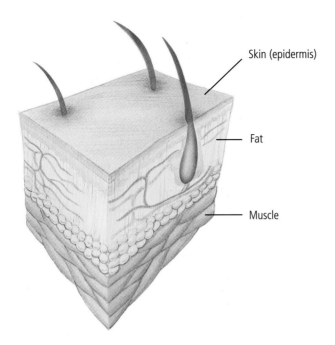

Figure 4–28 Layers of skin, fat and muscle protect underlying structures of the body.

Beneath the skin layers lies a layer of fat. This layer helps insulate the body to help maintain body temperature. The fat layer also stores energy. The amount of fat varies in different parts of the body and in different people.

The muscles lie beneath the fat layer and make up the largest portion of the body's soft tissues. Most soft tissue injuries involve the outer layers of tissue. However, deep burns or violent forces that cause objects to penetrate the skin can injure all the soft tissue layers. Although the muscles are considered soft tissues, muscle injuries are discussed more thoroughly in Chapter 13, with other musculoskeletal injuries.

Endocrine System

The endocrine system is one of the body's two regulatory systems. Together with the nervous system, it coordinates the activities of other systems. The endocrine system consists of several glands (Figure 4–29). Glands are

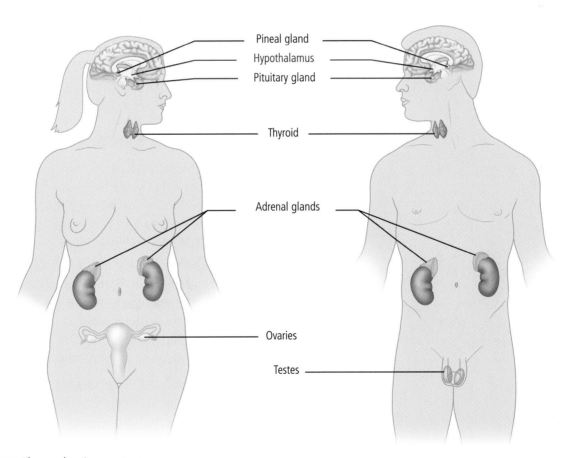

Figure 4–29 The endocrine system.

organs that release fluid and other substances into the blood or onto the skin. Some produce hormones, chemical messengers that enter the bloodstream and influence tissue activity in various parts of the body. For example, the thyroid gland makes a hormone that controls metabolism, the process by which all cells convert nutrients to energy. Other glands include the sweat and oil glands in the skin.

Problems in the endocrine system usually develop slowly and are seldom emergencies. Knowing how hormones work in general, however, helps you understand how some illnesses seem to develop suddenly, such as in the case of diabetic emergencies.

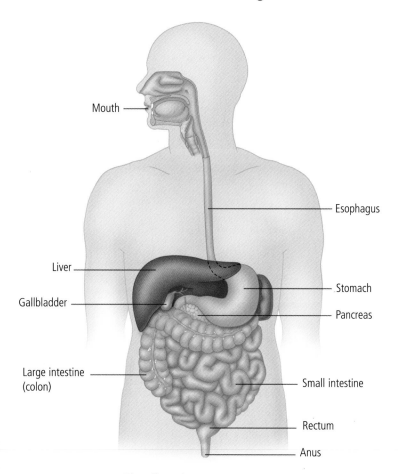

Mouth

Esophagus

Liver

Stomach

Gallbladder

Pancreas

Large intestine (colon)

Small intestine

Rectum

Anus

Figure 4–30 The digestive system.

Digestive System

The digestive system, also called the gastrointestinal system, consists of organs that work together to break down food and eliminate waste. Figure 4–30 shows the major organs of the digestive system. Food entering the system is broken down into a form the body can use. As food passes through the system, the body absorbs nutrients that can be converted for use by the cells. The unabsorbed portion continues through the system and is eliminated as waste.

Since most digestive system organs are in the unprotected abdominal cavity, they are very vulnerable to injury. Damaged organs may bleed internally, causing severe loss of blood, or spill waste products into the abdominal cavity.

Genitourinary System

The genitourinary system is made up of two organ systems: the urinary system and the reproductive system. The urinary system consists of organs that eliminate waste products filtered from the blood (Figure 4–31). The primary organs are the kidneys and the bladder. The kidneys are located behind the abdominal cavity just beneath the chest, one on each side. They filter wastes from the circulating blood to form urine. Urine is then stored in the bladder, a small muscular sac. The bladder stretches as it fills and then shrinks back when the urine is released.

The kidneys are partially protected by the lower ribs, making them less vulnerable to injury. But the kidneys may be damaged by a significant blow to the back just below the rib cage or a penetrating wound, such as a stab or gunshot wound. Because of the kidney's rich blood supply, such an injury may cause severe bleeding.

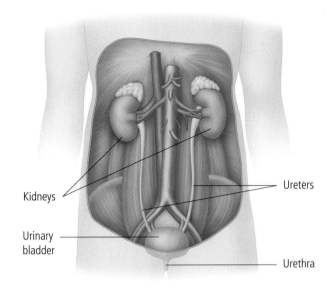

Kidneys

Urinary bladder

Ureters

Urethra

Figure 4–31 The urinary system.

The bladder is injured less frequently than the kidneys, but injuries to the abdomen can rupture the bladder, particularly when it is full. Bone fragments from a fracture of the pelvis can also pierce or rupture the bladder.

The male and female reproductive systems include the organs for sexual reproduction (Figure 4–32, a-b). Because these organs are close to the urinary system, injuries to the abdominal or pelvic area can injure organs in either system.

The female reproductive organs are smaller than many major organs and are protected by the pelvic bones. The soft tissue external structures are more susceptible to injury, although such injury is uncommon. The male reproductive organs are located outside the pelvis and are more vulnerable to injury.

The external reproductive organs, called genitalia, have a rich supply of blood and nerves. Injuries to these organs may cause heavy bleeding but are rarely life-threatening. Injuries to the genitalia are usually caused by a blow to the pelvic area but may be the result of sexual assault.

INTERRELATIONSHIPS OF BODY SYSTEMS

Each body system plays a vital role in survival. Body systems work together to help the body maintain a constant healthy state. When the environment changes, body systems adapt to the new conditions. For example, because your musculoskeletal system works harder when you exercise, your respiratory and circulatory systems must also work harder to meet your body's increased oxygen demands. Your body systems also react to the stresses caused by illness or injury.

Body systems do not work independently of each other. The impact of an injury or a disease is rarely restricted to

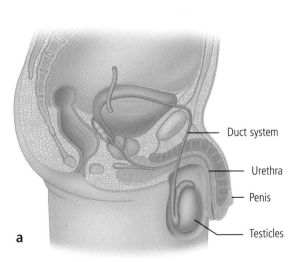

Duct system

Urethra

Penis

Testicles

a

Fallopian tubes

Ovaries

Uterus

Vagina

b

Figure 4–32, a-b The reproductive systems, **a**, male; **b**, female.

one body system. For example, a broken bone may result in nerve damage that may impair movement and feeling. Injuries to the ribs can make breathing difficult. If the heart stops beating for any reason, breathing will also stop.

In any significant illness or injury, body systems may be seriously affected. This may result in a progressive failure of body systems called shock. Shock results from the inability of the circulatory system to provide adequate oxygen to all body cells, especially those of the vital organs.

Generally, the more body systems involved in an emergency, the more serious the emergency. Body systems depend on each other for survival. In serious injury or illness, the body may not be able to keep functioning. In these cases, regardless of your best efforts, the patient may die.

SUMMARY

The body includes a number of systems, all of which must work together for the body to function properly. The brain, the centre of the nervous system, controls all body functions, including those of the other body systems. Knowing a few key structures, their functions, and their locations helps you understand more about these body systems. Knowing certain anatomical terms helps you communicate with more advanced medical personnel about any injury or illness you may encounter.

Illness or injury that affects one body system can have a serious impact on other systems. Fortunately, basic care is usually all you need to give to support injured body systems until more advanced medical care is available. By learning the basic principles of care described in later chapters, you may be able to make the difference between life and death.

As you get closer to the first woman, you see that she is clutching one side of her abdomen, near the top. Her passenger is holding his right hip and looks dazed. The driver of the van has shallow breathing and her pulse is weak. How will you describe their injuries and which body systems are involved?

Chapter 5

Assessment

During a basketball game, two players collide while diving for a loose ball. Both players fall to the ground. One player is holding her knee, screaming in pain. Her leg appears to be twisted to one side. The second player is lying still but is moaning. What do you do?

INTRODUCTION

In previous chapters, you learned how to prepare for an emergency, the precautions to take when approaching the scene, and how to recognize a dangerous situation. You also learned about your roles and responsibilities as a responder. You learned that you can make a difference in an emergency—you may even save a life. But to do this, you must learn how to provide care for a patient. More important, you need to learn how to set priorities for the care you provide.

When an emergency occurs, you must determine if the patient has any life-threatening conditions while conducting a primary survey, which includes assessing the patient's level of consciousness (responsiveness) and checking the patient's airway, breathing, and circulation. You can obtain more information about the patient through a secondary survey, which includes interviewing the patient and bystanders, monitoring vital signs, and conducting a physical exam.

In this chapter, you will learn a plan of action to guide you through any emergency (Figure 5–1). When an emergency occurs, at first you may feel confused. But you can train yourself to remain calm and to think before you act. Ask yourself, "What do I need to do? How can I help most effectively?" The following steps answer these questions. They are your plan of action for any emergency.

These principles, conducted in this order, can ensure your safety and that of the patient and bystanders. They will also increase the patient's chance of survival if he has a serious illness or injury.

Figure 5–1 Look for nearby clues as to what might have happened.

Scene Survey
Environment and Hazards Mechanism of Injury (MOI)/Chief Complaint Number of Patients Additional Resources

↓

Primary Survey
Introduce Self Level of Consciousness (LOC) Cervical Spine Airway Breathing Circulation

→ Circulation Check includes: Pulse Check Skin Check

↓

Oxygen Administration

↓

Rapid Body Survey*
Head/Neck Chest Abdomen Pelvis Lower Extremities Upper Extremities Back

↓

Transport Decision

↓

Secondary Survey
MOI/Chief Complaint SAMPLE OPQRST Quality of Vital Signs Glasgow Coma Scale Head-to-Toe Physical Examination

↓

Secondary Transport Decision

↓

Ongoing Survey

* Where legislation requires

SCENE SURVEY

Once you recognize that an emergency has occurred and decide to act, you must make sure the emergency scene is safe for you, the patient(s), and any bystanders. Take time to survey the scene and answer these questions:

Environment and Hazards

What are the potential hazards at the scene?
Weather conditions, people, animals, weapons, dangerous surfaces or objects, biohazards, tripping hazards, debris

---

Mechanism of Injury/Chief Complaint

What happened?
What is the mechanism of injury?

A fall (indicating a traumatic injury)? A sudden illness (indicating a medical emergency)? Were vehicles involved? Was there a collision? Are there pill containers? Are there bottles?

Number of Patients

How many people are ill or injured?

Additional Resources

What other resources might I need?
Law enforcement, Poison Control Centre, utilities, more advanced medical care, firefighters

---

Before You Approach the Patient

When you survey the scene, look for anything that may threaten your safety or that of bystanders or the patient. Examples of hazards that may be present are given in Chapter 2. Take the necessary precautions when working in a hazardous environment. If you are not properly trained and do not have the necessary equipment, do not approach the person. Summon the necessary personnel.

Nothing is gained by risking your safety. An emergency that begins with one ill or injured person could end up with two if you are hurt. If you suspect the scene is unsafe, wait and watch until the necessary personnel and equipment arrive. If conditions change, you may then be able to approach the person.

As You Approach the Patient

Try to find out what happened. Look around the scene for clues to what caused the emergency (the mechanism of injury) and the extent of the damage. Doing this will cause you to think about the possible type and extent of the person's injuries. You may discover a situation that requires you to act immediately. As you approach the patient, take in the whole picture and act appropriately. For example, if the mechanism of injury indicates a head and/or spine injury, approach the patient in a way that she can see you without having to turn her head. Nearby objects, such as shattered glass, a fallen ladder, or a spilled medicine container, may suggest what happened. If the patient is unconscious, surveying the scene may be the only way you can determine what happened.

When you survey the scene, always look carefully for more than one patient. You may not see everyone at first. For example, in a vehicle collision, an open door may be a clue that an injured person has left the car or was thrown from it. If one person is bleeding or screaming loudly, you may overlook another person who is unconscious. It is also easy in any emergency situation to overlook a baby or small child. Ask anyone present how many people may be involved. If you find more than one patient, ask bystanders to help you provide care.

Look for bystanders who can help. Bystanders may be able to tell you what happened or help in other ways. A bystander who knows the patient may know whether he has any medical conditions or allergies. Bystanders can meet and direct further personnel to your location, help keep the area free of unnecessary traffic, and help you provide care.

Once You Reach the Patient

Once you reach the patient, quickly survey the scene again to see if it is still safe. At this point, you may see other dangers, clues to what happened, and other injured people or bystanders that you did not notice before. Determine the level of risk and put on PPE if you have not done so already.

Forming a General Impression

Once you reach the patient and begin your assessment, you will be able to form a general impression of his condition. This includes determining:

- The patient's chief complaint or problem

- If the patient is injured or ill

- The patient's sex and approximate age

This general impression may alert you that the patient has a serious problem that requires additional resources or only a minor problem that you can easily care for. You will discover these problems by looking for any signs and symptoms that the patient may have. Signs are evidence of injury or illness that you can observe, such as bleeding or unusual skin appearance. Symptoms are what the patient tells you he is experiencing, such as pain, nausea, headache, or shortness of breath.

Do not move a patient unless there is an immediate danger, such as a fire, poisonous fumes, or an unstable structure. If the area is dangerous and the patient does not seem to be seriously injured, ask the patient to move to safety where you can help him. If the area is dangerous and the patient cannot move, you may try to move the patient as quickly as possible without making his condition worse. If there is no immediate danger, identify yourself, tell the patient not to move, and obtain consent to give care. If the mechanism of injury indicates a head and/or spine injury, initiate manual stabilization, as described in Chapter 14.

Throughout, try not to alarm the patient. Try to position yourself close to his eye level (Figure 5–2).

PRIMARY SURVEY

Check the Patient for Responsiveness and Obtain More Advanced Medical Care

Quality care begins with a primary survey. This is a check for conditions that are an immediate threat to the patient's life. The primary survey has several components:

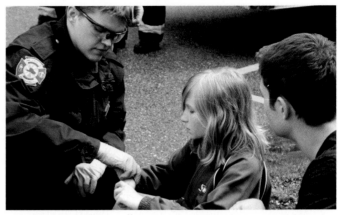

Figure 5–2 When talking to a patient, try to position yourself near eye level and speak in a calm and positive manner.

- Introducing self

- Assessing level of consciousness (LOC)

- Assessing cervical spine

- Assessing airway and breathing

- Assessing circulation (including pulse check and skin check)

- Distinguishing between trauma assessment and medical assessment

First, determine if the patient is responsive. Do this by gently tapping him on the shoulder and asking, "Are you okay?" (Figure 5–3). Do not jostle or move the patient. For a baby, instead of tapping on the shoulder, clap loudly and gently flick the bottom of the baby's feet. A patient who can speak or cry is conscious, is breathing, and has a pulse.

If the patient is unable to respond, he may be unconscious. Unconsciousness can indicate a life-threatening condition. When a patient is unconscious, the tongue relaxes and may fall to the back of the throat, blocking the airway. This can cause breathing to stop. Soon after, the heart will stop beating. With an unconscious patient, more advanced medical care is needed.

One of the most important indicators of a patient's condition is his LOC. A patient's LOC can range from being fully alert to being unconscious (Table 5–1). In describing a patient's LOC, a four-level scale is used. The letters **A**, **V**, **P**, and **U** each refer to a stage of awareness.

TABLE 5–1: LEVELS OF CONSCIOUSNESS

Level of Response	Characteristic Behaviour
Alert	Eyes are open; able to verbalize
Verbal	Responds to commands or questions
Painful	Facial grimace; flexion, extension, or withdrawal of body part; moan or groan
Unresponsive	No response

Figure 5–3 Determine if the patient is responsive by asking "Are you okay?" and gently tapping him.

A = Alert: If a patient is conscious and able to speak to you, this indicates the patient is alert. It is important to note that a patient can be deemed alert but still be confused or disoriented. If the patient is not alert, proceed to check his response to verbal stimuli.

V = Verbal: Sometimes a patient only reacts to sounds, such as your voice. This patient may appear to be lapsing into unconsciousness. State a command or ask a question. If the patient responds, the patient is said to be responsive to verbal stimuli. If the patient is not responsive to verbal stimuli, proceed to check response to painful stimuli.

P = Painful: If a patient responds only when someone inflicts pain, he is described as responding to painful stimuli. Pinching the nail bed or inside the arm is an example of a painful stimulus used to try to get a response. Avoid pinching anywhere above the collarbone as this could cause the patient to move his head.

U = Unresponsive: A patient who does not respond to any stimuli is considered to be unconscious, or unresponsive to stimuli.

Any change in the level of consciousness constitutes a possible life-threatening condition, and it is important to obtain more advanced medical care.

If your communication network is not directly linked to advanced medical personnel, you will need to use a telephone to call. If possible, ask another responder or a bystander to call the emergency number for you. Sending someone else to make the call will enable you to stay with the patient to provide care.

NOTE:

Obtain more advanced medical care if the primary survey determines a life-threatening condition and if you have not already called for help.

Whether placing the call yourself or sending someone to call, the following should be done:

1. Dial the local emergency number. This number is 9-1-1 in many communities. Sometimes the emergency number is on the inside front cover of telephone directories and on pay phones.

2. Be prepared to provide the dispatcher with the following information when asked:

   • Where the emergency is located—Give the exact address or location and the name of the city or town. It is helpful to give the names of nearby intersecting streets (cross streets), landmarks, the name of the building, the floor, and the room number.

- Telephone number from which the call is being made
- Caller's name
- What happened—for example, a motor vehicle collision, fall, or fire
- The number of patients involved
- Condition of the patient(s)—for example, chest pain, difficulty breathing (dyspnea), no pulse, bleeding
- Care being given

3. Hang up only when the dispatcher has told you to do so. It is important to make sure the dispatcher has all the information needed to send the appropriate help immediately.

If you must leave the patient for any reason, such as to call your emergency number, place him in the H.A.IN.E.S. recovery position to help keep the airway open (Figure 5–4). Place the patient on one side, bend the top leg, and move it forward to hold the patient in that position. Support the head so that it is angled toward the ground. In this position, if the patient vomits, the airway will stay clear.

Assessing the Patient's Airway, Breathing, and Circulation

If you can, try to check the ABCs in whatever position you find the patient, especially if you suspect he has a head and/or spine injury. Sometimes, however, the patient's position prevents you from checking the ABCs. In this case, you may roll the patient gently onto his back, keeping the head and spine in as straight a line as possible.

Check A: Airway

Be sure the patient has an open airway, the pathway for air from the mouth and nose to the lungs. If a patient is speaking or crying, he has an open airway, is breathing, and has a pulse. If a patient is unconscious, it may be difficult to tell if he has an open airway. Open an unconscious patient's airway by tilting the head back and lifting the chin. These two complementary motions, called the head-tilt/chin-lift, move the tongue and epiglottis, opening the airway. If there is any possibility of a head and/or spine injury, open the airway by using the two-handed jaw thrust technique (Figure 5–5). After opening the airway, check for breathing.

Sometimes opening the airway does not result in a free passage of air. This happens when a patient's airway is blocked by liquid, food, or other objects. In this case, you will need to remove the obstruction. Chapter 6 describes how to care for an obstructed airway.

Check B: Breathing

Position yourself so that you can hear and feel air from the patient's nose and mouth. At the same time, watch the chest rise and fall. If the patient is breathing normally, you will observe the rise and fall of the chest, ease of breathing, and approximate respiratory rate. If there is only an occasional gasp of air (agonal respiration), the patient is not breathing normally. Someone who is having trouble breathing may have the following signs and symptoms:

Figure 5–4 The H.A.IN.E.S. recovery position.

Figure 5–5 The jaw thrust.

Figure 5–6 Look, listen, and feel for breathing for no more than 5 to 10 seconds.

Figure 5–7 The location of the radial artery.

- Inadequate rise and fall of the chest

- Increased effort on respiration

- Decreased LOC

- Difficulty breathing (dyspnea)

- Blue or grey colour to the skin, lips, or nail beds (cyanosis)

- Very slow or fast breathing rates

Check for normal breathing for a maximum of 5 to 10 seconds (Figure 5–6). A patient with a breathing difficulty (dyspnea) needs oxygen immediately (see Chapter 7). By assessing the quality of respirations, you can determine if this is needed.

If the patient is not breathing or is not breathing adequately, you must breathe for him. Begin by giving two breaths, each lasting one second in length. Each breath should be given just until the chest starts to rise. This will get air into the patient's lungs. The longer someone goes without oxygen, the more likely he is to die. This process of breathing for the patient is called rescue breathing. You will learn rescue breathing in Chapter 6.

Check C: Circulation

The last step in the primary survey is checking for blood circulation. If the heart has stopped, blood will not circulate throughout the body. If blood does not circulate, the patient will die in just a few minutes because the brain will not get any oxygen.

If the patient (adult or child) is conscious and breathing, check his pulse using the radial artery on the thumb side of his wrist (Figure 5–7). If the adult or child is unconscious or not breathing, or you cannot feel a radial pulse, check the pulse at either of the carotid arteries located in the neck. You can also look for any movement of the patient, normal breathing (more than an occasional gasp), coughing, and appropriate skin colour.

To find the pulse, feel for the Adam's apple at the front of the neck and then slide your fingers into the groove at the side of the neck closest to you (Figure 5–8). Sometimes the pulse may be difficult to find since it may be slow or weak. If at first you do not find a pulse, relocate the Adam's apple and again slide your fingers into place. If after a maximum of 5 to 10 seconds you are not certain there is a pulse, start CPR.

Figure 5–8 The location of the carotid artery.

Figure 5–9 The location of the brachial artery.

To find a baby's pulse, place one or two fingers over the brachial artery, located on the underside of the baby's arm, halfway between the elbow and the shoulder (Figure 5–9).

If you do not observe signs of circulation, you need to keep oxygen-rich blood circulating. This involves doing rescue breathing to get oxygen into the patient's lungs and chest compressions to circulate the oxygen to the brain.

This procedure is called cardiopulmonary resuscitation (CPR) and is described in Chapter 8.

Checking circulation also means looking for severe bleeding. Bleeding is severe when blood spurts from the wound or cannot be controlled, and it is life-threatening. Check for severe bleeding by doing a quick visual check of the patient from head to toe, then quickly feel each major part of the body for signs of severe external bleeding. Inspect your gloves often for blood. This is also known as a "rapid body survey." Severe bleeding must be controlled before you provide any further care as, if left untreated, it can become fatal. Techniques for controlling severe bleeding are described in Chapter 9.

NOTE:

At this point, it may be appropriate to administer oxygen and treat for shock (see Chapter 10).

RAPID BODY SURVEY

The rapid body survey (RBS) is a hands-on check that is completed quickly, unless intervention is required. In carrying out the RBS, you are looking for life-threatening injuries and conditions. The information you gain from the RBS is used to determine your transport decision. The RBS includes checking the head/neck, chest, abdomen, pelvis, lower extremity, upper extremity, and back.

Initiate care for life-threatening emergencies as required, based on the primary assessment. If you are trained to do so, transport should also be initiated at this point, indicating that this patient is in a rapid transport category. Otherwise, begin the secondary survey. Information regarding care for life-threatening emergencies and transport is found later in this text.

TRANSPORT DECISION

Load-and-Go Emergencies

If a life-threatening condition is found, this constitutes a "load-and-go" response. Do not waste further time at the scene.

Load-and-go emergencies include:

- Seriously injured patients with multiple or severe traumas
- Instability or absence of the ABCs or neurological status
- Decreased level of consciousness (LOC) or unconsciousness
- Ongoing seizures
- Chest pain (if disorder or heart attack suspected)
- Burns with signs of inhalation injury
- Extensive burns
- Abdominal distension and tenderness
- Unstable pelvic injury
- Fractured femur(s)
- Amputation(s)
- Pregnancy-related conditions
- Conditions related to environmental mishaps (e.g., severe hypothermia, venomous animal bites, lightning strikes, diving emergencies)

In all cases of a load-and-go situation:

- Conduct a primary survey and perform intervention as necessary.
- Transfer and secure the patient to the appropriate equipment.
- Load and secure the patient in the transportation vehicle.
- Perform further assessment and management en route.
- If you are not trained for transport, contact EMS/9-1-1 and continue care.

NOTE:

When possible, take any patient medications with the patient to the hospital.

The Golden Period is a term sometimes used to describe the critical period (typically the first hour) after a life-threatening traumatic injury. Providing early interventions and advanced medical care during this time offers patients the best chance of survival. The danger of dying from shock or bleeding is highest during this period, so immediate care for these conditions is required. A severely injured patient requiring surgery has the best chance of survival if the surgery is performed as soon as possible (i.e., within an hour). Trauma is a physical injury, wound, or shock caused by an agent, force, or mechanism. The trauma patient requires rapid assessment and care of the conditions found.

SECONDARY SURVEY

If you are certain the patient has no life-threatening conditions, you can begin the secondary survey. The secondary survey is a systematic method of gathering additional information about injuries or conditions that may need care. These injuries or conditions are not immediately life-threatening but could become so if not cared for. For example, you might find possible broken bones, minor bleeding, or a specific medical condition, such as diabetes. The secondary survey is made up of the following three steps:

1. Interview the patient and bystanders.
2. Check vital signs.
3. Do a head-to-toe physical examination.

As you do the secondary survey, try not to move the patient. Most injured patients will find the most comfortable position for themselves. For example, a patient with a chest injury who is having trouble breathing may be sitting up and supporting the injured area. Let the patient continue to do this. Do not ask him to change positions unless it is necessary.

Interview the Patient and Bystanders

Begin by asking the patient and bystanders simple questions to learn more about what happened and the patient's condition. Asking about existing conditions and the incident itself, as well as what the chief complaint is (what is bothering the patient), is commonly known as obtaining a patient's "history." This should not take much time. You are looking not only for signs of the patient's condition but also for symptoms. A symptom is something the patient tells you about his condition, such as "I am dizzy" or "my head hurts." A sign is any evidence you can see of injury or illness, such as bleeding or unusually pale skin colour.

NOTE:

The chief complaint may have been determined during the scene survey.

If you have not done so already, remember to identify yourself and to get the patient's consent before helping. Begin the interview by asking the patient's name. Using his name will make the patient more comfortable. First ask what happened and whether the patient feels any pain. Use the acronym **SAMPLE** to remember to ask the following questions:

S = Signs and symptoms (What things are bothering you?)

A = Allergies (What allergies do you have?)

M = Medications (What medications do you take?)

P = Past medical history (What medical conditions do you have?)

L = Last meal (When did you last eat or drink? What did you last eat or drink?)

E = Events before the incident (What happened to cause the problem?)

TABLE 5–2: QUESTIONS ABOUT PAIN: OPQRST

Mnemonic	Question to Ask
Onset	Did it start suddenly?
Provoke	What provokes the pain or causes it to get worse?
Quality	What does the pain feel like? (Sharp, dull, stabbing, moving, etc.)
Region (or Radiate)	Where exactly is the pain located? Does it radiate to other areas?
Severity	How bad is the pain?
Time	When did the pain begin?

If the patient has pain, ask him to describe it. You may use the mnemonic OPQRST to remember the questions to ask (Table 5–2). You can expect to get descriptions such as burning, throbbing, aching, or sharp pain. Ask when the pain started. Ask how bad the pain is.

Sometimes the patient will be unable to give you the information. This is often the case with a child or with an adult who momentarily lost consciousness and may not be able to recall what happened or is disoriented. These patients may be frightened. Be calm and patient. Speak normally and in simple terms. Offer reassurance. Ask family members, friends, or bystanders what happened. They may be able to give you helpful information, such as telling you if the patient has a medical condition you should be aware of. They may also be able to help calm the patient if necessary.

Check Vital Signs

The first set of vital signs is considered to be the baseline vital signs. These may include:

- Level of consciousness
- Breathing
- Pulse
- Skin characteristics
- Blood pressure
- Pupils

Assessing a Conscious Child or Baby

Be aware that babies and young children might not be able to respond to methods used to assess the level of consciousness in adults. For example, they may not be able to respond to your questions because of an inability to speak or understand your questions, fear of a stranger, or they are crying. If possible, assess a baby or small child in his parent's or caregiver's arms or lap. When assessing a baby or child:

- Approach the baby or child slowly.

- Kneel so that you are at eye level with the baby or child.

- Give the baby or child a few minutes to get used to you, if possible.

- Use the child's name.

- Demonstrate what you are going to do on a stuffed animal or doll, if possible.

- Allow a child to inspect items such as bandages.

- Let a school-aged child know if you are going to do anything painful.

These vital signs can tell you how the body is responding to injury or illness. Look for changes in vital signs. Note anything unusual. Recheck vital signs every five minutes. Subsequent vital signs taken may depend on the conditions presented by the patient.

Level of Consciousness

You learned how to assess a patient's LOC earlier in the chapter using the AVPU scale. Another measure, typically used for assessing patients with head trauma, is the Glasgow Coma Scale.

Glasgow Coma Scale

The Glasgow Coma Scale (GCS) is a standardized system used to determine a patient's level of consciousness and is considered a good indicator of eventual clinical outcome for head trauma. The scale is often performed on patients with neurological damage. The assessment process involves assigning a score based on the patient's motor and verbal responses and his ability to open his eyes. This scale is divided into three sections. The sections are scored individually and then added together (Table 5–3). To assess the patient using the GCS, do the following:

Eye Opening

If a patient spontaneously opens his eyes, he receives a score of 4. If he does not spontaneously open his eyes, give a verbal command, such as "Open your eyes." If he still does not open his eyes, apply a painful stimulus, as with the AVPU assessment.

Best Verbal Response

Ask a question. If the patient responds coherently, he receives a score of 5. If the answer is not coherent, or the patient does not respond, the response (or lack of response) can be put into one of the other categories and the appropriate score assigned.

Best Motor Response

Give the patient a command, such as "wiggle your fingers." If he responds to your command, a score of 6 is given. If he does not follow your command, apply a painful stimulus, as described earlier, and score the response accordingly. If he pushes away the stimulus, this is localizing the pain.

TABLE 5–3: GLASGOW COMA SCALE

Eye Opening	E
spontaneous	4
to voice	3
to pain	2
no response	1
Best Verbal Response	**V**
oriented and converses	5
disoriented and converses	4
inappropriate words	3
incomprehensible sounds	2
no response	1
Best Motor Response	**M**
To Verbal Command:	
obeys command	6
To Painful Stimulus:	
localizes pain	5
withdrawal	4
abnormal flexion	3
abnormal extension	2
no response	1

E + V + M = 3 to 15

A score of 13 to 15 is associated with mild head injury; 8 to 12, moderate head injury; and less than 8, severe head injury.

Breathing

A healthy person breathes regularly, quietly, and effortlessly. The normal breathing rate for an adult is between 12 and 20 breaths per minute. However, some people breathe slightly slower or faster. Excitement, fear, and exercise cause breathing to increase and

TABLE 5–4: AVERAGE* VITAL SIGNS BY AGE

Age	Pulse	Respirations	Blood Pressure
Up to 28 days	120–160	40–60	80/40
1–12 months	100–120	30–40	80/40
1–8 years	80–120	16–24	90/50
Over age 8	60–100	12–20	120/80

These values vary among individuals and should not be considered "normal" values. They are averages for each age group.

become deeper. Certain injuries or illnesses can also cause both the breathing rate and quality to change.

During the secondary survey, watch and listen for any changes in breathing. Abnormal breathing may indicate a potential problem. The signs and symptoms of abnormal breathing include:

• Gasping for air

• Noisy breathing, including whistling sounds, crowing, gurgling, or snoring

• Excessively fast or slow breathing

• Painful breathing

In the primary survey, you are concerned with whether a patient is breathing at all, whereas in the secondary survey, you are concerned with the rate, rhythm, and volume of breathing. Look, listen, and feel again for breathing. Look for the rise and fall of the patient's chest or abdomen. Listen for sounds as the patient inhales and exhales. Count the number of times a patient breathes (inhales or exhales) in 15 seconds and multiply that number by four. This is the number of breaths per minute. As you check for the rate and volume of breathing, try to do it without the patient's knowledge. If a patient realizes that you are checking his breathing, he may change his breathing pattern without being aware of doing so. Maintain the same position you would be in when you are checking the pulse.

Pulse

With every heartbeat, a wave of blood moves through the blood vessels. This creates a beat called the pulse. You

can feel it with your fingertips in arteries near the surface of the skin. In the primary survey, you are concerned only with whether a pulse is present. To determine this, you check the carotid arteries. In the secondary survey, you are trying to determine pulse rate, rhythm, and quality. This is most often done by checking the radial pulse located on the thumb side of the patient's wrist.

When the heart is healthy, it beats with a steady rhythm. This beat creates a regular pulse. A normal pulse for an adult is between 60 and 100 beats per minute. A well-conditioned athlete may have a pulse of 50 beats per minute or lower. Table 5–4 lists average pulses at different ages. If the heartbeat changes, so does the pulse. An abnormal pulse may be a sign of a potential problem. These signs include:

• Irregular pulse

• Weak and hard-to-find pulse

• Excessively fast or slow pulse

When severely injured or unhealthy, the heart may beat unevenly, producing an irregular pulse. The rate at which the heart beats can also change. The pulse speeds up when a person is excited, anxious, in pain, losing blood, or under stress. It slows down when a person is relaxed. Some heart conditions can also speed up or slow down the pulse rate. Sometimes changes may be very subtle and difficult for you to detect. The most important change to note is a pulse that changes from being present to no pulse at all.

Checking a pulse is a simple procedure. It involves placing two fingers on top of a major artery where it is

Figure 5–10, a-c Checking for: **a**, the carotid pulse; **b**, the radial pulse; and **c**, the brachial pulse.

located close to the skin's surface. Pulse sites that are easy to locate are the carotid arteries in the neck, the radial artery in the wrist, and, for babies, the brachial artery in the upper arm (Figure 5–10, a-c). There are other pulse sites you may use. Figure 5–11 shows these sites. To check the pulse rate, count the number of beats

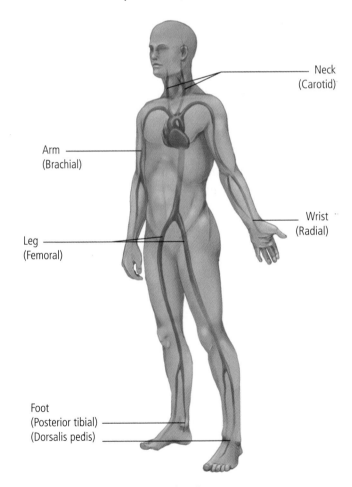

Figure 5–11 Easily located pulse sites.

in 15 seconds and multiply that number by four. The number you get is the number of heartbeats per minute. If you find the pulse is irregular, you may need to check it for more than 15 seconds.

A patient's pulse may be hard to find. If you have trouble finding a pulse, keep checking periodically. Take your time. Remember, if a patient is breathing, his heart is also beating. However, there may be a loss in circulation to the injured area, causing a loss of pulse. If you cannot find the pulse in one place, check it in another major artery, such as in the other wrist.

Pulse Oximetry

Purpose

Pulse oximetry is a simple, rapid, safe, and non-invasive method used to measure the percentage of oxygen saturation in the blood. The reading is taken by a pulse oximeter. A pulse oximeter is a device that measures the percentage of red blood cells that are saturated with oxygen. To ensure that the instrument is measuring arterial and not venous oxygenation, pulse oximeters are designed to assess only pulsating blood vessels. The pulse oximeter will also measure the pulse.

The reading from the oximeter appears as a percentage of hemoglobin saturated with oxygen. Normal saturation is approximately 97 to 100%. The reading is recorded as "95 to 99% SpO_2" A 100% saturation measurement means all the red blood cells are oxygenated; 80% saturation means only 80% of the red blood cells are carrying oxygen. A healthy, non-smoking adult should have oxygen saturation on room air around

95 to 100%. Smokers can have oxygen saturation on room air around 94 to 96%. People with chronic lung disease may have oxygen saturation on room air as low as 90% when they are not ill. See Table 5–5.

Oxygen saturation below 80% is considered insufficient to support life. At extreme elevations, such as on Mount Everest, oxygen saturations are often in the high-70% to low-80% range, and although people can climb to the top without supplemental oxygen, their body is actually slowly dying while they are at that altitude.

Pulse oximetry is also used to assess the adequacy of oxygen delivery during positive pressure ventilation and the impact of other medical care provided.

When monitoring a conscious patient's oxygen saturation levels using a pulse oximeter, you may reduce the flow of oxygen and, if needed, change to a lower-flowing delivery device if the patient's oxygen level reaches 100%.

The percent of oxygen saturation should always be documented when vital signs are recorded and in response to therapy to correct hypoxia. A reading below 94% may indicate hypoxia. Pulse oximetry should be used as an added tool for patient evaluation, as it is possible for patients to show a normal reading but have trouble breathing or to have a low reading but appear to be breathing. When treating the patient, all symptoms should be assessed along with the data provided by the device. The pulse oximeter reading should never be used to withhold oxygen from a patient who appears to be in respiratory distress or when it is the standard of care to apply oxygen despite good pulse oximetry readings, such as in a patient with chest pain. **WHEN IN DOUBT, LOOK AT THE PATIENT**. Remember, treat the patient, not the pulse oximeter.

Indications

Give oxygen when it is indicated by your physical assessment findings. Pulse oximetry should be applied whenever a patient's oxygenation is a concern and for the following situations:

- All patients with neurologic, respiratory, or cardiovascular complaints
- All patients with abnormal vital signs
- All patients who receive respiratory depressants (morphine, diazepam, midazolam)
- Multi-system trauma patients

Continue high-concentration oxygen delivery in all patients suspected of carbon monoxide (CO) poisoning regardless of the saturation readings.

Pulse oximetry should be taken and recorded with vital signs for stable patients at least every 15 minutes and reassessed and recorded every five minutes for unstable patients.

Consider tapering and discontinuing supplemental oxygen if the patient is not distressed and the saturation is greater than 96% on room air.

TABLE 5–5: PULSE OXIMETRY

Range	Value	Treatment
Normal	95 to 100%	None
Mild hypoxia	91 to 94%	Administer emergency oxygen using a nasal cannula or resuscitation mask.
Moderate hypoxia	86 to 90%	Administer emergency oxygen using a non-rebreather mask or bag-valve-mask resuscitator.
Severe hypoxia	85%	Administer emergency oxygen using a non-rebreather mask or bag-valve-mask resuscitator with positive pressure.

Procedure

When using a pulse oximeter, refer to the manufacturer's directions to ensure you use it properly. In general, the procedure for measuring pulse oximetry is the same.

Once the machine is turned on, allow for self-tests. Select a highly vascular site. Usually, the fingertip is the most convenient site; otherwise, use an earlobe or toe (if a proper probe is available).

If the patient is wearing nail polish, remove it using an acetone wipe, as it can block the sensor light and interfere with the reading. Then apply the probe to the patient's finger. The manufacturer may also recommend using alternative measuring sites, such as measuring first on the finger and then the earlobe for the next measurement.

Pediatric Considerations

The manufacturer may recommend alternative measuring sites for pulse oximetry in babies, such as the foot.

The machine will register the oxygen saturation level. Once it begins to register, record the time and the initial saturation percent, if possible, on the pre-hospital care report. Compare the patient's pulse rate on the oximeter to the actual pulse of the patient. Be sure to monitor critical patients continuously until more advanced medical personnel are available. If you are recording a one-time reading, be sure to monitor the patient for a few minutes, as oxygen saturation can vary. As mentioned above, document the percent of oxygen saturation whenever vital signs are recorded and in response to therapy to correct hypoxia.

Limitations

Some factors may reduce the reliability of the pulse oximetry reading, including:

- Hypoperfusion (i.e., poor perfusion) or shock (fewer circulating red blood cells to carry oxygen)
- Decreased circulation to the extremities (insufficient blood flow to obtain an accurate reading)
- Cardiac arrest (absent perfusion to fingers)
- Excessive motion of the patient during the reading
- Fingernail polish

- Carbon monoxide poisoning (carbon monoxide binds to hemoglobin more easily than to oxygen and saturates hemoglobin)
- Hypothermia or other cold-related illness
- Sickle cell disease or anemia (because there are fewer red blood cells to carry oxygen)
- Cigarette smokers (due to carbon monoxide)
- Edema (swelling)
- A delay in detecting respiratory insufficiency. (The pulse oximeter could warn too late of a decrease in respiratory function based on the amount of oxygen in circulation.)
- Hypotension

Consider applying supplemental oxygen to patients who, on first assessment, do not require oxygen but whose oxygen saturation is less than 95%.

Skin Characteristics

The colour, temperature, and condition of the skin often indicate something about the patient's condition. For example, a patient with a breathing problem may have a flushed or pale face.

The skin looks red when the body is forced to work harder. The heart pumps faster to get more blood to the tissues. This increased blood flow causes reddened skin and makes the skin feel warm. In contrast, the skin may look pale or bluish and feel cool and moist if the blood flow is directed away from the skin's surface. When a person with darker skin becomes pale, the skin turns ashen, a greyish colour. Illness and/or injury may also cause the skin to become dry, moist, or clammy, for example. Any changes in these skin characteristics may indicate a problem.

Blood Pressure

Blood pressure (BP) is the force exerted by the blood against the blood vessel walls as it travels throughout the body. Blood pressure is necessary to move the oxygen and nutrients in the blood to the body's organs and muscles. It is also necessary to move waste products, such as carbon dioxide, to various parts of the body for removal. Blood pressure is a good indicator of how the circulatory system is functioning.

Blood pressure is created by the pumping action of the heart. The pumping action involves two phases: the working (contracting) phase and the resting (refilling) phase. During the working phase, the ventricles (lower chambers) of the heart contract. This causes blood to be pumped through the arteries to all parts of the body. During the resting phase, the ventricles relax and refill with blood before the next contraction.

Stress, excitement, illness, and injury often affect blood pressure. When a patient is ill or injured, a single blood pressure measurement is often of little value. A more accurate picture of a patient's condition immediately following an injury or the onset of an illness is whether his blood pressure changes over time while you provide care. For example, a patient's initial blood pressure reading could be uncommonly high due to the stress of the emergency. Providing care, however, usually relieves some of the fear, and blood pressure may return to a normal range. At other times, blood pressure will remain unusually high or low. For example, an injury resulting in severe blood loss may cause blood pressure to remain unusually low. You should be concerned about unusually high or low blood pressure whenever symptoms of injury or illness are present.

To accurately assess a patient's blood pressure, you need a blood pressure cuff. Cuffs come in sizes for small, average, and large arms. Inside the cuff is a rubber bladder, similar to an inner tube, that can be inflated. A pressure gauge, inflation bulb, and regulating valve are connected to the bladder by rubber tubing.

Blood pressure is measured in units called millimetres of mercury (mmHg). These units, written on the blood pressure gauge, range from 20 mmHg to 300 mmHg. In measuring blood pressure, two different numbers are usually recorded. The first number reflects the pressure in the arteries when the heart is working, or contracting. This pressure is called the systolic blood pressure. The second number reflects the pressure in the

Figure 5–12 To auscultate blood pressure, position the cuff, find the brachial pulse, and position the stethoscope over it.

arteries when the heart is at rest and refilling. This is called the diastolic blood pressure.

You report blood pressure by giving the systolic number first and then the diastolic (S/D). Write this as BP 120/80.

The process of using a blood pressure cuff and stethoscope to listen for characteristic sounds is called auscultation. To auscultate means to listen. This method allows you to get accurate systolic and diastolic pressures. To auscultate blood pressure, begin by determining the systolic pressure using the palpation method (described on next page). Next, locate the brachial pulse. Place the earpieces of the stethoscope in your ears and the other end, the diaphragm, over the spot where you found the brachial pulse (Figure 5–12). Close the valve and begin to inflate the cuff. Inflate the cuff to 20 mmHg above the approximate systolic blood pressure.

Slowly deflate the cuff at a rate of about 2 mmHg per second. As you deflate the cuff, listen carefully for the pulse. In some instances, it may sound like a tapping sound. The point at which the pulse is first heard is the systolic pressure.

As the cuff deflates, the pulse sound will fade. The point at which the sound disappears is the diastolic pressure. Release the remaining air quickly. Record the blood pressure as two numbers, such as 130/80. Also record whether the patient was sitting or lying down.

Figure 5–13 The centre of the cuff should be placed over the brachial artery, about 2.5 cm (1 in.) above the crease of the elbow.

Figure 5–14 Estimating a systolic blood pressure requires you to feel for a radial pulse.

To determine both the systolic and the diastolic pressure, you need a stethoscope. The stethoscope enables you to hear the pulsating sounds of blood moving through the arteries with each contraction of the heart. Sometimes you may not have a stethoscope or, because of noise, are unable to use one. You can still determine the systolic blood pressure through a method known as palpation. Palpation requires you to feel (palpate) the radial artery as you inflate the blood pressure cuff.

To determine blood pressure by palpation, begin by having the patient sit or lie down. Wrap the blood pressure cuff around the patient's arm so that the lower edge is about 2.5 cm (1 in.) above the crease of the elbow. The centre of the cuff should be over the brachial artery, the major artery of the arm (Figure 5–13). Next, locate the radial pulse (Figure 5–14). Close the regulating valve by turning the valve clockwise and begin to inflate the cuff. Inflate the cuff until you can no longer feel the radial pulse. Note the number on the gauge.

Continue to inflate the cuff for another 20 mmHg beyond this point. Slowly release the pressure in the cuff by turning the regulating valve counter-clockwise. Allow the cuff to deflate at a rate of about 2 mmHg per second. Continue to feel for the radial pulse as the cuff deflates. The point at which the pulse at the wrist returns is the approximate systolic blood pressure by palpation. The systolic pressure found using this method is on average 10 to 20 mmHg less than the systolic pressure found by auscultation. This blood pressure reading is expressed as one number only, such as 130/P. In this example, the systolic pressure is 130, and P refers to palpation. Once you know the approximate systolic pressure, quickly deflate the cuff. Record the systolic pressure and whether the patient was sitting or lying down when the blood pressure was taken.

Pulse Points

There are a number of pulse points on the body where the arteries are close to the surface of the skin and a pulse can be found. Some of these include radial, brachial, carotid, femoral, and pedal pulse points. These points can be used to estimate the systolic blood pressure, without the use of equipment. The further away from the core the pulse is found, the higher the systolic blood pressure will be.

Pupils

Look closely at the size of the pupils, as well as whether they react to light and are of equal size. You can check the reaction to light by shading each eye and then allowing light to enter. You can also check by shining a

Figure 5–15 Pupils that are unequal, fully dilated, fully constricted, or unresponsive to light may indicate a serious head injury or illness.

light into each eye and then removing the light. Pupils should be equal, round, and reactive to light.

Pupils that are unequal, fully dilated or constricted, or unresponsive to light may indicate a serious head injury or illness (Figure 5–15).

Blood Glucose Monitoring

Blood glucose monitoring refers to the measurement of blood sugar (glucose). Everyone's blood has some glucose in it because our bodies turn the food we eat into this form of sugar, which is transported throughout the body. Insulin, a hormone from the pancreas, helps get the glucose into our cells to be used for energy.

Without insulin (e.g., in people with Type 2 diabetes), the blood glucose level (BGL) rises, leading to long-term health complications if untreated. In people taking insulin, low blood glucose creates critical health risks that must be treated immediately.

Testing BGL With a Glucometer

People with diabetes check their BGLs regularly, often using a portable device called a glucometer. Monitoring can be done at any time using a glucometer.

The test requires obtaining a drop of blood by piercing the skin of a finger pad with a sharp sterile device such as a lancet or needle. The drop of blood is then placed on a test strip containing a chemical substance, which is then inserted into the glucometer.

Using a Glucometer

When using a glucometer, follow these steps:

1. Ensure your hands are clean and the glucometer is in good working order.

2. Prepare the lancet and lancet device.

3. Insert the test strip into the glucometer, matching the code number on the screen to that on the test strip vial. Read the owner's manual for the blood glucometer carefully, and *only use the test strips specified for that device*. Otherwise, the device may fail to give results or may generate an inaccurate reading.

4. Wipe the pad of the patient's finger with an alcohol swab, or clean the finger with soap and water. Allow the skin to dry completely. Force blood into the finger (by squeezing).

5. Using a sterile lancet, prick the side of the fingertip and gently squeeze out a drop of blood.

6. Drop the blood onto the test strip in the appropriate place.

7. Read and record the numerical result.

8. Bandage the patient's finger and document the findings.

9. Remove the test strip, put it in a biohazard bag, and dispose of the sharp appropriately.

What the Numbers Mean

Blood glucose is measured in millimoles per litre (mmol/L), and a normal BGL ranges from 4 mmol/L to 8 mmol/L. Hypoglycemia is most often defined as a BGL of less than 4 mmol/L, whereas hyperglycemia is defined as a BGL of greater than 8 mmol/L.

Although the result may vary depending upon the patient and the testing device used, it is generally accepted that the normal range before meals is 5 to 7.2 mmol/L and for after meals it is less than 10 mmol/L.

Use this reading, along with the patient's history and any signs found during assessment, to determine whether to treat the situation as a diabetic emergency. Only some jurisdictions allow the responder to use a glucometer.

Low blood glucose, also called hypoglycemia, requires immediate treatment. If the patient is conscious, provide 115 mL (4 oz.) of fruit juice or regular soft drink or two to five glucose tablets, and recheck glucose in 15 minutes. If the patient is unconscious, seek medical attention immediately.

Pediatric Considerations

Low blood sugar levels in children under seven years of age should be of concern. Young children require higher blood sugar levels than do adults (for brain development). Also, children's food intake and activity level tend to vary quite a bit from day to day, causing blood sugar levels to fluctuate, so they are more at risk of low blood sugar levels. Further, it may be difficult for very young children to report and describe symptoms of low blood sugar, so it may go undetected.

Also keep in mind that, before reaching puberty, children seem to be at lower risk of the complications of diabetes even when blood sugar levels are abnormally high. The American Diabetes Association recommends aiming for the safe adult range of BGL only when children grow older and can recognize the early symptoms of BGLs dropping too low.

Head-to-Toe Physical Examination

Once you are certain that the patient has no life-threatening injuries or medical conditions that require your care, you can begin the physical exam.

If you find life-threatening injuries or medical conditions, such as unconsciousness, no breathing, no pulse, or severe bleeding during the primary survey, do not waste time with the physical exam. Instead, focus your attention on providing care for the life-threatening conditions.

The physical exam is a systematic "head-to-toe" examination that helps you gather additional information about injuries or conditions that may need care. These injuries or conditions are not immediately life-threatening but could become so if not cared for. For example, you might find minor bleeding or possible broken bones as you conduct your examination of the patient. Begin the physical exam by telling the patient what you are going to do and asking her for consent.

The physical exam process involves the use of exposing and examining (inspection), listening (auscultation), and feeling (palpation). You may even smell something that you can gather as information, such as the smell of bleach on the breath, which may indicate poisoning. After telling the patient exactly what you are going to do and asking her to hold still, inspect and palpate each part of the body, starting with the head, before you move on to the next area. Always maintain the patient's dignity and privacy while conducting the exam.

Ask the patient to tell you if any areas hurt. Avoid touching any painful areas or having the patient move any area in which there is discomfort. Watch facial expressions; listen for a tone of voice that may reveal pain. Look for a MedicAlert® medical identification product such as a necklace or bracelet (Figure 5–16). This tag may help you determine what is wrong, whom to call for help, and what care to give.

As you do the head-to-toe examination, think about how the body normally looks and feels. Be alert for any sign of injuries—anything that looks or feels unusual. If you are uncertain whether your finding is unusual, check the other side of the body.

Chest Auscultation

When auscultating, listen for present and equal breath sounds in both lungs, at the top and bottom. To do this:

- Place the stethoscope below the clavicle at the mid-clavicular line. Listen to one full inhalation and exhalation on both sides of the chest.

- Place the stethoscope at the fourth or fifth intercostal space on the mid-axillary line. Listen to one full inhalation and exhalation on both sides of the chest.

Absent, diminished, or abnormal breath sounds may indicate abnormal or inadequate breathing. Your local protocol may indicate a specific auscultation pattern to follow.

Figure 5–16 There are many forms of MedicAlert® medical identification products.

Check the head. Look for blood or clear fluid in or around the ears, nose, and mouth. Blood or clear fluid can indicate a serious head injury. Check the level of consciousness again and note any change. Check the pupils again and note any changes.

To check the neck, look and feel for any abnormalities (Figure 5–17, a). If the patient has not suffered an injury involving the head or trunk and does not have any pain or discomfort in the head, neck, or back, then there is little likelihood of a spinal injury. You should proceed to check other body parts. If, however, you suspect a possible head and/or spine injury because of the mechanism of injury, such as a motor vehicle collision or a fall from a height, minimize movement to the patient's head and spine. If you suspect head and/or spine injuries, take care of these first. Do not be concerned about finishing the secondary survey. You will learn techniques for stabilizing and immobilizing the head and spine in Chapter 14.

If you do not suspect injury, check the collarbones and shoulders by feeling for deformity (Figure 5–17, b). Ask the patient to shrug her shoulders. Check the chest by asking the patient to take a deep breath and then blow the air out. Ask the patient if she is experiencing pain. Auscultate for lung sounds if you are trained to do so. Look and listen for more subtle signs of breathing difficulty, such as wheezing or diminished lung sounds. Feel the ribs for deformity (Figure 5–17, c).

Examine the back for any injuries by palpating both sides of the spine from the neck downward with your

a

b

c

d

e

f

g

Figure 5–17, a-g To do a secondary survey: **a**, check the neck; **b**, check the shoulders and collarbones; **c**, check the chest and the patient's breathing; **d**, check the back, only moving the patient if required and safe to do so. Apply light pressure to the abdomen, then check the four quadrants; **e**, check the hips and pelvis; **f**, check the legs, feet, and toes; and **g**, check the arms, hands, and fingers.

fingertips. Check for any reaction to pain. Look for discoloration, open wounds, or any signs of bleeding.

Next, ask if the patient has any pain in the abdomen. Expose the abdomen; look for discoloration, open wounds, or distension. Look at the abdomen for any pulsating. If there is no pulsating, apply slight pressure to each of the abdominal quadrants (Figure 5–17, d), avoiding any areas where the patient had indicated pain. The abdomen should be soft. If it is rigid, this indicates a problem. Check the hips, asking the patient if she has any pain. Place your hands on both sides of the pelvis and push in on the sides and down on the hips (Figure 5–17, e).

Next, look and feel each leg for any deformity (Figure 5–17, f). If there is no apparent sign of injury, ask the patient to move her toes, foot, and leg. Finally, determine if the patient has any pain in the arms or hands. Feel the arms for any deformity (Figure 5–17, g). It is best to check only one extremity at a time. If there is no apparent sign of injury, ask the patient to move her fingers, hand, and arm. Repeat this procedure on the other arm. Check for distal circulation and sensation in both arms and legs.

NOTE:

As you perform the physical exam, try not to move the patient. Most injured patients will find the most comfortable position for themselves. For example, a person with a chest injury who is experiencing difficulty with his breathing may be sitting up and supporting the injured areas.

If the patient can move all her body parts without pain or discomfort and there are no other apparent signs or symptoms of injury, have her attempt to rest for a few minutes in a sitting position. If more advanced help is not needed, continue to check the signs and symptoms and monitor the ABCs.

Take note of the information you find during the physical exam. Sometimes you may need to have a partner fill out the form with the information you gather. This will help you when it is time to give a verbal report to the next level of care as you transfer the patient.

SECONDARY TRANSPORT DECISION

For secondary transport decision, see "Transport Decision" (covered earlier in this chapter). Make your decision based on any additional information you learn during the secondary and ongoing survey. Update the hospital and medical direction of your plans and any care you provide.

ONGOING SURVEY

If you have completed the secondary survey and have given care for any injuries and illness, provide ongoing survey and care while you wait to obtain advanced medical care. The patient's condition can gradually worsen, or a life-threatening condition, such as respiratory or cardiac arrest, can occur suddenly. Do not assume that the patient is out of danger just because there were no serious problems at first. Keep watching the patient's level of consciousness, breathing, and skin colour. Appropriate vital signs should be checked every five minutes if the patient has a life-threatening emergency; otherwise, check vital signs every 15 minutes. The physical exam and history do not need to be repeated unless there is a specific reason to do so. If any life-threatening emergencies develop, stop whatever you are doing and provide appropriate care immediately.

Record additional findings and turn this information over to the next level of care.

While waiting for more advanced medical care (Table 5–6), help the patient stay calm and as comfortable as possible. The conditions in Table 5–6 by no means make a complete list. It is impossible to describe every possible condition since there are always exceptions. Trust your instincts. If you think there is an emergency, there probably is. It is better to obtain more advanced medical care than wait until it is too late to help.

TABLE 5–6: WHEN TO OBTAIN MORE ADVANCED MEDICAL CARE

Condition	Signs and Symptoms
Unconscious or decreased level of consciousness	Patient does not respond to tapping, loud voices, or other attempts to awaken
Difficulty breathing (dyspnea)	Noisy breathing, such as wheezing or gasping Patient feels short of breath Skin has a flushed, pale, or bluish appearance
No breathing	You cannot see the patient's chest rise and fall You cannot hear and feel air escaping from the nose and/or mouth
No pulse or signs of circulation	You cannot feel the carotid pulse in the neck or the pulses in the arms and legs
Severe bleeding	Patient has bleeding that spurts or gushes from the wound
Persistent pain or pressure in the chest or abdomen	Patient has persistent pain or pressure in the chest or abdomen that is not relieved by resting or changing positions
Vomiting blood or passing blood	You can see blood in vomit, urine, or feces
Suspected poisoning	Patient shows evidence of swallowed, inhaled, or injected poison, such as presence of drugs, medications, or cleaning agents Mouth or lips may be burned
Sudden illness requiring assistance	Patient has seizures, severe headaches, slurred speech, or changes in level of consciousness, unusually high or low blood pressure, or a known diabetic condition
Head, neck, or spine injuries	How the injury happened; for example, a fall, severe blow, or collision suggests a head injury Patient complains of severe headaches or neck or back pain Patient is unconscious Bleeding, clear fluid, or deformity of the scalp, face, or neck
Possible broken bones	How the injury happened; for example, a fall, severe blow, or collision suggests a fracture Evidence of damage to blood vessels or nerves, for example, slow capillary refill, no pulse below the injury, loss of sensation in the affected part Inability to move body part without pain or discomfort Fractures associated with open wounds

SUMMARY

A primary survey serves to determine if any life-threatening conditions are present so they can be treated rapidly. The secondary survey helps determine any other conditions that may not be a threat to life at the moment but still require care. Problems that are not an immediate threat to life can become serious if you do not recognize them and provide care. By following the appropriate steps when conducting primary and secondary surveys, you will give the patient with a serious illness or injury the best chance for survival.

As you approach the scene, you notice the second basketball player falls silent and appears to go limp. What do you do?

Chapter 6

Respiratory Emergencies

It's a beautiful summer day. You are called to a family having a picnic.
A three-year-old girl is gasping for air and has a panicked look on her face.
Her mother is crying and doesn't know what to do. "She was just eating
her lunch when this happened!" she cries. You survey the scene.
What do you do?

INTRODUCTION

In this chapter, you will learn how to care for respiratory, or breathing, emergencies. Because oxygen is vital to life, you must always ensure that the patient has an open airway and is breathing. You will often detect a breathing emergency during the primary survey. In a breathing emergency, a person's breathing is so impaired that life is threatened. This kind of emergency can occur in two ways: breathing becomes difficult or breathing stops. A person who is having difficulty breathing (dyspnea) is having a breathing emergency. A person who has stopped breathing is in respiratory arrest.

PATHOPHYSIOLOGY

Normal breathing occurs in ambient (surrounding) air, which contains all the necessary gases for normal respiration. People may suffer breathing difficulties because of an inadequate amount of oxygen breathed in during respiration. Breathing difficulties may also occur as a result of breathing in a low-oxygen environment or when poisonous gases are in the air. Other causes of breathing difficulties include infection of the lungs; illnesses like asthma, which narrows the airway and causes wheezing; excess fluid in the lungs or excess fluid between the lungs and blood vessels; and poor circulation.

Breathing difficulties may also develop due to upper-airway problems caused by swelling, obstruction, or trauma. Swelling of the upper airway can occur due to anaphylaxis (severe allergic reaction) or asthma. Choking, caused by airway obstruction, is one of the most common causes of breathing emergencies and can occur due to anatomical (the person's own body) or mechanical (a foreign object) obstruction. Trauma can occur due to a blow to the upper chest, a puncture, or a crush injury. Breathing problems may develop because of ineffective circulation. This can be the result of shock, an acute condition in which the circulatory system fails to adequately circulate oxygen-rich blood to all cells of the body, or cardiac arrest, when the heart stops functioning as a pump, often the result of a heart attack.

Sometimes the rate or depth of breathing is inadequate, leading to an insufficient volume of air moving into and out of the lungs. Respiration may be ineffective due to unconsciousness, altered level of consciousness, injury to the chest, poisoning, overdose, or diseases such as chronic obstructive pulmonary disease (COPD) or emphysema.

Oxygenation refers to the amount of oxygen in the bloodstream. Oxygen is exchanged between the alveoli of the lungs and the capillaries and, at the cellular level, between the capillaries and the cells. If an insufficient amount of oxygen is delivered to the cells, this is referred to as hypoxia, and it may result from an obstructed airway, shock, inadequate breathing, drowning, strangulation, choking, suffocation, cardiac arrest, head trauma, carbon monoxide poisoning, or complications of general anesthesia.

CHOKING

The two types of airway obstruction that cause choking are anatomical and mechanical.

An anatomical obstruction occurs when the airway is blocked by an anatomical structure, such as the tongue or swollen tissues of the mouth and throat. This type of obstruction may result from injury to the neck or a medical emergency such as anaphylaxis. The most common obstruction in an unconscious person is the tongue, which may drop to the back of the throat and block the airway. This occurs because muscles, including the tongue, relax when deprived of oxygen.

A mechanical obstruction occurs when the airway is blocked by a foreign object, such as a piece of food or a small toy, or fluids, such as vomit, blood, mucus, or saliva.

Common causes of choking include:

- Trying to swallow large pieces of poorly chewed food

- Drinking alcohol before or during meals (alcohol dulls the nerves that aid swallowing, making choking on food more likely)

- Wearing dentures (dentures make it difficult for you to sense whether food is fully chewed before you swallow it)

- Eating while talking excitedly or laughing or eating too fast

- Walking, playing, or running with food or objects in the mouth

A person whose airway is blocked by a piece of food or another object can quickly stop breathing, lose consciousness, and die. You must be able to recognize that the airway is obstructed and give care immediately. This is why checking the airway comes first in the ABCs of the primary survey.

A person who is choking may have either a mild or severe airway obstruction. A person with a severe airway obstruction is not able to pass a sufficient amount of air to maintain the breathing process. With a mild airway obstruction, the person's ability to breathe depends on how much air can get past the obstruction into the lungs.

Mild Choking

A person with a mild airway obstruction can still move air to and from the lungs. This air allows the person to cough, in an attempt to dislodge the object. The person may also be able to move air past the vocal cords to speak. The narrowed airway causes a wheezing sound as air moves in and out of the lungs. As a natural reaction to choking, the person may clutch at the throat with one or both hands. If the person is coughing forcefully, do not interfere with attempts to cough up the object. A person who has enough air to cough forcefully or speak also has enough air entering the lungs to breathe. Stay with the person and encourage her to continue coughing to clear the obstruction. If coughing persists, obtain more advanced medical care.

Severe Choking

A mild airway obstruction can quickly become a severe airway obstruction. A person with a severely blocked airway is unable to speak, cry, breathe, or cough effectively. Sometimes the person may cough weakly and ineffectively or make high-pitched noises. All of these signs tell you the person is not getting enough air to the lungs to sustain life. Act immediately. If you have not already done so, have a bystander call for more advanced medical care while you begin to give care.

PREVENTING CHOKING

Choking can usually be prevented if you are careful when eating. Follow these guidelines:

- Chew food well before swallowing; eat slowly and calmly.
- Avoid talking or laughing with food in your mouth.
- Minimize alcohol consumption before and during meals.
- Avoid walking or other physical activity with food in your mouth.
- Keep other objects out of your mouth. For example, do not hold a pen cap or nails in your mouth when your hands are busy.

Babies and children are particularly at risk of choking. Parents and other supervisors should follow these guidelines:

- Feed children only when they are seated in a high chair or a secure seat. Do not let children move about with food in their hands or mouth.
- Feed babies or young children appropriate soft food in small pieces. Constantly watch them when they eat.
- Check the environment and all toys to be sure there are no small objects or parts that babies or young children may put in their mouths.
- Keep young children away from balloons, which can burst into small pieces that can be easily inhaled.

Care for a Patient Who Is Choking

When someone is choking, you must try to reopen the airway as quickly as possible.

The method you use depends on whether the patient is conscious or unconscious and whether the patient is an adult, a child, or a baby. For patients who are conscious, variations are used for large patients, pregnant women, and patients in a seated position (e.g., a wheelchair).

Care for a Conscious Choking Adult or Child

Stand (or kneel for a small child) behind the patient and wrap one arm diagonally across the patient's chest.

Bend the patient forward at the waist until the patient's upper airway is at least parallel to the ground (Figure 6–1, a). With the heel of your other hand, deliver five firm back blows between the shoulder blades (Figure 6–1, b). If the object has not been dislodged, perform abdominal thrusts.

NOTE:
To deliver effective back blows, you may need to stand behind and slightly to the side of the patient rather than directly behind the patient.

Make a fist with one hand and place the thumb side against the middle of the patient's abdomen just above the navel and well below the lower tip of the breastbone (Figure 6–1, c). Grab your fist with your other hand and give five quick upward thrusts into the abdomen.

Abdominal thrusts compress the abdomen, increasing pressure in the lungs and airway. This simulates a cough, forcing trapped air in the lungs to push the object out of the airway like a cork from a bottle of champagne. Continue the cycle of five firm back blows and five abdominal thrusts until the object comes out or the patient begins to breathe or cough or becomes unconscious.

If the patient becomes unconscious, lower him to the floor, ensuring you protect the head. Have someone obtain advanced medical care if this has not already been done.

Care for an Unconscious Choking Adult or Child

During your primary survey, you may discover that an unconscious adult is not breathing. If this happens, begin the CPR sequence (30 chest compressions).

Chest compressions are performed just as they are in CPR (Figure 6–2) and are proven to be effective in dislodging an object in the throat. Many people who have an obstructed airway will also not have circulation, so chest compressions will not only be effective in dislodging the obstruction but will also provide necessary care for absence of circulation.

After giving 30 chest compressions, attempt to ventilate. If your breath goes in, give a second

Figure 6–1, a-c To care for a conscious choking adult: **a**, stand behind the patient, wrap one arm diagonally across his chest, and bend him forward at the waist until his upper airway is at least parallel to the ground; **b**, with the heel of your other hand, give five firm back blows between the shoulder blades; and **c**, place the thumb side of your fist against the middle of the patient's abdomen, grab your fist with your other hand and give five quick upward thrusts into the abdomen.

Figure 6–2 Chest compressions for an unconscious choking adult or child are done just as they are in CPR.

Figure 6–3 To do a finger sweep, grasp the tongue and lower jaw and lift, then sweep the object out.

breath. If the patient's chest does not rise after the first breath, reposition the head to adjust the airway and attempt to give another breath. If you are still not able to breathe air into the patient's lungs, repeat the CPR sequence, then look in the patient's mouth. If you see an object, carefully remove it. Grasp the tongue and lower jaw and lift, then sweep the object out using a finger sweep (Figure 6–3).

> **NOTE:**
>
> *After you have repositioned the head and attempted to give a second breath once, you do not need to repeat the repositioning step between chest compression cycles.*

If your first attempt to clear the airway is unsuccessful, do not stop. The longer the patient goes without oxygen, the more the muscles will relax, making it easier to clear the airway.

Repeat the sequence until the object is expelled, you can breathe into the patient, or other trained personnel take over.

Once you are able to breathe air into the patient's lungs, give two one-second breaths. Then complete the primary survey by checking the patient for signs of circulation and checking and caring for any severe bleeding. If there are no signs of circulation, have someone get an automated external defibrillator (AED) (if you don't already have one) and begin CPR

(see Chapter 8). If the patient has signs of circulation but is not breathing on his own, continue rescue breathing, which is discussed later in this chapter.

If the patient starts breathing on his own, continue to monitor the patient and provide care until you obtain more advanced medical care. Place the patient in the recovery position, as described in Chapter 5.

When to Stop Care

Stop immediately if the object is dislodged or if the patient begins to breathe or cough. Make sure the object is cleared from the airway and the patient is breathing freely again. Even after the object is coughed up, the patient may still have breathing problems that you do not immediately see. You should also realize that abdominal thrusts, chest compressions, and chest thrusts may cause internal injuries. Therefore, anytime this type of care is used to dislodge an object, you should obtain more advanced medical care for follow-up, even if he seems to be breathing without difficulty.

Special Considerations for a Patient Who Is Choking

In some instances, abdominal thrusts are not the best or only method of care for someone who is choking. Some patients who are choking need chest thrusts. For example, if you cannot reach far enough around the patient to give effective abdominal thrusts or the

Figure 6–4 Give chest thrusts if you cannot reach around the patient to give abdominal thrusts or if the person is noticeably pregnant.

Figure 6–5 To give yourself abdominal thrusts, press your abdomen onto a firm object, such as the back of a chair.

patient is noticeably pregnant, you should give chest thrusts along with firm back blows. For someone in a seated position, such as a wheelchair, alternate between abdominal thrusts and chest thrusts.

Care for a Larger or Pregnant Patient

Alternate between five firm back blows and five chest thrusts. To perform chest thrusts, stand behind the patient and wrap both of your arms around the patient's chest, just under the armpits (Figure 6–4). Make a fist and place the thumb side of your fist in the middle of the patient's chest. Place your other hand over your fist and pull straight back toward you. If the first couple of thrusts aren't effective, pull more sharply and deeply. Continue to alternate between five firm back blows and five chest thrusts until the object comes out or the patient begins to breathe or cough or becomes unconscious.

Care for Someone in a Seated Position

If the patient is in a wheelchair, first lock the wheels. Then kneel or crouch behind the patient. For the abdominal thrusts, wrap both of your arms around the patient's abdomen. Make a fist with one hand and place the thumb side of your fist just above the patient's belly button. Grasp your fist with your other hand. Pull sharply in and

up five times. For the chest thrusts, make a fist with one hand and place the thumb side of your fist in the middle of the patient's chest. Place your other hand over your fist and pull straight back toward you sharply five times. Continue alternating between abdominal thrusts and chest thrusts until the object comes out or the patient begins to breathe or cough or becomes unconscious.

For Someone Choking Alone

If you are alone and are choking, dial EMS/9-1-1 and leave the phone off the hook. This will tell the dispatcher to send help. If there are people nearby, move to a place where you can get noticed. Drop your abdomen onto a safe object with no sharp edges or corners, such as the back of a chair (Figure 6–5). Try to dislodge the object by using the safe object to do thrusts on the same area you would use for abdominal thrusts.

Babies

Choking emergencies are common in children and babies. Care for babies who are choking includes a combination of chest thrusts given with two fingers and firm back blows. Abdominal thrusts are not used for a choking baby because of their potential to cause injury.

a

b

Figure 6–6, a–b To care for a conscious choking baby: sandwich the baby between your forearms; **a**, turn the baby over so she is face down along your forearm on your lap; and **b**, give 5 firm back blows with the heel of your hand between the shoulder blades.

Care for a Conscious Choking Baby

If, during the primary survey, you determine that a conscious baby cannot breathe, cough, or cry, give care for a severe airway obstruction. Begin by giving five firm back blows followed by five chest thrusts.

Start by positioning the baby face up on your forearm. Place your other arm on top of the baby, using your thumb and fingers to hold the baby's jaw while sandwiching the baby between your forearms. Turn the baby over so that she is face down on your forearm. Lower your arm onto your thigh so that the baby's head is lower than her chest (Figure 6–6, a). Give

Figure 6–7 After giving 5 back blows, turn the baby onto her back, lower your arm onto your thigh, and give 5 chest thrusts.

five firm back blows with the heel of your hand between the shoulder blades (Figure 6–6, b). Maintain support of the head and neck by firmly holding the jaw between your thumb and forefinger.

To give chest thrusts, you will need to turn the baby back over. Start by placing your free hand and forearm along the baby's head and back so that the baby is sandwiched between your two hands and forearms. Continue to support the head between your thumb and fingers from the front while you cradle the back of the head with your other hand.

Turn the baby onto her back. Lower your arm that is supporting the back onto your thigh. The head should be lower than her chest. Give five chest thrusts (Figure 6–7).

To locate the correct place to give chest thrusts, place your two fingers in the middle of the chest, just below the nipple line.

Use the pads of the two fingers to compress the breastbone. Compress the breastbone at least 4 cm (1.5 in.) or 1/3 to 1/2 the depth of the chest and then let the breastbone return to its normal position. Keep your fingers in contact with the baby's breastbone. Compress five times. You can give back blows and chest thrusts effectively whether you stand up or sit. If the baby is large or your hands are too small to adequately support the baby, you may prefer to sit. Place the baby in your lap to give back blows and chest thrusts. The baby's head should be lower than the chest.

Keep giving back blows and chest thrusts until the object is coughed up, the baby begins to breathe or cough, or the baby becomes unconscious. Obtain more advanced medical care if you have not already done so. Even if the baby seems to be breathing well, she should be examined by more advanced medical personnel.

Care for an Unconscious Choking Baby

Begin with the CPR sequence (30 chest compressions). Next, open the airway and attempt to ventilate. If your breath goes in, give a second breath. If the baby's chest does not rise after the first breath, reposition the head to adjust the airway and attempt to give another breath. If you still cannot breathe air into the baby's lungs, repeat the CPR sequence, then look in the baby's mouth for a foreign object.

To do a foreign-body check (i.e., a finger sweep), open the baby's mouth using your hand that is nearer the baby's feet (Figure 6–8). Grasp both the tongue and lower jaw and lift. Look for an object. If you can see it, try to remove it by sweeping the object out using a finger sweep with the little finger (Figure 6–9).

If your first attempt to clear the airway is unsuccessful, do not stop. Repeat the CPR sequence until the object is expelled, you are able to get air in the baby's lungs, or other trained personnel take over.

Once you are able to breathe air into the baby's lungs, finish the primary survey. Give two one-second breaths and check the baby's signs of circulation. Next, check and care for any severe bleeding. If the baby has no signs of circulation, begin CPR, which you will learn in Chapter 8. If the baby has signs of circulation and is not breathing on her own, continue rescue breathing.

If the baby starts breathing on her own, continue to monitor the baby and provide care until you obtain more advanced medical care.

NOTE:

After you have repositioned the head and attempted to give a second breath once, you do not need to repeat the repositioning step between chest compression cycles.

Figure 6–8 To do a finger sweep on a baby, put your thumb into the baby's mouth and hold the tongue and lower jaw between the thumb and fingers. Lift the jaw upward.

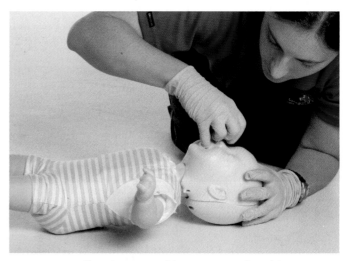

Figure 6–9 If you see an object, sweep the object out using your little finger.

BREATHING EMERGENCIES

Although breathing emergencies are often caused by injury, several other conditions can also cause them. These include anaphylaxis, chronic obstructive pulmonary disease (COPD), emphysema, chronic bronchitis, acute respiratory distress syndrome (ARDS), asthma, pneumonia, acute pulmonary edema, pulmonary embolism, and hyperventilation.

Signs and Symptoms of Breathing Emergencies

The signs and symptoms of breathing emergencies are usually obvious. People may look as if they cannot catch their breath, or they may gasp for air (Figure 6–10). Their breaths may be unusually fast, slow, deep, or shallow. They may be experiencing breathing difficulty (dyspnea). They may make unusual noises, such as wheezing or gurgling or high-pitched, shrill sounds.

The person's skin may also signal a breathing emergency. At first, the skin may be unusually moist and appear flushed. Later, it may appear pale or bluish as the oxygen level in the blood falls. When the person's skin, lips, or nail beds appear blue, the condition is called cyanosis.

The person may say he feels dizzy or lightheaded. He may feel pain in the chest and tingling in the hands and feet. He may be apprehensive or fearful (Figure 6–11). Any of these symptoms is a clue that the person may be having a breathing emergency. Table 6–1 lists the signs and symptoms of breathing emergencies.

Figure 6–10 People with breathing emergencies may look as if they cannot catch their breath, or they may gasp for air.

TABLE 6–1: SIGNS AND SYMPTOMS OF BREATHING EMERGENCIES

Conditions	Signs and Symptoms
Abnormal breathing	Breathing is unusually slow, rapid, deep, or shallow Person is gasping for breath Person is wheezing or gurgling or making high-pitched shrill noises
Abnormal skin appearance	Skin is unusually moist Skin has a flushed, pale or ashen, or bluish appearance
How the person feels	Short of breath Restless and anxious Dizzy or lightheaded Pain in the chest or tingling in hands and feet
How the person looks	Using accessory muscles to breathe, in the tripod position

Figure 6–11 There are many signs and symptoms of breathing emergencies.

Specific Types of Breathing Emergencies

Anaphylaxis

Anaphylaxis, also known as anaphylactic shock, is a severe allergic reaction. The air passages constrict and restrict the person's breathing. Anaphylaxis may be caused by insect bites or stings or contact with drugs, medications such as penicillin, food, and chemicals.

Anaphylaxis usually occurs suddenly, within seconds or minutes after contact with the substance. The skin or area of the body that came in contact with the substance usually swells and turns red (Figure 6–12). This breathing difficulty can progress to an obstructed airway as the tongue and throat swell. The person may also feel dizzy or confused. Other signs and symptoms include hives, itching, rash, weakness, nausea, vomiting, dizziness, and breathing difficulty that includes tightness in the chest and throat, coughing, and wheezing.

Anaphylaxis is a life-threatening emergency requiring advanced medical care. Death from anaphylaxis usually occurs because the person's breathing is severely impaired.

Figure 6–12 A person in anaphylaxis may have many signs and symptoms including swelling of the face.

If an unusual inflammation or rash is noticeable immediately after contact with a possible source, it could be an allergic reaction. Assess the patient's airway and breathing. If the patient has any breathing difficulty or complains that his throat is closing, obtain more advanced medical care immediately. Help the patient into the most comfortable position for breathing. Administer oxygen if available. Monitor the ABCs and try to keep the patient calm.

People who know they are extremely allergic to certain substances usually try to avoid them, although this is sometimes impossible. These people may carry an epinephrine auto-injector in case they have a severe allergic reaction (Figure 6–13). These are available most often by prescription. The injector contains a single dose of the drug epinephrine that can be injected into the body to counteract the reaction.

Figure 6–13 An epinephrine auto-injector.

How to Use an Epinephrine Auto-Injector

1. Make sure that you check the Six Rights of Medication (see Chapter 11).

2. Remove the safety cap.

3. Place the injection tip against the outer thigh and push the epinephrine auto-injector firmly against the thigh with a quick motion. You should hear a click. Hold for 10 seconds.

4. Remove the epinephrine auto-injector.

5. Make sure the used epinephrine auto-injector goes with the patient to the hospital.

There are epinephrine auto-injectors that have multiple doses in one injector. If a patient has an injector of this type, be very careful when handling it and have the patient recap the needle himself.

> **NOTE:**
>
> *See Chapter 11 for information regarding epinephrine.*

Chronic Obstructive Pulmonary Disease

Chronic obstructive pulmonary disease (COPD) is a disease of the airways that is characterized by a loss of lung function. This disease affects both men and women. The average Canadian with COPD is 65 years old and has a long history of smoking. However, the disease has been diagnosed in individuals as young as 40 years of age. COPD has also been reported to occur more often among people residing in urban centres compared with rural populations. The term COPD is used for emphysema or chronic bronchitis, two closely related diseases of the respiratory system.

People diagnosed with COPD may get colds or the flu often, and they also experience shortness of breath under conditions that do not tax most healthy people. Signs and symptoms of a person suffering from COPD are:

• Shortness of breath, gasping for air with sudden onset

• Sitting upright, leaning forward

• Barrel-chested

• Coarse rattling sounds in the lungs

• Distended neck veins

• Cyanosis

• Prolonged exhalation through pursed lips

• Person has oxygen system in his residence, either stationary or portable

Emphysema

Emphysema is a disease in which the alveoli lose their elasticity, become distended with trapped air, and stop working. This results in the lungs losing their ability to efficiently exchange carbon dioxide and oxygen. Emphysema is often caused by smoking and usually develops over many years.

People with emphysema suffer from shortness of breath. As the total number of alveoli decreases, breathing becomes more difficult. Exhaling is extremely difficult. They may cough and may have cyanosis or fever. People with advanced cases may be restless, confused, and weak and can go into respiratory or cardiac arrest. Emphysema can get worse over time.

Chronic Bronchitis

Bronchitis is a disease causing excessive mucous secretions and inflammatory changes to the bronchi. These secretions make breathing difficult. Bronchitis is often caused by prolonged exposure to irritants (most commonly, cigarette smoke).

People with bronchitis suffer from shortness of breath and the presence of a cough with sputum. Chronic bronchitis is characterized by a productive cough that has persisted for at least three months in a given year and over two consecutive years. There may also be narrowing of the large and small airways, making it more difficult for air to move in and out of the lungs. This disease gets worse over time.

People with emphysema and/or chronic bronchitis may eventually develop a hypoxic drive to breathe. In healthy individuals, the drive to breathe is from the amount of carbon dioxide in the blood. People with emphysema and/or chronic bronchitis build up high levels of carbon dioxide in the blood. Due to the consistently high levels, the body looks to the oxygen levels to determine the need to breathe. If oxygen levels are low, the breathing rate increases. People with COPD who are not acutely short of breath are usually receiving low concentrations of oxygen from their home oxygen unit.

In a person with COPD who has a true "hypoxic drive," increased levels of oxygen could signal the body to slow down or stop breathing entirely. However, this is rarely encountered in the field because EMS is usually called for a person who is acutely short of breath. In this case, you should administer high-flow oxygen to the patient.

Acute Respiratory Distress Syndrome

Acute respiratory distress syndrome (ARDS) is a serious lung disease caused by a variety of direct and indirect conditions. These conditions lead to an increase in the quantity of fluid between the alveolar membrane and the surrounding pulmonary capillaries, causing a decrease in the amount of oxygen the red blood cells can absorb. ARDS can develop within hours to days of the inciting event. The additional fluid volume makes the lungs feel heavy, requiring additional pressure when ventilating a patient with the syndrome.

Signs and symptoms of ARDS include:

- Rapid breathing (tachypnea)
- Shortness of breath
- Cyanosis (mottled, bluish skin)
- Possible pulmonary edema
- History of injury or illness involving the lungs

Asthma

Asthma is a condition that narrows the air passages and makes breathing difficult. During an asthma attack, the air passages become constricted or narrowed by a spasm of the muscles lining the bronchi or by swelling of the bronchi themselves. People may become anxious or frightened because breathing is difficult.

Asthma is more common in children and young adults. It may be triggered by an allergic reaction to food, pollen, a drug, cold weather, or an insect sting. Emotional distress may also trigger it. For some people, physical activity induces asthma. Normally, someone with asthma easily controls attacks with medication. These medications stop the muscle spasm, opening the airway and making breathing easier.

A characteristic sign of asthma is wheezing when exhaling due to constricted air passages. This also leads to air being trapped in the lungs. This trapped air may also make the person's chest appear larger than normal, particularly in small children.

How to Help Someone Use a Metered-Dose Inhaler

When assisting with a metered-dose inhaler (puffer), follow these steps:

1. Check the Six Rights of Medication before proceeding.
2. Tell the patient to shake the inhaler three or four times.
3. Help the patient remove the cap from the inhaler. If the patient uses a spacer and it has a cap, help the patient remove it.
4. Tell the patient to put the inhaler into the spacer, if applicable (Figure 6–14).
5. Tell the patient to breathe out, away from the inhaler and spacer.
6. For a child, bring the spacer or the inhaler to the child's mouth (Figure 6–15). Help to put the mouthpiece between the child's teeth and then tell the child to close her lips around it. For an adult, help bring the spacer or the inhaler to her mouth.
7. Tell the patient to press the top of the inhaler once. If the patient is unable to do this, you may do it instead if the patient asks you to.
8. Tell the patient to take one slow, full breath, hold it for as long as comfortable (up to 10 seconds), and then breathe out.[15]

Figure 6–14 An inhaler prescribed for asthma and a spacer.

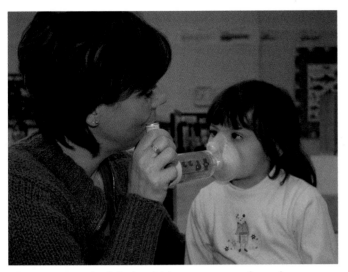

Figure 6–15 An inhaler with a spacer and mask.

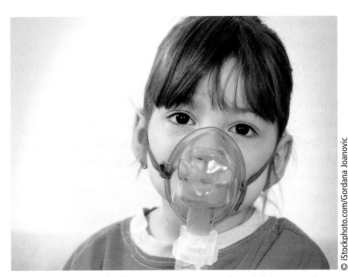

Figure 6–16 Nebulizers are common for children under the age of five.

Nebulization

A small-volume nebulizer is a special mask designed to administer aerosolized (mist) medication over a few minutes, ensuring the efficacy of drug delivery during treatment will not be jeopardized even if the patient takes a single ineffective breath. Nebulization is typically self-administered by patients. It allows medication to be delivered to the smaller airways by converting it from a liquid form to an aerosol by forcing oxygen through at a high velocity. Smaller particles penetrate further into the lung to reach target sites in the smaller airways.

Nebulizers are common for children under the age of five, those who have difficulty using inhalers, and those with severe asthma (Figure 6–16).

Typically, bronchodilators are administered to patients with acute shortness of breath/respiratory distress. Bronchodilators relax the bronchial muscles, making them smooth, which improves airflow during inhalation and exhalation.

Pneumonia

Pneumonia is a term used to describe a group of illnesses characterized by lung infection and fluid- or pus-filled alveoli, resulting in inadequate oxygen in the blood. Pneumonia is caused by bacteria or a virus but also can be caused by irritants, such as smoke, or aspirated materials, such as vomit. The type of illness caused by chemical irritation or aspiration is called pneumonitis. People with pneumonia may complain of fever and chills.

The following signs and symptoms may be found in a person suffering from pneumonia:

- Difficulty breathing (dyspnea)
- Rapid breathing (tachypnea)
- Pleuritic chest pain, usually worse with breathing
- Productive cough with pus in the sputum or mucus
- Fever, usually exceeding 38°C (100°F)
- Chills

There may be other symptoms as well, such as:

- Nausea
- Vomiting
- Headache
- Tiredness
- Muscle aches

Have the patient with a suspected case of pneumonia assume a comfortable position and administer supplemental oxygen.

Acute Pulmonary Edema

Pulmonary edema can be caused by heart or lung damage. For example, a number of heart disorders (e.g., heart attack, left-sided heart failure, dysrhythmias) can cause fluid to back up in the blood vessels (pulmonary veins) that carry blood away from the lungs to the heart. As a result of a buildup of pressure in these veins, excess fluid leaks out into the alveoli. Congestive heart failure (CHF) is the most common condition to cause pulmonary edema.

However, other causes include pneumonia, smoke or toxin inhalation, narcotic overdose, drowning, and high-altitude illness. You may find people with pulmonary edema sitting upright, leaning forward. If you find a person lying down, instruct her to sit up and dangle her legs to encourage fluid to pool in the legs.

As the fluid builds up in the lungs, the amount of oxygen entering the blood decreases (Figure 6–17). You should give high-flow oxygen to anyone with acute pulmonary edema. In some cases, you may need to assist the patient's ventilations.

Signs and symptoms of pulmonary edema are:

• Shortness of breath with sudden onset

• Rapid, laboured breathing

• Cyanosis

• Frothy sputum (later stage)

• Restlessness

• Anxiety

• Exhaustion

• Rapid pulse (tachycardia)

• Cool, clammy skin

Pulmonary Embolism

Pulmonary embolism is caused by a blockage (embolus) of a pulmonary artery by a clot or other foreign material that has travelled from another part of the circulatory system. It is a surprisingly common disorder that usually begins as a venous disease. It is most often caused by a blood clot (thrombus) breaking free in the large veins of the lower extremities but can also be caused by fat, air, amniotic fluid, or tumour tissue. The embolus flows to the right side of the heart. From there it enters the pulmonary arteries, obstructing blood supply to that part of the lung.

An embolus may range in size from small to massive; therefore, the signs and symptoms may be varied (Figure 6–18). They depend on the location of the blockage and the size of the clot and may include the following:

• Shortness of breath

• Cough

• Pain

Figure 6–17 Pulmonary edema is a buildup of fluid in the lungs.

Figure 6–18 A pulmonary embolus may range in size from small to massive; therefore, the signs and symptoms may be varied.

- Anxiety

- Fainting (syncope)

- Drop in blood pressure (hypotension)

- Cool, clammy skin

- Rapid pulse (tachycardia)

- Fever

- Distended neck vein

If you suspect a patient has a pulmonary embolism, help her to a comfortable position and administer high-flow oxygen. Definitive care requires hospitalization and thrombolytic or heparin therapy.

Hyperventilation

Hyperventilation occurs when someone breathes faster than normal. This rapid breathing (tachypnea) upsets the body's balance of oxygen and carbon dioxide. Hyperventilation is often the result of fear or anxiety and is more likely to occur in people who are tense and nervous. But it is also caused by injuries such as head injuries, by severe bleeding, or by conditions such as high fever, heart failure, lung disease, or diabetic emergencies. It can be triggered by asthma or exercise.

A characteristic sign of hyperventilation is shallow, rapid breathing (tachypnea). Despite their breathing efforts, people say that they cannot get enough air or that they are suffocating. Therefore, they are often fearful and apprehensive or may appear confused. They may say they feel dizzy or that their fingers and toes feel numb or tingly.

General Care for Breathing Emergencies

Recognizing the signs and symptoms of breathing emergencies and providing emergency care are often the keys to preventing other emergencies. Breathing emergencies may signal the beginning of a life-threatening condition. For example, it can be the first signal of a more serious breathing emergency or even a heart attack. Some breathing emergencies can lead to respiratory arrest, which, if not cared for, will result in death.

Many of the signs and symptoms of different kinds of breathing emergencies are similar. You do not need to know the specific cause to provide care. If the patient is breathing, you know the heart is beating. Make sure the patient is not bleeding severely. Help her rest in a comfortable position. Usually, sitting is more comfortable than lying down because breathing is easier. Open a window to provide more air if necessary. Provide ongoing survey and care. Have bystanders move back. Obtain more advanced medical care.

When you are able, do a secondary survey. Remember that a patient experiencing breathing difficulty may have trouble talking. Ask questions to any bystanders who may know about the patient's problem. The patient can confirm answers or answer yes-or-no questions by nodding. If possible, try to help reduce any anxiety; it may contribute to the patient's breathing difficulty. Help the patient take any prescribed medication for the condition if it is available. This may be oxygen or an inhalant (bronchial dilator). Continue to provide ongoing survey and care. Help maintain normal body temperature by preventing chilling or overheating. Administer oxygen if available and indicated.

If the patient's breathing is rapid and there are signs of an injury or an underlying illness, obtain more advanced medical care or transport immediately. If the patient's breathing is rapid and you suspect that it is caused by emotion, such as excitement, try to calm the patient to slow her breathing. Reassurance is often enough to correct hyperventilation. But you can also ask the patient to try to breathe with you. Breathe at a normal rate, emphasizing inhaling and exhaling.

If the condition does not improve, the patient may become unconscious. Obtain more advanced medical care if this has not already been done. Keep the patient's airway open and monitor breathing.

RESPIRATORY ARREST

Respiratory arrest is the condition in which breathing stops. It may be caused by illness, injury, or an obstructed airway. The causes of breathing emergencies can also lead to respiratory arrest. In respiratory arrest, the person gets no oxygen. The body can function for only a few minutes without oxygen before body systems begin to fail. Without oxygen, the heart muscle stops functioning. This causes the circulatory system to fail. When the heart stops, other body systems will also start to fail. However, you can keep the person's respiratory system functioning artificially with rescue breathing.

Rescue Breathing

Rescue breathing is a technique of breathing air into a patient to supply her with the oxygen needed to survive. Rescue breathing is given to patients who are not breathing but still have a pulse.

Rescue breathing works because the air you breathe into the patient contains more than enough oxygen to keep that patient alive. The air you take in with every breath contains about 21% oxygen, but your body uses only a small part of that. The air you breathe out of your lungs and into the lungs of the patient contains about 16% oxygen, enough to keep someone alive.

A responder should always use a resuscitation mask when giving rescue breaths. In this chapter, you will learn how to do rescue breathing. You will learn how to use a resuscitation mask as well as other ventilatory devices in Chapter 7.

You will discover whether you need to give rescue breathing during the first two steps of the ABCs in the primary survey, when you open the airway and check for breathing. If you cannot see, hear, or feel signs of breathing, give two one-second breaths immediately to get air into the patient's lungs. Then check for signs of circulation and look for severe bleeding. Obtain advanced medical care if you have not already done so.

If the patient is not breathing but has a pulse, begin rescue breathing. To give breaths, keep the airway open with the head-tilt/chin-lift. Next, using a mask, make a tight seal over the patient's mouth. If using a breathing barrier device that does not cover the nose, gently pinch the patient's nose shut with the thumb and index finger of your hand that is on the patient's forehead. Breathe into the patient just until you see his chest rise (Figure 6–19). Each breath should last one second, with a pause between breaths to let the air flow back out. Watch the patient's chest rise each time you breathe to make sure that your breaths are actually going in.

Figure 6–19 When giving a rescue breath, breathe into the patient just until you see his chest rise.

NOTE:

If you suspect a head injury, do a jaw thrust.

If you do not see the patient's chest rise and fall as you give a breath, you may not have the head tilted back far enough to open the airway adequately. Re-tilt the patient's head and attempt to ventilate again. If air still does not go in, the patient's airway is obstructed. You must provide care for an obstructed airway described earlier in this chapter.

Once you are able to give two breaths, check for signs of circulation. If the patient has signs of circulation but is not breathing, continue rescue breathing by giving one breath every five to six seconds (for an adult).

After two minutes of rescue breathing, recheck for signs of circulation and normal breathing to make sure the heart is still beating. If the patient still has circulation but is not breathing, continue rescue breathing. Check for signs of circulation every few minutes thereafter. Do not stop rescue breathing unless one of the following occurs:

• The patient begins to breathe on her own

• The patient has no signs of circulation—begin CPR (described in Chapter 8)

- Another responder with training equal to or greater than yours takes over
- You are too exhausted to continue
- The scene suddenly becomes unsafe

Special Considerations for Rescue Breathing

Air in the Stomach

When you do rescue breathing, air normally enters the patient's lungs. Sometimes air may enter the patient's stomach. There are several reasons why this may occur. First, breathing into the patient longer than for one second may cause extra air to fill the stomach. Do not overinflate the lungs. Stop the breath when the chest starts to rise. Second, if the patient's head is not tilted back far enough, the airway will not open completely. As a result, the chest may only rise slightly. This will lead you to breathe more forcefully, causing air to enter the stomach. Third, breaths given too quickly create more pressure in the airway, causing air to enter the stomach.

Air in the stomach is called gastric distension. Gastric distension can be a serious problem because it can make the patient vomit. When an unconscious patient vomits, stomach contents may get into the lungs, obstructing breathing. Taking such foreign material into the lungs is called aspiration. Because aspiration can hamper rescue breathing due to an airway obstruction, it may require the responder to perform CPR or unconscious choking techniques.

To avoid forcing air into the stomach, be sure to keep the patient's head tilted back far enough. Give one-second breaths, with just enough volume to make the chest start to rise. Pause between breaths long enough for the patient's lungs to empty and for you to take another breath.

Vomiting

When you give rescue breathing, the patient may vomit. If this happens, turn the patient's head and body together as a unit to the side. This helps prevent vomit from entering the lungs. Quickly wipe the patient's mouth clean, carefully reposition the patient on her back, and reassess ABCs.

Mouth-to-Nose Breathing

Sometimes you may not be able to make an adequate seal over a patient's mouth to perform rescue breathing. For example, the patient's jaw or mouth may be injured or shut too tightly to open, or your mouth may be too small to cover the patient's mouth. If so, provide mouth-to-nose rescue breathing as follows:

- Maintain the head-tilt/chin-lift position with one hand on the forehead. Use your other hand to close the patient's mouth, making sure to push on the chin, not on the throat.
- Seal your mouth tightly around the patient's nose, and breathe full breaths into the patient's nose (Figure 6–20). Open the patient's mouth between breaths, if possible, to let air escape.

As with other rescue breathing situations, use a resuscitation mask if you are able to seal it properly on the face.

Mouth-to-Stoma Breathing

Some people have had an operation to remove all or part of the larynx, the upper end of the windpipe. They breathe through an opening in the front of the neck called a stoma (Figure 6–21). Air passes directly into the trachea through the stoma instead of through the mouth and nose.

To give rescue breathing to someone with a stoma, you must give breaths through the stoma instead of

Figure 6–20 If giving mouth-to-nose breathing, seal your mouth around the patient's nose, and breathe in. Ensure the patient's mouth remains closed.

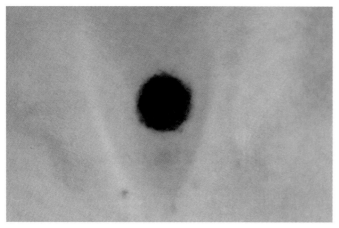

Figure 6–21 A stoma is an opening in the front of the neck that someone breathes through.

Figure 6–22 When giving rescue breaths to a patient with a stoma, breathe directly into the stoma.

the mouth or nose. Follow the same basic steps as in mouth-to-mask breathing, except:

1. Look, listen, and feel for breathing with your ear over the stoma.

2. Give rescue breaths into the stoma (Figure 6–22).

If the chest does not rise when you give rescue breaths, suspect that the patient may have had only part of the larynx removed. That means that some air continues to flow through the larynx to the lungs during normal breathing. When giving mouth-to-stoma breathing, air may leak through the nose and mouth, diminishing the amount of oxygen that reaches the lungs. If this occurs, you need to seal the nose and mouth with your hand to prevent air from escaping during rescue breathing.

People With Dentures

If you know or see the patient is wearing dentures, do not automatically remove them. Dentures help rescue breathing by supporting the patient's mouth and cheeks during mouth-to-mask breathing. If the dentures are loose, the head-tilt/chin-lift may help keep them in place. Remove the dentures only if they become so loose that they block the airway or make it difficult for you to give breaths.

Suspected Head and/or Spine Injuries

You should suspect head and/or spine injuries in patients who have suffered a violent force, such as that caused by a motor vehicle crash, a fall, or a diving or other sports-related incident. If you suspect the patient may have an injury to the head, neck, or spine, you should try to minimize movement of the head and neck when opening the airway. This requires you to change the way you open the airway.

Open the airway by placing your fingers under the angles of the jaw and lifting. Next, using a mask, make a tight seal over the patient's mouth and breathe (Figure 6–23). This technique allows you to open the airway and provide rescue breathing without moving the head. If using a face shield, use your cheek to block the nose. If you are unable to ventilate properly with a jaw thrust, perform a head-tilt/chin-lift.

Babies and Children

Rescue breathing for babies and children follows the same general procedure as that for adults. The minor differences take into account the baby's or child's undeveloped physique, moderately faster pulse, and breathing rate. Rescue breathing for babies and children uses less air in each breath, and breaths are delivered at a slightly faster rate.

You do not need to tilt a child's or baby's head as far back as an adult's to open the airway. Tilt the head back only far enough to allow your breaths to go in. Tipping the head back too far for a child or baby may cause injury that will obstruct the airway. Using a mask, give one breath every three to five seconds for both a child and a baby. Figure 6–24, a-b, shows rescue breathing for an adult or a child and a baby.

Figure 6–23 Use a jaw thrust when giving rescue breaths to a patient with a suspected head and/or spine injury.

If using a face shield, cover the baby's mouth and nose with your mouth. Remember to breathe slowly into the baby or child. Each breath should last about one second. Be careful not to overinflate a child's or baby's lungs. Breathe only until you see the chest start to rise. After two minutes of rescue breathing, recheck for signs of circulation and normal breathing.

SUMMARY

Because oxygen is vital to life, you must always ensure that the patient has an open airway and is breathing. You will often detect a breathing emergency during the primary survey. In a breathing emergency, a person's breathing is so impaired that life is threatened. This kind of emergency can occur in two ways: breathing becomes difficult or breathing stops. A person who is having difficulty breathing is having a breathing emergency. A person who has stopped breathing is in respiratory arrest.

The body requires a constant supply of oxygen for survival. The brain is the control centre for breathing. It adjusts the rate and depth of breaths according to the oxygen and carbon dioxide levels in the body. Breathing requires the respiratory, circulatory, nervous, and musculoskeletal systems to work together. Injuries or illnesses that affect any of these systems may cause breathing emergencies.

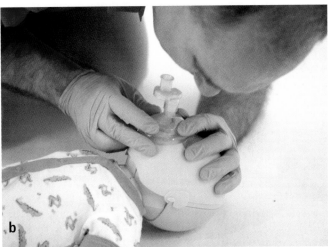

Figure 6–24, a-b Rescue breathing for **a**, an adult or a child; and **b**, a baby is similar. Often, the older the patient, the farther the head needs to be tilted back in order to open the airway.

Respiratory emergencies can be caused by choking, illness such as pneumonia, respiratory conditions such as emphysema and asthma, electrocution, shock, drowning, heart attack or heart disease, injury to the chest or lungs, allergic reactions such as to food or insect stings, drugs, and poisoning such as inhaling or ingesting toxic substances.

Recognizing the signs and symptoms of breathing emergencies and providing emergency care are often the keys to preventing other emergencies. Breathing emergencies may signal the beginning of a life-threatening condition. For example, it can be the first signal of a more serious breathing emergency or even a heart attack. Some breathing emergencies can lead to respiratory arrest, which, if not cared for, will result in death.

Many of the signs and symptoms of different kinds of breathing emergencies are similar. You do not need to know the specific cause to provide care. If the patient is breathing, you know the heart is beating. Make sure the patient is not bleeding severely. Help her rest in a comfortable position. Usually, sitting is more comfortable than lying down because breathing is easier. Open a window to provide more air if necessary. Provide ongoing survey and care. Have bystanders move back. Obtain more advanced medical care.

The little girl begins to make a high-pitched wheezing sound. What do you do?

Chapter 7

Airway and Ventilation

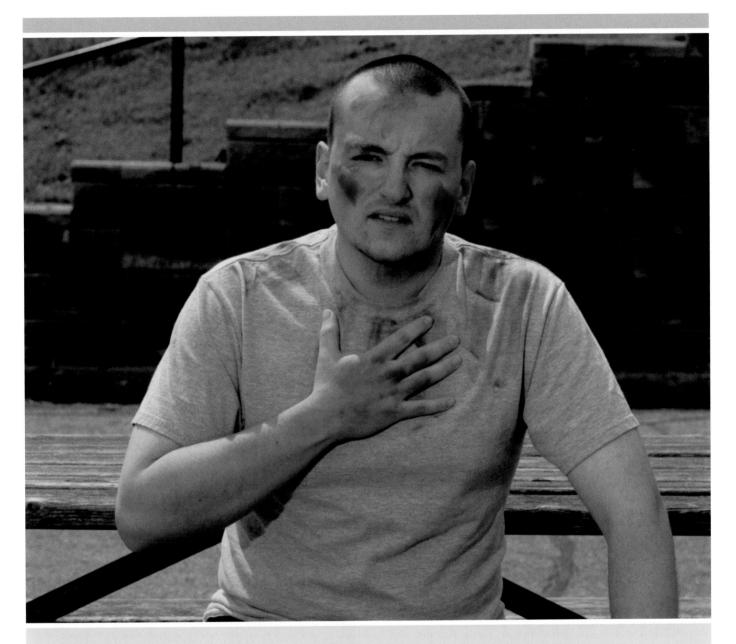

At the scene of an industrial fire, a young man is lucky to escape from the burning building. However, after he leaves the building, he finds that he has difficulty breathing. He clutches his chest and gestures to you for assistance. What do you do?

INTRODUCTION

Airway and ventilation management can contribute significantly to the survival and recovery of a seriously ill or injured person. A number of devices can help you maintain an open airway, perform rescue breathing, and increase the oxygen concentration in a patient's bloodstream. In addition, these devices also limit the potential for transmitting disease.

CLEARING THE AIRWAY

Sometimes injury or sudden illness results in foreign matter, such as mucus, vomitus, water, or blood, collecting in a patient's airway. The most appropriate initial method of clearing the airway is to roll the patient onto his side and sweep the foreign matter from the mouth. A more effective method is to suction the airway clear. Suctioning is the process of removing foreign matter by means of a mechanical or manual device. A variety of manual and mechanical devices are used to suction the airway.

Manual suction devices are lightweight, compact, and relatively inexpensive (Figure 7–1, a-b). Mechanical suction devices use either battery-powered pumps or oxygen-powered aspirators. These devices are normally found on ambulances. Attached to the end of any suction device is a suction tip. These come in various sizes and shapes. Some are rigid and others are flexible. A "tonsil tip" catheter can be used for clearing the mouth and throat of an unconscious adult, child, or baby, whereas a "French" catheter can be used to clear the nose.

Whether using a manual or mechanical suction device, follow these six steps:

1. Measure the distance of insertion, which is from the patient's earlobe to the corner of the mouth (Figure 7–2).

2. If the patient has an oropharyngeal airway (OPA) inserted (see "Oropharyngeal Airways" in this chapter) and it will interfere with suctioning the oral cavity, remove the OPA prior to suctioning.

3. With one hand, open the mouth using the crossed-finger technique (see page 115) and insert the suction tip into the mouth. Ensure that you only insert the tip as far as the measurement taken prior to insertion (Figure 7–3).

Figure 7–1, a-b Manual suction devices are lightweight and compact.

Figure 7–2 Measure the suction device from the patient's earlobe to the corner of their mouth.

Figure 7–3 Insert the suction tip into the back of the mouth.

4. Suction until the airway is clear.

5. If required, reinsert the OPA.

6. Apply supplemental oxygen.

NOTE:

If a mechanical suction device will not adequately clear the airway, you should turn the head to one side (if the patient does not have a suspected head and/or spine injury) or roll the patient into the recovery position and sweep the oral cavity with your finger.

NOTE:

For suctioning a baby's mouth, you can use a bulb syringe. When using a bulb syringe, ensure you deflate the device before you insert it into the baby's airway.

NOTE:

If a patient has a tracheostomy, or a stoma, suction through the tube, or hole, as this is where the patient's air passes. Do not insert the suction tip more than 5 cm (2 in.) beyond the lower edge of the opening.

OROPHARYNGEAL AIRWAYS

The tongue is the most common cause of airway obstruction in an unconscious patient. An oropharyngeal airway (OPA) is a device that is inserted into the mouth of an unconscious patient and positioned to assist in keeping the tongue off of the back of the throat. An improperly placed airway device can compress the tongue into the back of the throat, further blocking the airway.

The OPA is an adjunct and will not secure or maintain the airway on its own; the responder may still be required to maintain the airway manually.

OPAs come in a variety of sizes (Figure 7–4). The curved design fits the natural contour of the mouth and throat. Once you have positioned the device, you can use a resuscitation mask or bag-valve-mask (BVM) resuscitator to ventilate a non-breathing patient.

If you have determined the patient is unconscious, based on finding no response to painful stimuli, the

Figure 7–4 Oropharyngeal airways (OPAs) come in a variety of sizes.

person should be able to have an OPA inserted without causing a gag reflex.

Proper Sizing and Insertion of an OPA

Measure the device on the patient to see that it extends from his earlobe to the corner of the mouth (Figure 7–5). Open the patient's mouth using the crossed-finger technique, then insert the OPA with the curved end along the roof of the mouth (Figure 7–6). As the tip of the device approaches the back of the throat, rotate it a half-turn (Figure 7–7). If the patient begins gagging as the device is positioned in the back of the throat, remove the device. The OPA should drop into the throat without resistance. The flange end should rest on the patient's lips (Figure 7–8).

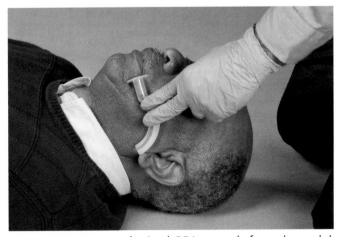

Figure 7–5 A properly sized OPA extends from the earlobe to the corner of the mouth.

Figure 7–6 To insert the OPA, open the patient's mouth using the crossed-finger technique. Insert the OPA with the curved end along the roof of the mouth.

180°

Figure 7–7 As the tip of the device approaches the back of the throat, rotate it a half-turn.

Figure 7–9 You may attempt to insert the OPA by pointing the tip of the device toward the cheek, then rotating it 90°.

Figure 7–8 The flange end of the OPA should rest on the patient's lips.

An Alternate Way to Open the Airway: The Crossed-Finger Technique

One method of opening the mouth to assess the airway, insert an OPA, or suction the patient's mouth is known as the crossed-finger technique.

1. Cross the thumb and index finger of one hand.

2. Place the thumb on the patient's lower front teeth and the index finger on the upper front teeth.

3. Open the mouth using a scissor motion.

OPAs in Children and Babies

Younger children and babies have delicate airways, so caution must be taken when inserting an airway to avoid damage. Also, you must be careful not to overextend the neck, which could close or even damage the airway. When inserting an OPA in a baby, place some padding under the baby's shoulders to properly open the airway.

On rare occasions, such as when inserting an OPA into a child's mouth, you may not be able to insert the OPA using the technique described above. As a secondary method, you can attempt to insert with the tip of the device pointing toward the cheek and then rotating it 90° to place it into the throat (Figure 7–9).

For babies, it may be required that you insert the OPA directly into position, without rotating it, by using a tongue depressor to open the back of the oral cavity. As always, follow local protocol.

Figure 7–10 Lubricate a nasopharyngeal airway (NPA) with a water-soluble lubricant.

NASOPHARYNGEAL AIRWAYS

A nasopharyngeal (nasal) airway (NPA) is used to assist in maintaining an airway in an unconscious adult. An NPA may also be used on responsive adults who need help keeping the tongue from obstructing the airway. Nasal airways are available in a variety of sizes.

Inserting an NPA

When using an NPA, determine the correct size by measuring the device on the patient to see that it extends from his earlobe to the tip of the nose. Also make sure the diameter of the NPA is not larger than the diameter of the nostril.

Lubricate the airway with a water-soluble lubricant (Figure 7–10). Insert the NPA into the patient's right nostril, with the bevel toward the septum. Advance the airway gently, straight in, not upward, until the flange rests on the nose (Figure 7–11, a-b). If you feel even minor resistance, do not try to force the airway. If you cannot get the airway to pass easily, remove it and try the other nostril. Unlike the OPA, the NPA should not cause the patient to gag. Do not use an NPA on someone with a suspected skull fracture, active bleeding from the nose, or facial fractures. Insertion of an NPA may cause nosebleeds (epistaxis).

OXYGEN DELIVERY DEVICES

Many different oxygen delivery devices are commonly used in the pre-hospital setting. Which devices are routinely available to you will depend on your local standards and protocols. This section focuses on those

Figure 7–11, a-b a, Advance the airway gently, straight in, not upward; **b**, until the flange end rests on the nose.

devices that you are likely to have immediately available or be asked to assist with in providing care. You should not delay care because a specific device is not available. Instead, you should start basic care, adding any devices when they become available.

Some of these devices include resuscitation masks and BVM resuscitators. They provide several advantages. They can help you:

- Maintain an open airway
- Perform rescue breathing
- Limit the potential for disease transmission
- Increase the oxygen concentration in a patient's bloodstream

With all delivery devices, give the same number of ventilations as you would for CPR, or rescue breathing.

Resuscitation Masks

One of the most readily available, simple ventilation devices for responders is the resuscitation mask. Resuscitation masks are pliable, dome-shaped devices that fit over a patient's mouth and nose, aiding ventilation (providing oxygen to the lungs). Several types of resuscitation masks are available, varying in size, shape, and features.

Resuscitation masks offer you several advantages. These include:

- Increasing the flow of air to the lungs by permitting air to travel through a patient's mouth and nose at the same time
- Providing an adequate seal for ventilation, even when a patient has facial injuries

- Providing an effective and easily accessible alternative to other methods of ventilation
- Permitting easy delivery of supplemental oxygen to either a breathing or a non-breathing patient
- Reducing the possibility of disease transmission by providing a barrier between the responder and the patient

Selecting a Resuscitation Mask

For a resuscitation mask to be most effective, it should meet the following criteria (Figure 7–12):

- Be made of a transparent, pliable material that allows you to make a tight seal on the patient's face when you perform rescue breathing or supply supplemental oxygen
- Have a one-way valve for redirecting a patient's exhaled air
- Have an inlet for the delivery of supplemental oxygen

Figure 7–12 A resuscitation mask should meet specific criteria.

Figure 7–13 A resuscitation mask should be positioned over the mouth and nose, with the lower rim placed between the patient's lower lip and chin.

a

b

Figure 7–14, a-b To use a resuscitation mask: **a**, position yourself behind the patient's head and hold the two sides tightly against the face or; **b**, position yourself beside the patient and hold the mask in place.

• Work well under a variety of environmental conditions, such as extreme heat or cold

• Be easy to assemble and use

Using a Resuscitation Mask

When using a resuscitation mask, begin by attaching the one-way valve to the mask. Next, place the mask so that it covers the patient's mouth and nose. Position the lower rim of the mask between the patient's lower lip and chin. The opposite end of the mask should cover the nose. Figure 7–13 shows how to position the resuscitation mask.

When you use a resuscitation mask to give rescue breathing, you must maintain a good seal to prevent air from leaking at the edges of the mask. Use both hands to hold the mask in place and to maintain an open airway. You do this by:

1. Tilting the patient's head back

2. Lifting the jaw upward

Figure 7–14, a-b, shows two methods for using a resuscitation mask.

If you suspect the patient has a head and/or spine injury, use the two-handed jaw thrust technique without a head-tilt (Figure 7–15).

Bag-Valve-Mask Resuscitators

There may be times when you will have a bag-valve-mask (BVM) available or be asked to assist with one. A BVM is a hand-held device, like the resuscitation mask, primarily used to ventilate a non-breathing patient. It is also used to assist ventilation of someone who is breathing too slowly or too quickly.

The device has three main components: a bag, a valve, and a mask. The bag is self-inflating. Once compressed, it reinflates automatically. The one-way valve allows air to move from the bag to the patient but prevents his exhaled air from entering the bag. The mask is similar to the resuscitation masks described earlier in this chapter. An oxygen reservoir bag should be attached to the BVM when supplemental oxygen is administered (Figure 7–16).

Figure 7–15 If you suspect a head and/or spine injury, use the two-handed jaw thrust technique and hold the mask to the face without tilting the head.

Figure 7–17 When using a BVM, one responder maintains a tight seal of the mask on the patient's face, and a second responder provides ventilations.

The principle of the BVM is simple. By placing the mask on the patient's face and squeezing the bag, you open the one-way valve, forcing air into the patient's lungs. When you release the bag, the valve closes and air from the atmosphere refills the bag. At approximately the same time, the patient exhales. This exhaled air is diverted into the atmosphere through the closed one-way valve.

Using a Bag-Valve-Mask Resuscitator

In the hands of a well-practised rescue team, the BVM is effective. For this reason, using a BVM is a two-rescuer skill whenever possible. When using a BVM on a non-breathing patient, make sure an OPA or NPA is in place.

When using a BVM, one responder positions the mask and opens the patient's airway. This is done in the same way as previously described for resuscitation masks. While the first responder maintains a tight seal with the mask on the patient's face, the second responder

provides ventilations by squeezing the bag just until the patient's chest starts to rise (Figure 7–17). The bag should always be squeezed smoothly, not forcefully. This two-person technique maintains an open airway and a tight mask seal, while a second responder provides ventilations.

Using the BVM has distinct advantages and disadvantages:

Advantages

- It delivers a higher concentration of oxygen than that delivered during mouth-to-mask rescue breathing.

- It limits the potential for disease transmission.

BVMs for Children and Babies

Some BVMs are designed specifically for children and babies. These devices have a smaller mask, and the bag is designed to hold a smaller volume of air, for a better fit on the face, and to limit the amount of air able to be squeezed into the lungs. The mask of the BVM should extend from the bridge of the nose to the cleft of the chin, which will ensure a proper seal on the face. A number of these BVMs also include a valve that stops the forced entrance of air once a certain pressure has been reached, avoiding overinflation of the lungs. As always, ventilate just until the chest starts to rise.

Figure 7–16 A bag-valve-mask (BVM).

Disadvantages

- Without regular practice, you cannot stay proficient.
- It may take longer to assemble than other ventilation devices.

> **NOTE:**
>
> *If someone has a tracheostomy tube, it may be possible to attach the BVM directly to it.*

Supplemental Oxygen

The normal concentration of oxygen in the air is approximately 21%, which is what we inhale. Under normal conditions, this is more than enough oxygen to sustain life. However, when serious injury or sudden illness occurs, the body does not function properly and can benefit from additional, or supplemental, oxygen. Without adequate oxygen, hypoxia will result. Hypoxia is a condition in which insufficient oxygen reaches the cells. Hypoxia causes increased breathing and heart rate, cyanosis, changes in consciousness, restlessness, and chest pain.

For example, delivery of a higher concentration of oxygen may reduce breathing discomfort and chest pain caused by a heart attack or angina. Someone with shortness of breath or chest pain should always receive supplemental oxygen. Supplemental oxygen delivered to the patient's lungs may help meet the increased demand for oxygen for all body tissues.

If a patient who has had a heart attack suddenly suffers cardiac arrest, then, in combination with chest compressions, you must use rescue breathing to supply air into his lungs. When you perform rescue breathing using the mouth-to-mask method, the oxygen concentration you deliver to the patient is only 16%. This is adequate to sustain life in a healthy person, but since chest compressions only circulate one third of normal blood flow under the best of conditions, some body tissues will not receive the oxygen required for short-term survival.

Using a BVM alone only improves this situation slightly since it delivers atmospheric air (21% oxygen). Administering supplemental oxygen allows a substantially higher oxygen concentration, in some cases nearly 100%, to be delivered to the patient (Figure 7–18).

To deliver supplemental oxygen, you must have:

- An oxygen cylinder
- A pressure regulator with flowmeter
- A delivery device

Figure 7–19 shows an oxygen cylinder, pressure regulator, and flowmeter.

Oxygen Cylinder

It is easy to recognize an oxygen cylinder because of its distinctive green or white colour and yellow diamond marking that says oxidizer. These cylinders are made of steel or an alloy. Depending on their size, those used in the pre-hospital setting can hold between 350 and 625 litres of oxygen. These cylinders have internal pressures

Figure 7–18 Administering supplemental oxygen allows a substantially higher oxygen concentration to be delivered to the patient.

Figure 7–19 An oxygen cylinder, pressure regulator, and flowmeter.

of approximately 2,000 pounds per square inch (psi). Oxygen cylinders should never be left free-standing.

Pressure Regulator with Flowmeter

The pressure inside the oxygen cylinder is far too great for you to simply open the cylinder and administer the oxygen. Instead, a device must be attached to the cylinder to reduce the delivery pressure of the oxygen to a safe level. This regulating device is called a pressure regulator. The pressure regulator reduces the pressure from approximately 2,000 psi inside the cylinder to a safe pressure range of 30 to 70 psi.

A pressure regulator has a gauge that indicates how much pressure is in the cylinder. By checking the gauge, you can determine if a cylinder is full (2,000 psi), nearly empty (200 psi), or somewhere in between.

NOTE:

For more information on indications and contraindications of oxygen, see Chapter 11.

A pressure regulator has two metal prongs that fit into the valve at the top of the oxygen cylinder. To ensure a

tight seal between the regulator and the tank, a gasket, commonly called an O-ring, must be used.

A flowmeter controls the amount of oxygen administered in litres per minute (lpm). Flowmeters normally deliver from 1 to 25 lpm.

Using Oxygen Delivery Devices

Some oxygen delivery devices can deliver oxygen to either breathing or non-breathing patients. Two devices, the resuscitation mask and the BVM, can deliver oxygen to both. For this reason, these devices are the most appropriate for you to use. Regardless of the device being used, a section of tubing is attached to the device at one end and to the flowmeter at the other end to create an oxygen-enriched environment for the patient.

A resuscitation mask is capable of delivering approximately 50% oxygen to a breathing patient when delivered at 6 lpm or more. This is substantially higher than the normal 21% that the patient would get from the atmosphere. Some resuscitation masks have elastic straps attached to the mask. The elastic strap can be placed over the patient's head and tightened to help keep the mask securely in place (Figure 7–20, a). If the mask does not have a strap, either you or the patient can hold it in place. When a resuscitation mask is used on a non-breathing patient, it will deliver an oxygen concentration of approximately 35%. The oxygen concentration is reduced because oxygen mixes with your exhaled air as you perform mouth-to-mask rescue breathing.

The BVM resuscitator with an oxygen reservoir bag is capable of supplying a minimum oxygen concentration of 90% when used at 10 lpm or more.

The BVM can be held against the patient's face, allowing a breathing patient to inhale the supplemental oxygen (Figure 7–20, b). A patient breathing at a rate of less than 10 breaths per minute, or more than 30 breaths per minute, should have his breathing assisted. For someone breathing less than 10 times per minute, squeeze the bag each time the patient breathes and once in-between each breath. To assist a patient breathing more than 30 times per minute, squeeze the bag on every second breath.

The high-concentration non-rebreather mask (or partial non-rebreather mask) needs to have a flow rate of 10 lpm or more to ensure the proper reservoir bag

Figure 7–20, a-c Common oxygen delivery devices include: **a**, a resuscitation mask; **b**, a BVM; and **c**, a non-rebreather mask.

Figure 7–21 A nasal cannula.

inflation. This device allows the patient to inhale air from the bag and exhale through the holes in the sides of the mask (Figure 7–20, c). The non-rebreather mask is used only on a breathing patient.

Some devices, such as the nasal cannula, can be used only to administer oxygen to breathing patients. A nasal cannula is a device that delivers oxygen through the person's nostrils (Figure 7–21). It is a plastic tube with two small prongs that are inserted into the nose. The use of a nasal cannula is limited since it is normally used at a flow rate of 1 to 4 lpm. Under these conditions, it delivers a peak oxygen concentration of only approximately 36%. Flow rates above 4 lpm are not commonly used because of the tendency to quickly dry out mucous membranes. This can cause nosebleeds (epistaxis) and headaches.

NOTE:

Adding moisture to oxygen, by attaching an oxygen humidifier to the regulator, can help decrease irritation to the respiratory tract, which can result from using oxygen over a long period of time. The oxygen is forced through sterile water in a container, which allows it to pick up moisture before being delivered to the person. Generally, a humidifier is not used in a pre-hospital setting, although it may be used during a long transfer or, possibly, with someone with asthma.

TABLE 7–1: OXYGEN DELIVERY DEVICES

Device	Common Flow Rate	Oxygen Concentration	Function
Nasal cannula	1–4 lpm	24–36%	Breathing patients only
Resuscitation mask	6+ lpm	35–55%	Breathing and non-breathing patients
Bag-valve-mask resuscitator	10+ lpm	90+%	Breathing and non-breathing patients
Non-rebreather mask	10+ lpm	90+%	Breathing patients only

Because of its limitations, the nasal cannula is commonly used for patients with only minor breathing difficulty. This device is not appropriate for patients experiencing a serious breathing emergency since they are generally breathing through their mouth and need a device that can supply a greater concentration of oxygen. In addition, the nasal cannula can be ineffective if the patient has a nasal airway obstruction, nasal injury, or bad cold causing blocked sinus passages. It should, however, be used if the patient cannot tolerate a mask over his face.

Table 7–1 provides an overview of each of the delivery devices presented.

Administering Oxygen

Begin by examining the cylinder to be certain that it is labelled "Oxygen" (Figure 7–22, a). Next, check to see that the cylinder is full. Full cylinders come with a protective covering over the tank opening. Remove this covering and save the "O-ring." While pointing the cylinder away from you, open the cylinder for one second (Figure 7–22, b). This will remove any dirt or debris from the cylinder valve. Position the gasket (Figure 7–23, a).

Next, examine the pressure regulator. Check to see that the pin index corresponds to an oxygen tank (Figure 7–23, b). Attach the pressure regulator to the cylinder, seating the prongs inside the holes in the valve

Figure 7–22, a-b a, An oxygen cylinder is usually green or white, with a yellow diamond indicating oxygen; **b**, open the cylinder for one second, pointing it away from you.

Figure 7–24 After turning on the flowmeter to the desired rate, check to ensure the oxygen is flowing into the delivery device.

stem (Figure 7–23, c). Hand-tighten the screw until the regulator is snug (Figure 7–23, d). Open the cylinder one full turn and listen for leaks.

Check the pressure gauge to determine how much pressure is in the cylinder (Figure 7–23, e). A full cylinder should have approximately 2,000 psi. Attach the chosen delivery device to the oxygen port near the flowmeter. Attach the device to the tank using the appropriate tubing. Turn on the flowmeter to the desired flow rate. Listen and feel to make sure that oxygen is flowing into your delivery device. If using a reservoir bag, ensure it is full before placing the device on the patient (Figure 7–24). Finally, place the delivery device on the patient.

Figure 7–23, a-e To attach the pressure regulator to the cylinder: **a**, insert the gasket into the pressure regulator; **b**, check to see that the pin index corresponds to an oxygen tank; **c**, seat the prongs of the regulator inside the cylinder; **d**, hand-tighten the screw until the regulator is snug; and **e**, turn on the oxygen and check how much pressure is in the cylinder.

Precautions

When administering oxygen, safety is a primary concern. Remember the following precautions:

- Do not operate oxygen equipment around an open flame or sparks or in close proximity to an AED. Oxygen causes fire to burn more rapidly.

- Do not stand oxygen cylinders upright unless they can be well secured. If the cylinder falls, it could damage the regulator or possibly loosen the cylinder valve.

- Do not use grease, oil, or petroleum products to lubricate any pressure regulator parts. Oxygen does not mix with these products, and a severe chemical reaction could cause an explosion.

SUMMARY

Although they are not required, oxygen delivery devices can make the emergency care you provide safer, easier, and more effective. OPAs and NPAs help maintain an open airway by elevating the tongue away from the back of the throat. Suction equipment helps clear the airway of substances such as water, blood, saliva, or vomitus. The use of supplemental oxygen can relieve pain and breathing discomfort. The resuscitation mask and BVM are the most appropriate devices for responders. They can significantly increase the oxygen concentration that a patient needs, help ventilate a non-breathing patient, and reduce the likelihood of disease transmission.

Oxygen delivery devices are appropriate for almost all types of injury or illness in which breathing may be impaired. Knowing how to use these devices will enable you to provide effective care until more advanced medical care has been obtained.

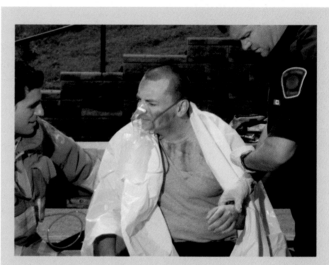

The man's breathing gets worse. What do you do?

Chapter 8

Circulatory Emergencies

A 59-year-old woman is experiencing chest pain. She states that it started about 30 minutes ago as a mild, squeezing sensation. Now the pain is severe, and she is gasping for breath. You recognize that these signs and symptoms suggest a serious condition. While waiting to obtain more advanced medical care, what do you do?

INTRODUCTION

In this chapter, you will learn how to recognize and provide care for circulatory emergencies. You will learn the care for someone with persistent chest pain and for someone whose heart stops beating, as well as for someone who has had a stroke. The condition in which the heart stops, known as cardiac arrest, sometimes results from a heart attack. To provide care for someone with cardiac arrest, you need to learn how to perform cardiopulmonary resuscitation (CPR). Properly performed, CPR can keep someone's vital organs supplied with oxygen-rich blood until more highly trained personnel arrive to provide advanced medical care.

This chapter also identifies the important risk factors for cardiovascular disease. It is as important to prevent stroke, heart attack, and cardiac arrest as it is to learn how to recognize them when they occur and provide appropriate care. You will also learn to modify your behaviour to prevent cardiovascular disease.

PATHOPHYSIOLOGY OF THE CIRCULATORY SYSTEM

Cardiovascular disease is an abnormal condition that affects the heart and blood vessels. It is one of the leading causes of death in Canadians; about 80,000 deaths in Canada each year are attributed to cardiovascular disease.

The most common conditions caused by cardiovascular disease include coronary heart disease (CHD), also known as coronary artery disease (CAD), and stroke, also called a brain attack.

CHD occurs when the arteries that supply blood to the heart muscle become hardened and narrowed, a process called atherosclerosis. This damage occurs gradually, as cholesterol and fatty deposits called plaque build up on the inner artery walls. As this buildup worsens, the arteries become narrower, reducing the amount of blood that can flow through them and preventing the heart from getting the blood or oxygen it needs (Figure 8–1). Patients who suffer from acute myocardial ischemia (reduced blood flow to the cardiac muscle) suffer chest pain, which usually results from CHD and is referred to as acute coronary syndrome (ACS). This reduced blood and oxygen supply

Figure 8–1 In atherosclerosis, a buildup of cholesterol and fatty deposits on inner artery walls results in hardened, narrowed arteries.

to the heart can cause symptoms of angina pectoris or a heart attack.

A heart attack, or myocardial infarction (MI), occurs when coronary blood vessels become blocked by plaque buildup or when a blood clot blocks one of the arteries supplying the heart. This may lead to an irregular heartbeat (arrhythmia), which then causes the pumping action of the heart to work less efficiently. A heart attack can also lead to a cardiac arrest, where the heart ceases to function as a pump.

As the reduction of blood flow or blockage progresses, some people experience symptoms such as chest pain, pressure, or discomfort, which are early warning signs that the heart is not receiving enough oxygen-rich blood. Others may suffer a heart attack or even cardiac arrest without any warning signs or symptoms. If a blockage in an artery of the heart is not treated quickly, the affected heart muscle tissue will die.

PREVENTING CARDIOVASCULAR DISEASE

Although a heart attack seems to strike suddenly, the conditions that lead to it may develop over years. Many people's lifestyle may gradually be endangering their heart, which can eventually result in cardiovascular disease. Potentially harmful behaviours frequently begin early in life.

Risk Factors of Heart Disease

Scientists have identified many factors that increase a person's chances of developing heart disease. These are known as risk factors. Some risk factors for heart disease cannot be changed. For instance, men have a higher risk for heart disease than do women. Having a history of heart disease in your family also increases your risk.

But people can control many risk factors for heart disease. Smoking, diets high in fats, high blood pressure, obesity, and a lack of routine exercise are all linked to an increased risk of heart disease (Table 8–1). When one risk factor, such as high blood pressure, is combined with other risk factors, such as obesity or cigarette smoking, the risk of heart attack or stroke is greatly increased.

Controlling Risk Factors

Smoking

Cigarette smokers are more likely to have a heart attack than non-smokers and are also more likely to have cardiac arrest. The earlier a person starts using tobacco, the greater the risk to her future health. Giving up smoking will rapidly reduce the risk of heart disease. After a number of years, the risk becomes the same as if the person had never smoked. If you do not smoke, do not start. If you do smoke, quit. Living and working in a smoke-free environment will also control your risk of heart disease.

Diet

Eating healthy fats, such as omega-3 fats, will help combat the buildup of fatty materials in the arteries. Some cholesterol in the body is essential. The amount of cholesterol in the blood is determined by how much your body produces and by the food you eat. Foods high in cholesterol include egg yolks, shrimp, lobster, and organ meats such as liver.

A more important contributor to an unhealthy blood cholesterol level is saturated fat. Saturated fats raise the blood cholesterol level by interfering with the body's ability to remove cholesterol from the blood. Saturated fats are found in beef, lamb, veal, pork, ham, whole milk, and whole milk products.

TABLE 8–1: CARDIOVASCULAR DISEASE RISK FACTORS

Uncontrollable	Controllable
Sex Males have a higher risk than do females.	**Smoking** Smokers are twice as likely to have a heart attack.
Family History A history of heart disease in the family increases the risk.	**Diet** A diet high in saturated fats and cholesterol increases the risk of atherosclerosis.
Age The risk of heart attack increases with age.	**Blood Pressure** High blood pressure can damage blood vessels throughout the body.
	Weight Individuals who are overweight have a significantly higher risk of fatal heart attack.
	Exercise Level Low exercise levels lead to increased weight and decreased muscle tone.

Rather than eliminating saturated fats and cholesterol from your diet, limit your intake. This is easier than one may think. Moderation is the key. Make changes whenever possible by substituting low-fat milk or skim milk for whole milk and margarine for butter, trimming visible fat from meats, and broiling or baking rather than frying. Read labels carefully. A "cholesterol-free" product may be high in saturated fat.

Blood Pressure

You can often control high blood pressure by losing excess weight and by changing your diet. When these are not enough, medications can be prescribed. It is important to have regular checkups to guard against high blood pressure and its harmful effects.

Weight and Exercise

Two additional ways to help prevent heart disease are to control your weight and exercise regularly. You store excess calories in your diet as fat. In general, overweight people have a shorter life expectancy.

Routine exercise has many benefits, including increased muscle tone and weight control. Exercise can also help you survive a heart attack because the increased circulation of blood through the heart develops additional channels for blood flow. If the primary channels that supply the heart are blocked during a heart attack, these additional channels can supply the heart tissue with oxygen-rich blood.

Routine exercise will often decrease stress and reduce your risk of heart disease. You can also develop a new hobby, set realistic goals for yourself, practise relaxation exercises, and avoid caffeinated products.

Results of Managing Risk Factors

Managing the risk factors for cardiovascular disease really works. Over the past number of years, deaths from cardiovascular disease have decreased substantially.

Why did deaths from these causes decline? Probably as a result of improved detection and treatment as well as lifestyle changes. People are becoming more aware of their risk factors for heart disease and are taking action to control them. If you do this, you can improve your chances of living a long and healthy life. If you suffer a cardiac arrest, your chances of survival are poor. Begin today to reduce your risk of cardiovascular disease.

DID YOU KNOW?

Did you know that second-hand smoke…

- Can lead to heart disease?
- Can cause the formation of blood clots that can lead to heart attacks and stroke?
- Raises your heart rate?
- Damages your heart muscle?
- Lowers the level of protective cholesterol in your blood?

DID YOU KNOW?

Too often we take our hearts for granted. The heart is extremely reliable. It beats about 70 times each minute, or more than 100,000 times a day. During the average lifetime, the heart will beat nearly three billion times. The heart moves about four litres (four quarts) of blood per minute through the body. This is about 160 million litres in an average lifetime. The heart moves blood through about 100,000 kilometres (62,000 miles) of blood vessels.

ANGINA

Some people with coronary artery disease may experience chest pain or pressure that comes and goes and is not generally caused by a heart attack. This type of pain is called angina pectoris, a medical term for pain in the chest. Angina pectoris, commonly referred to as angina, develops when the heart needs more oxygen-rich blood than it gets, such as during physical activity or emotional stress. This lack of oxygen can cause a constricting chest pain that may spread to the neck, jaw, and arms.

Pain associated with angina usually lasts less than 10 minutes. Someone who knows she has angina will often have a prescribed medication to help relieve the pain. Reducing the heart's demand for oxygen, such as by stopping physical activity, and taking prescribed medication often relieve angina. Administering oxygen to someone experiencing angina may help relieve chest pain.

Figure 8–2 The heart is located in the middle of the chest, behind the lower half of the sternum.

Sternum (breastbone)

Ribs

Lung

Heart

Diaphragm

■ = Oxygen-poor blood pumped from the body to the lungs

■ = Oxygen-rich blood pumped from the lungs to the body

Figure 8–3 The heart has four chambers and is separated into right and left halves. The right side of the heart receives blood from the body and sends it to the lungs. The left side of the heart receives blood from the lungs and pumps it out through the body. One-way valves direct the flow of blood through the heart.

HEART ATTACK

The heart is a muscular organ about the size of your fist, which functions like a pump. It lies between the lungs, in the middle of the chest, behind the lower half of the sternum (breastbone). The heart is protected by the ribs and sternum in front and by the spine in back (Figure 8–2). It has four chambers and is separated into right and left halves. Oxygen-poor blood enters the right side of the heart and is pumped to the lungs, where it picks up oxygen. The now oxygen-rich blood returns to the left side of the heart, from where it is pumped to all parts of the body. One-way valves direct the flow of blood as it moves through each of the heart's four chambers (Figure 8–3). For the circulatory system to be effective, the respiratory system must also be working so that the blood can pick up oxygen in the lungs.

Like all living tissue, the cells of the heart need a continuous supply of oxygen. The coronary arteries supply the heart muscle with oxygen-rich blood (Figure 8–4, a). If heart muscle tissue is deprived of this blood, it dies, and the person often develops certain signs and symptoms. When a great deal of tissue is deprived of oxygen and dies, it is called a heart attack.

To upper body

From upper body

Aorta

To lung

To lung

From lung

From lung

Right atrium

Left atrium

Right ventricle

Left ventricle

From lower body (inferior vena cava)

To lower body (descending aorta)

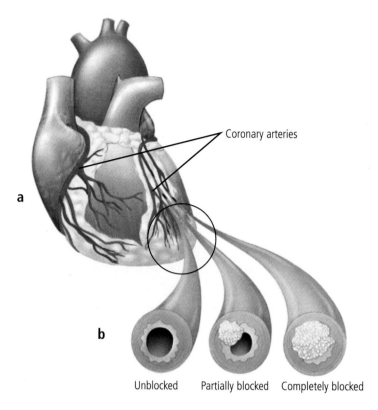

Figure 8–4, a-b a, The coronary arteries supply the heart muscle with blood; **b**, buildup of material on the inner walls of these arteries reduces blood flow to the heart muscle and may cause a heart attack.

A heart attack interrupts the heart's electrical system. This may result in an irregular heartbeat, which prevents blood from circulating effectively.

Common Causes of Heart Attack

Heart attacks usually result from cardiovascular disease. Half of all deaths in Canada that are attributed to cardiovascular disease are due to heart attack, and most of them are sudden deaths.

When coronary arteries narrow, a common form of coronary artery disease, a heart attack may occur (Figure 8–4, b).

Because atherosclerosis develops gradually, it can go undetected for many years. Even with significantly reduced blood flow to the heart muscle, there may be no signs and symptoms of heart trouble. Most people

with atherosclerosis are unaware of it. Some may suffer a heart attack or even cardiac arrest without any previous warning. Fortunately, this process can be slowed or stopped by lifestyle changes, such as forming healthy eating habits.

Arteriosclerosis is the thickening, loss of elasticity, and calcification of the walls of arteries. This results in a decrease in blood flow. Most commonly affected are the cerebrum and the lower extremities.

Signs and Symptoms of a Heart Attack

The most prominent symptom of a heart attack is persistent chest pain or discomfort (Figure 8–5). However, it may not always be easy for you to distinguish between the pain of a heart attack and chest pain caused by indigestion, muscle spasms, or other conditions. Brief, stabbing chest pain or pain that feels more intense when the person bends or breathes deeply is usually not caused by a heart attack.

The pain of a heart attack can range from mild discomfort to an unbearable crushing sensation in the chest. The person may describe it as an uncomfortable pressure, squeezing, tightness, aching, constricting, or heavy sensation in the chest. Often the person feels pain in the centre of the chest behind the sternum. It may spread to

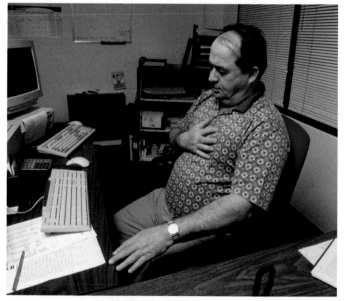

Figure 8–5 The most prominent symptom of a heart attack is persistent chest pain.

the shoulder, arm, neck, or jaw (Figure 8–6). The pain is constant and usually not relieved by resting, changing position, or taking oral medication. Any severe chest pain, chest pain that lasts longer than 10 minutes, or chest pain that is accompanied by other heart attack signs and symptoms should receive immediate emergency medical care.

Although a heart attack is often dramatic, someone experiencing a heart attack can have relatively mild symptoms. The person often mistakes the symptoms for indigestion. Sometimes the person feels little or no chest pain or discomfort. During a heart attack, many women, older adults, and people with diabetes tend to experience "soft signs," including tiredness, gastric discomfort, flu-like symptoms, and mild unfocused chest discomfort that comes and goes, gets better with rest, gets worse with activity, and starts mild and gets continually stronger.

Another sign of a heart attack is difficulty breathing (dyspnea). The person may be breathing faster than normal because the body tries to get much-needed oxygen to the heart. Depending on the person's general condition, her pulse may be faster or slower than normal or irregular. The person's skin may be pale or bluish, particularly around the face. The face may also be moist from perspiration. Some people with a heart attack sweat profusely. These signs result from the stress the body experiences when the heart does not work effectively. Nausea and vomiting may also occur.

Since any heart attack may lead to cardiac arrest, it is important to recognize and act on these signs and symptoms. Prompt action may prevent cardiac arrest. Most people who die from a heart attack die within one to two hours after the first signs and symptoms appear. Many could have been saved if bystanders or the person herself had been aware of the signs and symptoms of a heart attack and acted promptly. Many people who have had a heart attack delay seeking care. Nearly half of them wait two or more hours before going to the hospital. Often they do not realize they are having a heart attack. They may dismiss the symptoms as indigestion or muscle soreness.

Since most heart attacks result from blood clotting within arteries, early treatment of an attack with

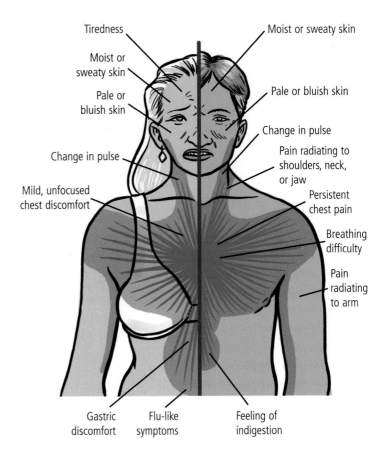

Figure 8–6 Signs and symptoms of a heart attack may be different for men and women.

medication that dissolves clots has been helpful in minimizing damage to the heart.

Remember, the key symptom of a heart attack is persistent chest pain. If the person states that chest pain is severe or chest discomfort has been present for more than 10 minutes, obtain more advanced medical care immediately and begin to care for the person.

A "silent MI" (myocardial infarction) is a heart attack that is not recognized; therefore, advanced medical care is not obtained. This can happen to anyone but occurs most often in those who experience "soft signs," such as women, people with diabetes, and older adults.

Figure 8–7 Many people having a heart attack find it easier to breathe when they are sitting.

Figure 8–8 Nitroglycerin spray is one of the common forms this medication comes in.

Care for a Heart Attack and Angina

The most important step in providing care is to recognize the signs and symptoms of a heart attack. You must take immediate action if any of these appear. Someone having a heart attack will probably deny the seriousness of the symptoms she is experiencing. Do not let this influence you. If you think there is a possibility that the patient is having a heart attack, you must act. First, have the patient stop what she is doing and rest comfortably. Many people having a heart attack find it easier to breathe while sitting (Figure 8–7). Second, obtain more advanced medical care.

Continue with your secondary survey. Talk to the patient and bystanders, if possible, to get more information. If the patient continues to experience chest pain, ask her SAMPLE and OPQRST questions (see Chapter 5).

You may assist the patient in taking her prescribed nitroglycerin, if needed, after checking the Six Rights of Medication. If under medical direction to do so, you may administer nitroglycerin.

NOTE:

For further information on nitroglycerin, refer to the drug profile in Chapter 11.

Nitroglycerin is a medication often prescribed for angina, which may come in pill or spray form (Figure 8–8). Once absorbed into the body (under the tongue), nitroglycerin enlarges the blood vessels to make it easier for blood to reach heart muscle tissue, which results in a drop in blood pressure. Because of this, it is important to take a blood pressure before and after the patient takes nitroglycerin. Nitroglycerin may relieve the pain because the heart does not have to work so hard and it increases oxygen delivery to the heart.

NOTE:

Locol protocol may dictate that it is not recommended that a patient take nitroglycerin if the systolic blood pressure is too low, often below 100 mmHg, and/or pulse is below 60 bpm. In all cases, the patient should be resting, preferably in a supine position, before taking nitroglycerin. As always, follow local protocol.

A patient will often know when he should take his prescribed nitroglycerin. If the patient answers "yes" when you ask, "Would you normally take your medication at this time?" (taking into consideration his signs and symptoms), this is a good indication that this circumstance warrants use of his nitroglycerin.

Before suggesting that the patient take nitroglycerin, ask if he has taken Viagra® or Levitra® in the past 24 hours or Cialis® in the past 48 hours for erectile dysfunction. If the patient has, advise him not to take the nitroglycerin because the combination can cause a fatal lowering of blood pressure.

The nitroglycerin dose may be repeated every five minutes until the pain is relieved or until a maximum of three doses has been administered. If the patient doesn't carry nitroglycerin, or the first dose does not make the pain go away, suggest that the person chew a minimum of 160 mg up to a maximum of 325 mg of acetylsalicylic acid (ASA), depending on what is available. Do not repeat the dosage. ASA is an anti-clotting agent that will reduce the formation of a clot in the coronary artery at the site of the blockage. This will possibly decrease the damage to the heart muscle. Administer oxygen if it is available.

Obtain more advanced medical care. Surviving a heart attack often depends on how soon the patient receives advanced medical care (that being the special equipment and medications needed for someone experiencing a cardiac emergency).

Be calm and reassuring when caring for someone experiencing a heart attack. Comforting the patient helps reduce anxiety and eases some of the discomfort.

Provide ongoing survey and care until you can obtain advanced medical care. Watch for any changes in appearance or behaviour. Since the heart attack may lead to cardiac arrest, be prepared to perform CPR. Table 8–2 summarizes the care for a heart attack and angina.

TABLE 8–2: CARE FOR A HEART ATTACK AND ANGINA

- Recognize the signals of a heart attack.
- Convince the patient to stop activity and rest.
- Help the patient to rest comfortably.
- Try to obtain information about the patient's condition.
- Comfort the patient.
- Administer oxygen if available.
- Obtain more advanced medical care.
- Assist with medication.
- Monitor vital signs.
- Be prepared to perform CPR.

CONGESTIVE HEART FAILURE

Congestive heart failure (CHF) is an abnormal condition in which the heart loses its pumping ability. This may be the result of a heart attack (acute myocardial infarction, or MI), valvular disease, ischemic heart disease, or any disease that affects the heart muscle or myocardium (cardiomyopathy). The result is that fluids and blood back up into the lungs or body tissues.

In acute MI, usually the left ventricle is damaged. Also, in chronic hypertension, the left ventricle suffers the long-term effects of having to pump against restricted arteries in the extremities (peripheral arteries). As a result, the left ventricle doesn't pump as effectively and can't pump with enough force to push enough blood through the body. Blood coming into the left chamber of the heart from the lungs backs up, causing fluid to leak into the lungs, which causes fluid in the lungs (pulmonary edema).

Signs and symptoms of left-sided heart failure may include:

- Shortness of breath

- Increased respiratory rate
- History of severe shortness of breath at night when the person is lying down, which gets better when standing
- Cyanosis
- Coughing up foamy sputum (sometimes blood-tinged)
- Increased heart rate
- Wheezing
- Pale, cool, clammy skin
- Panic, restlessness, agitation
- Normal to high blood pressure
- Confusion and disorientation

RIGHT-SIDED HEART FAILURE

Right-sided heart failure usually occurs due to left-sided failure. When the left ventricle fails, increased fluid pressure is transferred back through the lungs. Eventually, the right side is unable to keep up with the increased workload, it becomes damaged, and heart failure results. Right-sided heart failure may also occur as a result of a pulmonary embolism, long-standing COPD, or MI. When the right side fails and loses its pumping power, blood backs up into the body's veins. This usually causes pooling of fluid in the tissues, resulting in swelling of the extremities (peripheral edema). This will be most noticeable in the feet when the person is sitting or standing or in the lower back if the person is bedridden.

Signs and symptoms of right-sided heart failure may include:

- Shortness of breath
- Swelling of feet and ankles
- Urinating more frequently at night
- Pronounced neck veins (also known as jugular venous distension [JVD])
- Heart palpitations
- Irregular fast heartbeat
- Weakness and fatigue
- Fainting

Figure 8–9 Biological death is the irreversible damage caused by brain cell death.

Right-sided heart failure by itself is seldom a life-threatening emergency. A change in lifestyle and possibly medications are the definitive treatments for this condition.

CARDIAC ARREST

What Is Cardiac Arrest?

Cardiac arrest occurs when the heart stops beating or beats too irregularly or too weakly to circulate blood effectively. Without a heartbeat, breathing soon ceases. The condition when the heart stops beating and breathing stops is referred to as clinical death.

Cardiac arrest is a life-threatening emergency because the body's vital organs, including the brain, are no longer receiving oxygen-rich blood. The irreversible damage caused by brain cell death is known as biological death (Figure 8–9). Every year, tens of thousands of Canadians die of cardiac arrest before reaching a hospital.

Common Causes of Cardiac Arrest

Cardiovascular disease is the most common cause of cardiac arrest. Other causes include drowning, suffocation, certain drugs, severe injuries to the chest, severe blood loss, and electrocution. Stroke and other types of brain damage can also stop the heart.

Signs of Cardiac Arrest

Someone in cardiac arrest is not breathing and does not have a pulse. The person's heart has either stopped beating or is beating so weakly or irregularly that it cannot produce a pulse. The signs of cardiac arrest include unconsciousness, no signs of normal breathing, and a lack of pulse. If you cannot feel a carotid pulse, no blood is reaching the brain. The person will be unconscious, and breathing will stop.

Although cardiac arrest can result from a heart attack, cardiac arrest can also occur suddenly, from other causes. Therefore, the person may not have shown the signs and symptoms of a heart attack before the cardiac arrest.

Care for Cardiac Arrest

Someone in cardiac arrest needs cardiopulmonary resuscitation (CPR). The term "cardio" refers to the heart, and "pulmonary" refers to the lungs. CPR is a combination of rescue breathing and chest compressions. Chest compression is a method of making the blood circulate when the heart is not beating. Given together, rescue breathing and chest compressions artificially take over the functions of the lungs and heart.

For the patient in cardiac arrest, CPR increases the chances of survival by keeping the brain supplied with oxygen until she receives advanced medical care. Without CPR, the brain will begin to die within four to six minutes. Be aware that, at best, CPR generates only about one third of the normal blood flow to the brain.

CPR alone is not enough to help someone survive cardiac arrest. Advanced medical care is needed immediately. Trained emergency personnel can provide advanced cardiac life support (ACLS). Acting as an extension of a hospital emergency department, some responders can administer medications or use a defibrillator as part of their emergency care.

A defibrillator is a device that sends an electric shock through the chest to allow the heart to resume its normal rhythm. Defibrillation given as soon as possible is the key to helping some patients survive cardiac arrest. Immediate CPR must be combined with early defibrillation and other forms of ACLS to give the patient in cardiac arrest the best chance for survival.

Responders in some communities are trained to use defibrillators called automated external defibrillators (AEDs). Today, AEDs are available for use by individuals in places such as factories, stadiums, airports, recreation facilities, casinos, and other places where large numbers of people gather. The use of defibrillators is described later in this chapter.

In all cases of cardiac arrest, it is very important to start CPR promptly and continue it until a defibrillator is available. When a defibrillator is not available, CPR should be continued. Effective rescue breathing and chest compressions can help keep the brain, heart, and other vital organs supplied with oxygen-rich blood. Any delay in starting CPR, or unnecessary delay in continuing it, reduces the patient's chance for survival.

Starting CPR and defibrillation promptly, as well as ensuring advanced medical care is obtained, greatly increases the chance for survival.

> **NOTE:**
>
> *Use two hands to compress a child's chest, unless the child is very small in comparison with the responder. With a small child, using two hands may create too much pressure. If this is the case, compress with only one hand.*

CPR FOR ADULTS AND CHILDREN

Chest Compressions

Chest compressions create pressure within the chest cavity that moves blood through the circulatory system. For compressions to be most effective, the patient should be flat on her back, on a firm surface.

Finding the Correct Hand Position

Placing your hands in the middle of the patient's chest allows you to give the most effective compressions without causing injury.

- Once the heel of your hand is in position on the chest, place your other hand directly on top of it.
- Use the heel of your hand to apply pressure on the sternum.

If you have arthritis or a similar condition in your hands or wrists, you may use an alternative hand position. Find the correct hand position, as above; then grasp the wrist of the hand on the chest with the other hand (Figure 8–10).

Figure 8–10 An alternate hand position for compressions can be done by grasping the wrist of the hand on the chest with the other hand.

If you can position your hands without removing thin clothing, such as a T-shirt, do so. The patient's clothing will not necessarily interfere with your ability to position your hands on the chest.

Position of the Responder

Your body position is important when giving chest compressions. Compressing the chest straight down provides the best blood flow. The correct body position is also less tiring for you.

Kneel at the patient's chest with your hands in the correct position. Straighten your arms and lock your

Figure 8–11 When doing compressions, your arms should be straightened and locked so your shoulders are directly over your hands.

> **NOTE:**
>
> *For a child, compress 1/3 to 1/2 the depth of the chest.*

elbows so that your shoulders are directly over your hands (Figure 8–11). When you press down in this position, you are pushing straight down onto the patient's sternum. Locking your elbows keeps your arms straight and prevents you from tiring quickly.

Compressing the chest requires less effort in this position. When you press down, the weight of your upper body creates the force needed to compress the chest. Push with the weight of your upper body, not with the muscles of your arms. Push straight down. Do not rock back and forth. Rocking results in less effective compressions and uses unnecessary energy. If your arms and shoulders tire quickly, you are not using the correct body position. After each compression, release the pressure on the chest without losing contact with it and allow the chest to return to its normal position before you start the next compression (Figure 8–12).

Compression Technique

Each compression should push the sternum of an adult down at least 5 cm (2 in.). The downward and upward movement should be smooth, not jerky. Maintain a steady down-and-up rhythm and do not pause between compressions. When you press down, the chambers of the heart empty. When you come up, release all pressure on the chest, which lets the chambers of the heart fill with blood between compressions.

Give compressions at the rate of at least 100 per minute and "Push hard. Push fast." You should be able to do the 30 compressions in about 18 seconds. Even though you are compressing the chest at a rate of at least 100 times per minute, you will not actually perform 100 compressions in a minute. This is because you must take the time to do rescue breathing, giving two breaths between each group of 30 compressions.

Figure 8–12 When doing compressions, push straight down, then release, allowing the chest to return to its normal position.

Compression/Breathing Cycles

When you perform CPR, do cycles of 30 compressions and two breaths. You should be positioned midway between the chest and the head to move easily between compressions and breaths. For each cycle, do 30 chest compressions; then open the airway and give two one-second breaths, with just enough volume to make the chest start to rise.

After doing five cycles (2 minutes) of continuous CPR, recheck for signs of circulation and normal breathing. Tilt the patient's head to open the airway and take no more than 5 to 10 seconds to check for signs of circulation. If there are no signs of circulation or you are unsure, continue CPR, beginning with compressions. Check circulation and breathing again every few minutes. If the patient has a pulse but is not breathing, give rescue breaths. If the patient is breathing, keep her airway open and provide ongoing survey and care.

CPR for Pregnant Women

When performing CPR on a visibly pregnant woman, putting a blanket or cushion under her right hip will help blood return to the heart. However, do not interrupt CPR to find an object.

When to Stop CPR

Once you begin CPR, do not interrupt the blood flow you are creating artificially. However, you can stop CPR if:

- The patient's heart starts beating.

- Another responder with training equal to or greater than yours takes over. (Continue to assist by obtaining advanced medical care if this has not already been done.)

- You are too exhausted to continue.

- The scene suddenly becomes unsafe.

Disturbances in Heart Rhythm

The healthy adult heart usually displays normal sinus rhythm (NSR), the normal conduction of electrical impulses without any disturbances, on the electrocardiogram (ECG). Disturbances or variations in the conduction of electrical impulses within the heart are called dysrhythmias. Although dysrhythmias can either be benign or have serious consequences, there are three major conduction disturbances that are immediately life-threatening: asystole, ventricular tachycardia (VT), and ventricular fibrillation (VF).

Asystole

Asystole is the absence of electrical activity in the heart. AEDs are not able to shock this rhythm (Figure 8–13).

Ventricular Tachycardia

VT is a rhythm of fast-paced contractions of the heart's ventricles. The contractions are too rapid to allow the ventricles to fill with blood to pump an adequate supply of blood to the body (Figure 8–14). Someone experiencing this type of dysrhythmia can still have a pulse.

Ventricular Fibrillation

VF is a chaotic discharge of electrical activity that causes the heart muscle to quiver (Figure 8–15). Patients with this dysrhythmia have no pulse. VF will deteriorate to asystole within a few minutes if not treated promptly.

Correcting the Problem

In over 80% of all sudden cardiac arrests, the initial rhythm is VT or VF, which are the only two rhythms an AED will shock.

Figure 8–13 Asystole.

Figure 8–14 Ventricular tachycardia.

Figure 8–15 Ventricular fibrillation.

Studies show that early CPR and defibrillation are most likely to improve the survival of adults in cardiac arrest. Each minute that defibrillation is delayed, the chance of survival is reduced by about 7 to 10%.

During defibrillation, an electrical shock is delivered to the heart. The shock is intended to briefly stop the abnormal electrical activity (e.g., VF or pulseless VT) long enough to allow the heart to develop an effective rhythm on its own.

Because the treatment of choice for both of these rhythms in cases of cardiac arrest is CPR along with defibrillation, early response with an AED is important. Unfortunately, defibrillation does not correct asystole, and CPR must continue until more advanced help is obtained. CPR may cause an unshockable rhythm to become a shockable rhythm. The successful resuscitation of patients in cardiac arrest with a shockable dysrhythmia (i.e., VF or VT) depends greatly on how much time has passed from the start of the dysrhythmia until defibrillation is initiated, as well as whether CPR was initiated. The availability of AEDs to a wider range of responders could greatly reduce the time from collapse to defibrillation, thereby increasing the chance for survival.

Using an AED

In a situation involving a cardiac arrest, an AED should be put to use as soon as it is available. To defibrillate someone in cardiac arrest by using an AED, take the following steps.

1. Confirm cardiac arrest. Check for responsiveness and ABCs.

2. Place the AED beside the patient in a safe position. Turn on the AED.

3. Expose and prepare the chest. Wipe the patient's chest dry and shave it if needed.

4. Attach the electrode pads to the chest. Place one pad on the upper-right side of the chest and the other pad on the lower-left side of the chest (Figure 8–16).

5. Plug the electrode pads into AED, if needed.

6. Let the AED analyze the heart rhythm (or push the "analyze" button if required).

7. Make sure no one is touching the patient.

8. Deliver a shock if indicated by the AED.

   • Say "I'm clear, you're clear, everybody's clear"; ensure that no one is touching the patient.

   • Deliver a shock by pushing the "shock" button when prompted by the AED.

   • After the shock, the AED will prompt you to provide five cycles (two minutes) of CPR.

   • After the two minutes, the AED will analyze again.

If the AED advises no shock is needed:

   • If there are no signs of circulation, do five cycles of CPR (two minutes).

   • Follow the prompts of the AED.

Responders using AEDs may fall under medical direction provided on a local, regional, or province/territory-wide basis. You must follow local protocols that establish how many shocks are delivered, the energy setting of each shock, and how CPR and other lifesaving measures are used.

Special Resuscitation Situations

Some situations require responders to pay special attention when using an AED. It is important that responders be familiar with these situations and be able to respond appropriately.

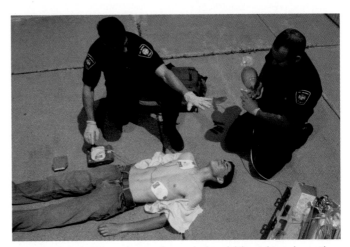

Figure 8–16 One electrode pad should be placed on the upper-right side of the chest and the other pad on the lower-left side of the chest.

Hypothermia

Check the pulse of a patient suffering from severe hypothermia for up to 45 seconds. If AED is indicated, give only one shock. Following the shock, continue with the CPR sequence. Follow local protocol.

Transdermal Medications

AED electrodes should not be placed over a transdermal medication patch (e.g., a patch of nitroglycerin, nicotine, pain medication, hormone replacement therapy, or antihypertensive medication) as the patch may block the transfer of the energy to the heart and may cause small burns to the skin. With a gloved hand, remove any patches from the chest and wipe the area before attaching the electrode pads.

Implanted Pacemakers and Implanted Cardioverter-Defibrillators

The patient may have a pacemaker or implanted cardioverter-defibrillator (ICD) implanted in the chest area where one of the electrode pads is intended to go. If you observe a small scar and a matchbox-sized lump on the chest, reposition the electrodes at least 2.5 cm (1 in.) away. If an ICD is already in shock sequence (e.g., the patient's muscles contract in a manner similar to that observed during external defibrillation), allow 30 to 60 seconds for the ICD to complete the treatment cycle before delivering a shock from the AED.

NOTE:

Someone is considered to be a child from the age of one year until the onset of puberty, except when using an AED. In the case of an AED, someone is considered to be a child when between the ages of one and eight. A baby is up to one year of age. Both babies and children can be defibrillated. For a baby, use baby electrode pads; if unavailable, use child or adult pads. For a child, use child electrode pads; if unavailable, use adult pads. Follow the directions for electrode pad placement. If there is less than 2.5 cm (1 in.) between the electrode pads when on the chest, place one on the front of the chest (anterior) and one on the back (posterior).

Body Jewellery

If a necklace or other body jewellery is in the way or within 2.5 cm (1 in.) of electrode pad placement, remove the jewellery before AED use.

Trauma to the Torso

Place electrode pads on the chest if the trauma does not interfere with the placement.

AEDs Around Water

If the patient is in freestanding water, remove the patient before defibrillation. A shock delivered in water could conduct to rescuers or bystanders. Once you have removed the patient from the water, be sure there are no puddles of water around you, the patient, or the AED. Remove wet clothing for proper pad placement, if necessary. Dry the patient's chest and attach the AED pads.

If it is raining, ensure that the patient is as dry as possible and sheltered from the rain. Wipe the patient's chest dry. Minimize delaying defibrillation when taking steps to provide for a dry environment. The electrical current of an AED is very directional between the pads. AEDs are quite safe, even in rain and snow, when all precautions and the manufacturer's operating instructions are followed.

Maintenance

For defibrillators to perform optimally, they must be maintained like any other machine. The AEDs available today require minimal maintenance. These devices have various self-testing features. However, it is important that operators are familiar with any visual or audible warning or prompts that the AED may feature to warn of a malfunction or low battery. It is important to read the operator's manual thoroughly and check with the manufacturer to obtain all necessary information regarding maintenance.

Other Precautions

The following precautions must be taken when using an AED:

- As alcohol is flammable, avoid using alcohol pads to clean the chest before attaching the pads.

- Stand clear of the patient while analyzing and defibrillating.

- Do not analyze the heart rhythm or defibrillate in a moving vehicle.

- Do not defibrillate a patient in the presence of flammable materials (e.g., gasoline).

- Avoid radio transmissions while defibrillating, including cellphones within two metres (six feet) of the patient.

- Keep breathing devices with free-flowing oxygen away from the patient during defibrillation.

- Avoid the use of supplemental, free-flowing oxygen while using an AED in a confined space.

CARDIAC EMERGENCIES IN BABIES AND CHILDREN

A child's heart is usually healthy. Unlike adults, children do not often initially suffer a cardiac emergency. Instead, the child suffers a respiratory emergency, which can lead to a cardiac emergency.

Common causes of cardiac emergencies for both babies and children include injuries from drowning, smoke inhalation, burns, poisoning, airway obstruction, and falls.

	ADULT	CHILD	BABY
HAND POSITION:	Two hands on middle of chest	One or two hands on middle of chest	Two fingers on middle of chest (just below nipple line)
COMPRESS:	At least 5 cm (2 in.)	At least 5 cm (2 in.) or $1/3$ to $1/2$ of chest depth	At least 4 cm (1.5 in.) or $1/3$ to $1/2$ of chest depth
BREATHE:	Until chest starts to rise (about 1 second per breath)	Until chest starts to rise (about 1 second per breath)	Slowly, until chest starts to rise (about 1 second per breath)
CYCLE:	30 compressions 2 breaths	30 compressions 2 breaths	30 compressions 2 breaths
COMPRESSION RATE:	At least 100 per minute (with no breaths)	At least 100 per minute (with no breaths)	At least 100 per minute (with no breaths)

Figure 8–17 The technique for chest compressions is very similar for adults, children, and babies.

Most cardiac emergencies in babies and children are preventable. One way to prevent them in this age group is to prevent injuries. Another is to make sure that babies and children receive proper medical care. A third is to recognize the early signs of a breathing emergency. These signs include:

- Agitation

- Drowsiness

- Change in skin colour (to pale blue or grey)

- Difficulty breathing (dyspnea)

- Increased heart and breathing rates

If you recognize that a baby or child is having a breathing emergency, provide necessary care. If the baby or child is in cardiac arrest, start CPR immediately. In either event, obtain more advanced medical care.

CPR FOR BABIES

The CPR technique for babies is similar to that for adults. As in rescue breathing, you need to modify the

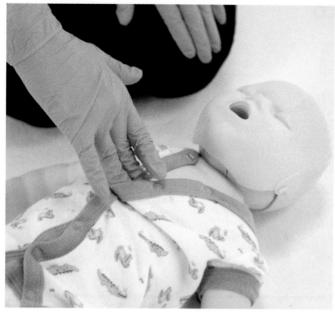

Figure 8–18 When doing compressions on a baby, use the pads of two fingers. Allow the chest to return to its normal position between compressions.

Figure 8–19 Continue cycles of 30 compressions and two breaths.

techniques to accommodate the smaller body size and faster breathing and heart rates. Figure 8–17 compares the adult, child, and baby CPR techniques.

To find out if a baby needs CPR, begin with a primary survey to check the ABCs. To check the pulse in a baby, locate the brachial pulse in the arm. If the baby has no signs of circulation, including lack of a brachial pulse, begin CPR.

Position the baby face up on a firm, flat surface. Stand or kneel facing the baby from the side. Keep one hand on the baby's head to maintain an open airway. Use your other hand to give compressions.

To find the correct place to give compressions, place your two fingers in the middle of the chest, just below the nipple line.

Use the pads of two fingers to compress the chest (Figure 8–18). Compress the chest at least 4 cm (1.5 in.) or 1/3 to 1/2 the depth of the chest and then let the sternum return to its normal position. When you compress, push straight down. The down-and-up movement of your compressions should be smooth, not jerky. Keep a steady rhythm. Do not pause between compressions. When you are coming up, release pressure on the baby's chest completely but do not let your fingers lose contact with the chest. Keep your fingers in the compression position. Use your other hand to keep the airway open using a head-tilt.

When you give CPR, do cycles of 30 compressions and two breaths (Figure 8–19). Compress at a rate of at least 100 compressions per minute. When you complete 30 compressions, give two one-second breaths, with just enough volume to make the chest start to rise, covering the baby's nose and mouth with your mask. Keep repeating cycles of 30 compressions and two breaths.

Recheck for signs of circulation and breathing after about five cycles (two minutes) of continuous CPR. Check for signs of circulation for no more than 5 to 10 seconds with the hand that was giving compressions. If there are no signs of circulation or you are unsure, continue CPR, starting with compressions. Recheck circulation and breathing every few minutes.

If the baby has a pulse but is not breathing, give rescue breaths. If the baby is breathing, keep the airway open and provide ongoing survey and care.

Figure 8–20 When two responders are doing CPR, they share the responsibility of performing rescue breathing and chest compressions.

Figure 8–21 For baby CPR with two responders, the responder doing compressions circles his hands around the baby's chest, with the fingers at the back, and the thumbs on the lower half of the baby's breastbone.

TWO-RESCUER CPR

When two professional responders are available, they give two-rescuer CPR. They share the responsibility for performing rescue breathing/ventilations and chest compressions (Figure 8–20).

Two-Rescuer CPR for an Adult or Child

One responder begins CPR while the second responder calls EMS/9-1-1 and gets an AED. When the second responder returns, one responder performs chest compressions and gives rescue breaths/ventilations. The other responder maintains the head-tilt/chin-lift and/or jaw thrust with the BVM.

For an adult, use the same technique and ratios as in adult CPR with one responder (30 compressions to two breaths/ventilations). For a child, when there are two responders, use a ratio of 15 compressions to two breaths/ventilations.

The responder giving breaths (the ventilator) checks the effectiveness of the compressions by feeling for the carotid pulse while the compressor is giving chest compressions. If the patient has lost a significant amount of blood, a carotid pulse may not be felt even though compressions are effective.

The ventilator also checks for signs of circulation after the five cycles (two minutes) of compressions and repeats the check every few minutes after that to determine if circulation has returned. The ventilator does this by communicating that he is performing a circulation check; then the compressor stops after the 30th compression. The ventilator checks for signs of circulation for no more than 5 to 10 seconds. If there is no circulation or he is unsure, CPR is continued, starting with compressions.

Two-Rescuer CPR for a Baby

One responder encircles the baby's chest with both hands, spreading his fingers around the baby's back and placing both thumbs on the lower half of the baby's breastbone (Figure 8–21). Compressions are performed by compressing the sternum with the hands in this position. The other responder monitors the baby's pulse to check whether the compressions are effective and gives rescue breaths/ventilations. For a baby, if there are two responders, use a ratio of 15 compressions to two breaths. In two minutes, 10 cycles of CPR should be done.

When Two Responders Arrive on the Scene at the Same Time

If CPR is not being performed when you arrive, one responder should do a primary survey and, if appropriate, begin CPR. The other responder should manage other responsibilities at the scene and get an AED if available; then she can assist with CPR and AED. If both responders begin CPR at the same time, the first responder does a primary survey. While the first responder is doing the primary survey, the second responder gets into position to give chest compressions. She should begin chest compressions when the first responder communicates that there are no signs of circulation. Both responders continue CPR together.

When CPR Is in Progress by One Responder

When a responder is giving CPR and a second responder arrives, that responder should ask whether more advanced medical care has been obtained. If not, she should call, or send someone else to call, and have the person get an AED if available. Then the second responder should either replace the first responder or assist in giving two-rescuer CPR by providing ventilations or compressions.

Changing Positions

It is recommended that responders change every two minutes (between cycles) to maintain quality CPR. When the responders change, the responder at the person's head completes two breaths and then moves immediately to the chest. The responder at the chest moves immediately to the head. Both responders move quickly into position without changing sides. The person who is now at the chest begins compressions immediately.

STROKE AND TRANSIENT ISCHEMIC ATTACK (TIA)

Prevention of Stroke and TIA

The risk factors for stroke and transient ischemic attack (TIA) are similar to those for heart disease. Some risk factors are beyond your control, such as age, sex, or a family history of stroke, TIA, or diabetes. To prevent

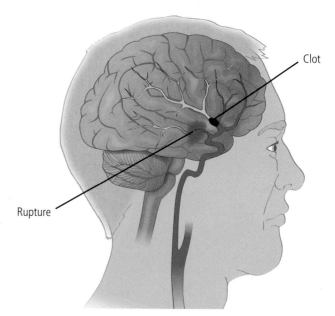

Figure 8–22 A stroke can be caused by a clot or rupture.

stroke, follow the same guidelines as those for preventing cardiovascular disease.

TIA

A TIA is a temporary episode that is like a stroke. TIAs are sometimes called "mini-strokes." Like a stroke, a TIA is caused by reduced blood flow to part of the brain. Unlike a stroke, the signs and symptoms of a TIA disappear within a few minutes or hours, although the person is not out of danger. Someone who experiences a TIA has a significantly increased risk of having a stroke in the future.

Stroke

A stroke, also called a cerebrovascular accident (CVA), is a disruption of blood flow to a part of the brain that is serious enough to damage brain tissue (Figure 8–22).

There are three causes of stroke. Two of these are caused by a moving blood clot that forms or lodges in the arteries that supply blood to the brain, and the third is a rupture of the arteries.

1. *Embolic strokes.* A mass known as an embolus—which could be a solid, liquid or gas—can be carried to a blood vessel from another site in the body. The most common type is a clot coming from diseased carotid blood vessels or from abnormally contracting chambers in the heart.

2. *Thrombotic strokes.* A thrombus is a gradually developing blood clot that leads to an obstruction of a cerebral artery. Plaque deposits forming on the inner walls of arteries causes a narrowing of the arteries and reduces blood flow.

3. *Bleeding from a ruptured artery in the brain.* A head injury, high blood pressure or a weak area in an artery wall can result in this type of stroke.

Less commonly, a tumour or swelling from a head injury may cause a stroke by compressing an artery.

Signs and Symptoms of Stroke and TIA

As with other sudden illnesses, the primary signs and symptoms of stroke or TIA are looking or feeling ill, changes in consciousness, and abnormal behaviour.

Others signs and symptoms may include:

- Sudden weakness and/or numbness of the face, arm, or leg, usually only on one side of the body
- Difficulty talking or understanding speech
- Blurred or dimmed vision
- Pupils of unequal size
- Sudden, severe headache
- Dizziness
- Confusion
- Changes in mood
- Ringing in the ears
- Unconsciousness or temporary loss of consciousness
- Loss of bowel or bladder control

Remember FAST:

FACE – facial numbness and/or weakness, especially on one side (Figure 8–23)

ARM – arm numbness and/or weakness, especially on one side

SPEECH – slurred speech or difficulty speaking or understanding

TIME – time is critically important; obtain more advanced medical care immediately

Figure 8–23 Weakness or numbness, often on one side of the face, is a sign of stroke.

Assessing Someone Who Has Had a Suspected Stroke

To assess facial droop, arm weakness, and speech abnormalities, responders can use a tool such as the Cincinnati Pre-hospital Stroke Scale (CPSS).

Facial droop: Have the patient show her teeth or smile.

If both sides of the face move equally, this is normal.

If one side of the face does not move as well as the other side, this is abnormal.

Arm weakness: Have the patient close both eyes and hold her arms out straight for 10 seconds.

If both arms move the same or both arms do not move at all, this is normal.

If one arm does not move or one arm drifts down compared with the other, this is abnormal.

Speech abnormalities: Have the patient say, "You can't teach an old dog new tricks."

If the patient uses the correct words and does not slur, this is normal.

If the patient uses the incorrect words, slurs the words, or does not speak at all, this is abnormal.

Care for Stroke and TIA

If the patient is unconscious, make sure she has an open airway and care for any life-threatening conditions that may occur. If the patient is unable to protect her own airway, position her on one side to allow fluids to drain out. You may have to use a finger sweep to remove some of the material from the mouth. Obtain more advanced medical care.

A stroke can make the patient fearful and anxious; therefore, it is important to comfort and reassure the patient. Often she does not understand what has happened. Have the patient rest in a comfortable position. Do not give her anything to eat or drink. Rapid access to advanced medical care is very important. Provide ongoing survey and care.

SUMMARY

It is important to recognize signs and symptoms that may indicate a circulatory emergency. If you think someone is suffering from a circulatory emergency or if you are unsure, obtain more advanced medical care without delay. Provide care by helping the patient to rest in the most comfortable position and administering oxygen. If you are qualified to transport the patient, do so safely and efficiently.

When heartbeat and breathing stop, it is called cardiac arrest. Someone who suffers a cardiac arrest is clinically dead since no oxygen is reaching the cells of vital organs. Irreversible brain damage will occur from a lack of oxygen. By starting CPR immediately, you can help keep the brain supplied with oxygen. By obtaining more advanced medical care rapidly, you can increase the chances for survival for the patient in cardiac arrest.

If the patient does not have signs of circulation, start CPR. Once you start CPR, do not stop unnecessarily. Continue CPR until you are relieved by another trained responder, you are exhausted, the scene suddenly becomes unsafe, the patient's heart starts beating, you obtain more advanced medical care and they take over, or an AED is available.

When blood flow to the brain is interrupted, either due to a blockage or rupture of an artery in the brain, this is called a stroke. The part of the brain that was supplied by that artery is starved of oxygen and suffers damage. This can cause muscle weakness or numbness, difficulty speaking, or a range of other problems throughout the body. It is critical to obtain advanced medical care immediately as there are steps that will minimize that damage or even prevent it.

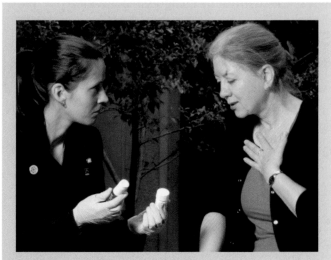

You find out that she has medication in her purse for this type of emergency. What do you do?

Chapter 9

Bleeding

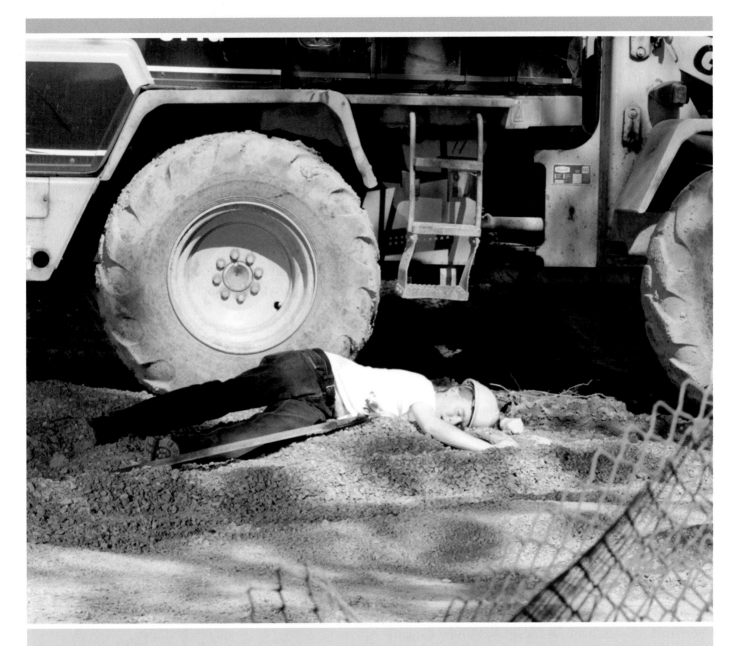

You are called to the scene of a construction site. A worker has fallen from some heavy equipment and has been impaled by a sharp metal fence post. He is bleeding profusely from a wound in his side. He's pale and his skin is moist. His voice is weak and he's starting to lose consciousness. What do you do?

INTRODUCTION

Bleeding is the loss of blood from arteries, veins, or capillaries. A large amount of bleeding occurring in a short time is called a hemorrhage. Bleeding is either internal or external. Internal bleeding is often difficult to recognize. External bleeding is usually obvious because it is typically visible. Uncontrolled bleeding, whether internal or external, is a life-threatening emergency.

Severe bleeding can result in death. Check for and control severe bleeding during the primary survey once you have checked for a pulse. You may not identify internal bleeding, however, until you perform a more detailed check during the secondary survey. In this chapter, you will learn how to recognize and care for both internal and external bleeding.

BLOOD AND BLOOD VESSELS

Blood Components

Blood consists of liquid and solid components and comprises approximately 8% of the body's total weight, to a volume of approximately five litres (five quarts). The liquid part of the blood is called plasma. The solid components are the red and white blood cells and cell fragments called platelets.

Plasma makes up about half of the blood volume circulating within the body. Composed mostly of water, plasma maintains the blood volume that the circulatory system needs to function normally. Plasma also contains nutrients essential for energy production, growth, and cell maintenance and carries waste products for elimination.

White blood cells are a key disease-fighting component of the immune system. They defend the body against invading micro-organisms. They also aid in producing antibodies that help the body resist infection.

Red blood cells account for most of the solid components of the blood. They are produced in the marrow in the hollow centre of large bones such as the large bone of the arm (humerus) and of the thigh (femur). Red blood cells number nearly 260 million in each drop of blood. The red blood cells transport oxygen from the lungs to the body cells and carbon dioxide from the cells to the lungs. Red blood cells outnumber white blood cells about 1,000 to 1.

Platelets are disc-shaped cells in the blood. Platelets are an essential part of the blood's clotting mechanism because they tend to bind together. Clotting is the process by which whole blood thickens at a wound site. Platelets help stop bleeding by forming blood clots at wound sites. Blood clots form the framework for healing. Until blood clots form, bleeding must be controlled.

Blood Functions

The blood has three major functions:

1. Transporting oxygen, nutrients, and wastes

2. Protecting against disease by producing antibodies and defending against germs

3. Helping to maintain constant body temperature by circulating throughout the body

Blood Vessels

Blood is channelled through blood vessels. There are three major types of blood vessels: arteries, capillaries, and veins (Figure 9–1). Arteries carry blood away from the heart. Arteries become narrower the farther they extend from the heart until they connect to the capillaries. Capillaries are microscopic blood vessels linking arteries and veins that transfer oxygen, nutrients, and carbon dioxide. The veins carry blood back to the heart. Waste products from the cells move through the blood to the organs that eliminate waste from the body, such as the kidneys and lungs.

Figure 9–1 Blood flows through the three major types of blood vessels: arteries, capillaries, and veins.

Blood in the arteries travels faster and is under greater pressure than blood in the capillaries or veins. Blood flow in the arteries pulses with the heartbeat; blood in the veins flows more slowly and evenly.

WHEN BLEEDING OCCURS

When bleeding occurs, the body begins a complex chain of events. The brain, heart, and lungs immediately attempt to compensate for blood loss to maintain the flow of oxygen-rich blood to the body, particularly to the vital organs.

Other important reactions also occur. Platelets collect at the wound site in an effort to stop blood loss through clotting. White blood cells try to prevent infection by attacking micro-organisms that commonly enter through breaks in the skin. The body manufactures extra red blood cells to help transport more oxygen to the cells.

Blood volume is also affected by bleeding. Normally, excess fluid is absorbed from the bloodstream by the kidneys, lungs, intestines, and skin. However, when bleeding occurs, this excess fluid is reabsorbed into the bloodstream as plasma. This helps maintain the critical balance of fluids needed by the body to keep blood volume constant.

Bleeding severe enough to critically reduce the blood volume is life-threatening. Severe bleeding can be either external or internal (Figure 9–2, a-b).

EXTERNAL BLEEDING

External bleeding occurs when a blood vessel is opened externally, such as through a tear in the skin. You can usually see this type of bleeding. Most external bleeding you will encounter will be minor. Minor bleeding, such as small cuts, usually stops by itself within 10 minutes, when the blood clots. Sometimes the damaged blood vessel is too large or the blood is under too much pressure for effective clotting to occur. In these cases, you will need to recognize and control bleeding promptly. Look for severe bleeding during the check for circulation as part of the primary survey.

Recognizing Severe External Bleeding

The signs of severe external bleeding include:

- Blood spurting or flowing freely from a wound
- Blood that fails to clot after you have taken all measures to control bleeding

Each type of blood vessel bleeds differently. Bleeding from arteries is often rapid and profuse and is life-threatening. This is because arterial blood is under direct pressure from the heart, so it usually spurts from the wound, making it difficult for clots to form. Because clots do not form rapidly in arteries, this type of bleeding is harder to control than bleeding from veins and capillaries. Its high concentration of oxygen gives arterial blood a bright red colour.

Figure 9–2, a-b Severe bleeding can be: **a**, external; or **b**, internal.

Veins are damaged more often than arteries because they are closer to the skin's surface. Bleeding from veins (venous bleeding) is easier to control than arterial bleeding. Venous blood is under less pressure than arterial blood and flows from the wound at a steady rate without spurting. Only damage to veins deep in the body, such as those in the trunk or thigh, produces profuse bleeding that is hard to control. Because it is oxygen poor, venous blood is dark red or maroon.

Capillary bleeding is usually slow because the vessels are small and the blood is under low pressure. It is often described as "oozing" from the wound. Clotting occurs easily with capillary bleeding. The blood from capillaries is usually dark red in colour.

Controlling External Bleeding

External bleeding is usually easy to control. Generally, you can control it by applying a pressure dressing with your gloved hand directly on the wound. This is called applying direct pressure. Pressure on the wound restricts the blood flow through the wound and allows normal clotting to occur. You can maintain pressure on a wound by snugly applying a bandage to the injured area.

In a few cases, direct pressure may not control severe bleeding. In these cases, other measures may have to be taken such as using a tourniquet.

To control external bleeding, follow these general steps:

1. Place direct pressure on the wound with a sterile gauze pad or any clean cloth, such as a washcloth, towel, or handkerchief. Using gauze or a clean cloth keeps the wound free from germs. Place a gloved hand over the gauze pad and apply firm pressure (Figure 9–3, a). If gauze or cloth is not available, apply pressure with your gloved hand or, if necessary, have the patient apply pressure with his own hand.

2. Have the patient sit or lie down and rest.

3. Apply a pressure bandage. This bandage will hold the gauze pads or cloth in place while maintaining direct pressure (Figure 9–3, b). If blood soaks through, add additional dressings and bandages with additional direct pressure. Do not remove any blood-soaked dressings or bandages.

Figure 9–3, a-c To control external bleeding: **a**, place direct pressure on the wound; **b**, apply a pressure bandage; and **c**, apply a tourniquet if bleeding continues.

4. If bleeding continues, apply a tourniquet above the injury to slow the flow of blood (Figure 9–3, c).

Tourniquets

A tourniquet, a tight band placed around an arm or leg to constrict blood vessels to stop blood flow to a wound, can be used as a last resort to control severe external bleeding. Tourniquets should be made with a wide material (e.g., a triangular bandage or blood pressure cuff). You should only use tourniquets if you are trained to do so. Tourniquets should be used in combination with direct pressure whenever possible.

Assess the patient's distal circulation and neurovascular status before and after application. Apply the tourniquet 5 to 10 cm (2 to 4 in.) above the injury and above any joint in this range. If using a blood pressure cuff, inflate the cuff to approximately 30 mmHg above the systolic pressure, until the bleeding stops. Continue to apply direct pressure to the wound, if possible.

Document the time the tourniquet was applied and tightened as well as any release times. Reassess the patient's distal circulation. After 10 minutes, you may slowly remove the tourniquet. Check that the previously applied pressure bandage is secure and controlling the bleeding. If the bleeding reoccurs, reapply the tourniquet.

The removal of a tourniquet should include appropriate medical direction, unless extreme circumstances exist where the delivery of the patient to more advanced medical care is delayed.

Continue to monitor the patient's airway and breathing. Observe him closely for signs that indicate a worsening condition. If bleeding is severe, administer supplemental oxygen to the patient if available. More advanced medical care must be obtained if not already done.

INTERNAL BLEEDING

Internal bleeding is the escape of blood from arteries, veins, or capillaries into spaces in the body. Capillary bleeding, indicated by mild bruising, is just beneath the skin and is not serious. Deeper bleeding, however, involves arteries and veins and may result in severe blood loss.

Severe internal bleeding usually occurs in injuries caused by a violent blunt force, such as when the driver is thrown against the steering wheel in a car crash or when someone falls from a height. Internal bleeding may also occur when a sharp object, such as a knife, penetrates the skin and damages internal structures.

Recognizing Internal Bleeding

Because internal bleeding is more difficult to recognize than external bleeding, you should always suspect internal bleeding in any serious injury. For example, if you find a motorcycle rider thrown from a bike, you may not see any serious external bleeding, but you should consider that the violent forces involved indicate the likelihood of internal injuries. Internal bleeding can occur from a fractured bone that ruptures an organ or blood vessels.

NOTE:
Major fractures, such as those involving the pelvis, femur, chest, and abdomen, can result in a significant amount of internal bleeding.

The body's inability to adjust to severe internal bleeding will eventually produce signs and symptoms that indicate shock. These signs and symptoms are less obvious and may take time to appear. They include:

- Discoloration of the skin (bruising) in the injured area
- Soft tissues that are tender, swollen, or firm
- Anxiety or restlessness
- Rapid, weak pulse
- Rapid breathing (tachypnea)
- Skin that feels cool or moist or looks pale or bluish
- Nausea and vomiting
- Excessive thirst
- Declining level of consciousness
- Drop in blood pressure

Shock is discussed in detail in Chapter 10.

Controlling Internal Bleeding

How you control internal bleeding depends on the severity and site of the bleeding. For minor internal bleeding, such as a bruise on an arm, apply ice or a chemical cold pack to the injured area to help reduce pain and swelling. When applying ice, always remember to place something, such as a gauze pad or a towel, between the source of cold and the skin to prevent skin damage due to freezing.

If you suspect internal bleeding caused by serious injury, you must obtain more advanced medical care. There is little you can do to control bleeding effectively. The patient must be transported rapidly to the hospital. The patient will often need immediate surgery to correct the problem. While awaiting more advanced medical care, treat the patient for shock and provide ongoing survey and care.

Because of the nature of the injury, you suspect internal bleeding as well. What do you do?

SUMMARY

One of the most important things you can do in any emergency is to recognize and control severe bleeding. External bleeding is easily recognized and should be cared for immediately. Check and care for severe bleeding during the primary survey. Severe external bleeding is life-threatening. Although internal bleeding is less obvious, it also can be life-threatening. Recognize when a serious injury has occurred and suspect internal bleeding. You may not identify internal bleeding until you perform the secondary survey. When you identify or suspect severe bleeding, you must obtain advanced medical care.

Shock

You are dispatched to a motor vehicle collision in a parking lot. You arrive to see that a car has been hit head-on by a minivan. The passenger door of the car is jammed and the young passenger, who appears to be breathing, is not responding to the bystander. As you survey the scene, the driver of the minivan says he is fine. He is agitated and directs you to help the driver of the car, who appears to be unconscious. What do you do?

INTRODUCTION

Both medical emergencies and injuries can cause life-threatening conditions, such as cardiac and respiratory arrest and severe bleeding. Medical emergencies and injuries also can become life-threatening as a result of shock. When the body experiences injury or sudden illness, it responds in a number of ways. Survival depends on the body's ability to adapt to the physical stresses of illness or injury. When the body's measures to adapt fail, the patient can progress into a life-threatening condition called shock. Shock complicates the effects of injury or sudden illness. In this chapter, you will learn to recognize the signs and symptoms of shock and to provide care to minimize it.

SHOCK

What Is Shock?

Shock is a condition in which the circulatory system fails to adequately circulate oxygen-rich blood to all cells of the body. When vital organs such as the heart, lungs, brain, and kidneys do not receive oxygen-rich blood, they fail to function properly. This triggers a series of responses that produces specific signs and symptoms known as shock. These responses are the body's attempt to maintain adequate blood flow to the vital organs, preventing their failure.

When the body is healthy, three conditions are necessary to maintain adequate blood flow:

1. The heart must be working well.

2. An adequate amount of blood must be circulating in the body.

3. The blood vessels must be intact and able to adjust blood flow.

Injury or sudden illness can interrupt normal body functions. In cases of minor injury or illness, this interruption is brief because the body is able to compensate quickly. With more severe injuries or illnesses, however, the body may be unable to adjust. When the body is unable to meet its demands for oxygen because the blood fails to circulate adequately, shock occurs.

How Shock Develops

There are different types of shock, as shown in Table 10–1. Although the responder does not have to be able to identify each of these different types of shock, it may

TABLE 10–1: TYPES OF SHOCK

Type	Cause
Anaphylactic	Life-threatening allergic reaction to a substance; can occur from insect stings or from foods or drugs
Cardiogenic	Failure of the heart to effectively pump blood to all parts of the body; occurs with heart attack or cardiac arrest
Hypovolemic	Severe lack of blood and fluid in the body
Neurogenic	Failure of nervous system to control size of blood vessels, causing them to dilate; occurs with brain or nerve injuries
Psychogenic	Factors such as emotional stress cause blood to pool in the body in areas away from the brain because of vessels dilating
Respiratory	Failure of the lungs to transfer sufficient oxygen into the bloodstream; occurs with breathing emergencies or respiratory arrest
Septic	Poisons caused by severe infections that cause blood vessels to dilate

be helpful to know that there are different ways in which people can develop shock. Each causes a decrease in the amount of blood that effectively circulates in the body. Regardless of the cause, when the body cells receive inadequate oxygen, it triggers shock.

You learned in Chapter 4 that the heart pumps blood by contracting and relaxing in a consistent, rhythmic pattern. The heart adjusts its speed and the force of its contractions to meet the body's changing demands for oxygen. For instance, when a person exercises, the heart beats faster and more forcefully because the working muscles demand more oxygen (Figure 10–1).

NOTE:

Hypovolemic shock is also commonly caused by dehydration and is the most common cause of shock in children.

Similarly, when someone suffers a severe injury or sudden illness that affects the flow of blood, the heart beats faster and stronger at first, to adjust to the increased demand for more oxygen.

Because the heart is beating faster, breathing must also speed up to meet the body's increased demands for oxygen. You can detect these changes by feeling the

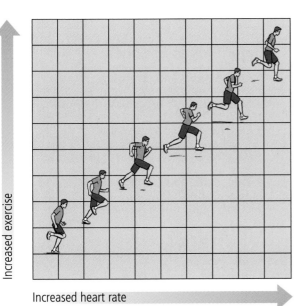

Figure 10–1 The heartbeat changes to meet the body's demand for oxygen.

pulse and listening to breathing when you check vital signs during the secondary survey.

For the heart to do its job properly, an adequate amount of blood must circulate within the body. The body can compensate for some decrease in blood volume. Consider what happens when you donate blood. You can lose 500 mL (17 oz.) of blood over a 10- to 15-minute period without any real stress to the body. Fluid is reabsorbed from the kidneys, lungs, and intestines to replace lost fluid. The body immediately begins to manufacture the blood's solid components. With severe injuries involving greater or more rapid blood loss, the body may not be able to adjust adequately. Body cells do not receive enough oxygen, and shock occurs.

For the circulatory system to function properly, blood vessels must remain intact to maintain blood volume. Normally, blood vessels decrease or increase the flow of blood to different areas of the body by constricting (decreasing their diameter) or dilating (increasing their diameter). This ability ensures that blood reaches the areas of the body that need it most, such as the vital organs. Injuries or illnesses, especially those that affect the brain and spinal cord, can cause blood vessels to lose this ability to change size, causing a drop in blood volume (Figure 10–2). Blood vessels can also be affected if the nervous system is damaged by infections, drugs, or poisons.

Regardless of the cause, a significant decrease in blood volume affects the function of the heart. The heart will eventually fail to beat rhythmically. The pulse will become irregular or be absent altogether. With some irregular heart rhythms, blood does not circulate at all.

When shock occurs, the body attempts to prioritize its needs for blood by ensuring adequate flow to the vital organs. The body does this by reducing the amount of blood circulating to the less important tissues of the arms, legs, and skin. This is why the skin of a person in shock appears pale and feels cool. When checking capillary refill, you may find it to be slow. In later stages of shock, the skin, especially on the lips and around the eyes, may appear blue from a prolonged lack of oxygen. Increased sweating is also a natural reaction to stress caused by injury or illness, which makes the skin feel moist.

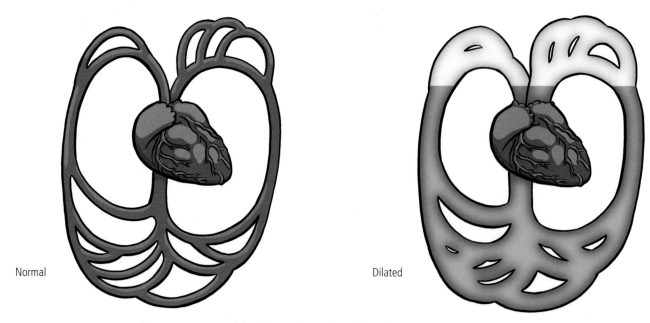

Normal   Dilated

Figure 10–2 Injury or illness can cause blood vessels to lose their ability to change size, causing a drop in blood volume.

Signs and Symptoms of Shock

Although you may not always be able to determine the cause, remember that shock is a life-threatening condition. You should learn to recognize its signs and symptoms (Figure 10–3).

People in shock usually show many of the same signs and symptoms. A common one is restlessness or irritability. This is often the first indicator that the body is experiencing a significant problem. More clearly recognizable signs are pale, cool, moist skin; rapid breathing (tachypnea); a rapid and weak pulse; and changes in the level of consciousness. Often a recognizable symptom is nausea. Conditions that affect blood volume or cause the blood vessels to work improperly can cause significant changes in blood pressure.

Later Stages of Shock

- Listlessness and confusion
- Slow, shallow, irregular breathing
- Decreasing blood pressure
- Rapid but weak and irregular pulse
- Pale, cold, and clammy skin
- Lower than normal blood pressure
- Dilated pupils

Figure 10–3 The signs and symptoms of shock may not be obvious immediately.

Shock: The Domino Effect

- An injury causes severe bleeding.

- The heart attempts to compensate for the disruption of blood flow by beating faster, which causes a rapid pulse in the injured person. This causes more blood to be lost, and as blood volume drops, the pulse becomes weak or hard to find.

- The increased workload on the heart results in an increased oxygen demand. Therefore, breathing becomes faster.

- To maintain circulation of blood to the vital organs, blood vessels in the arms and legs and in the skin constrict. Therefore, the skin appears pale and feels cool. In response to the stress, the body perspires heavily and the skin feels moist.

- Since tissues of the arms and legs are now without oxygen, cells start to die. The brain now sends a signal to return blood to the arms and legs in an attempt to balance blood flow between these body parts and the vital organs.

- Vital organs are now without adequate oxygen. The heart tries to compensate by beating even faster. More blood is lost, and the person's condition worsens.

- Without oxygen, the vital organs fail to function properly. As the brain is affected, the person becomes restless and drowsy and eventually loses consciousness. As the heart is affected, it beats irregularly, resulting in an irregular pulse. The rhythm then becomes chaotic, and the heart fails to pump blood. There is no longer a pulse. When the heart stops, breathing stops.

- The body's continuous attempt to compensate for severe blood loss eventually results in death.

If the patient does not show the telltale signs and symptoms of specific injury or illness, such as the persistent chest pain of heart attack or obvious external bleeding, it can be difficult to know what is wrong. Remember, you do not have to identify the specific nature of illness or injury to provide care that may help save the patient's life. If the signs and symptoms of shock are present, assume that there is a potentially life-threatening injury or illness.

Care for Shock

After your scene survey, do a primary survey by checking the ABCs. Caring for life-threatening conditions, such as severe bleeding, will minimize the effects of shock. If you do not find any life-threatening conditions, perform a secondary survey. During the secondary survey, the signs and symptoms of shock will most likely become evident. Always follow the general care steps you learned in Chapter 5 for any emergency:

- Assess the ABCs and provide care for any airway, breathing, or circulation problem you find (Figure 10–4, a).

- Provide care for specific conditions.

- Help the patient rest comfortably. This is important because pain can intensify the body's stress and accelerate the progression of shock. Helping the patient rest in a more comfortable position may minimize the pain. Often having the patient lay down will increase blood flow to the vital organs, especially the brain.

- Help the patient maintain normal body temperature (Figure 10–4, b).

- Provide ongoing survey and care.

The general care you provide in any emergency will always help the patient's body adjust to the stresses imposed by any injury or illness, thus reducing the effects of shock.

Figure 10–4, a-b Care for shock includes: **a**, providing care for the ABCs; and **b**, helping the patient maintain a normal body temperature.

You can further help the patient manage the effects of shock if you:

• Control any external bleeding as soon as possible to minimize blood loss.

• Administer oxygen if the equipment is available.

• Avoid giving the patient anything to eat or drink, even though she is likely to be thirsty. The patient's condition may be severe enough to require surgery, in which case, it is better for her to have an empty stomach.

• Obtain more advanced medical care. Shock cannot be managed effectively by emergency care alone.

SUMMARY

Do not wait for shock to develop before providing care to a patient with an injury or sudden illness. Always provide prompt care to minimize the effects of shock. Care for life-threatening conditions, such as breathing problems or severe external bleeding, before caring for lesser injuries. Remember that the key to managing shock effectively begins with recognizing a situation in which shock may develop and giving appropriate care.

Remember that shock is a factor in serious injuries and illnesses, particularly if there is blood loss or if the normal function of the heart is interrupted. You cannot always prevent shock by administering emergency care, but you can usually slow its progress. Advanced medical care must be obtained immediately if there are signs and symptoms of shock.

While you are assisting the driver, the passenger starts to vomit. What do you do?

Chapter 11

Pharmacology

You arrive at the home of a six-year-old girl. Her mother tells you that she has asthma and has been having difficulty breathing all afternoon. You can hear wheezes on exhalation and see that she is getting worse. The girl appears frightened. When you assess her, you find she has very low oxygen saturation and her chest appears larger than normal. Her mother hands you her inhaler and tells you it's her Ventolin®. What do you do?

INTRODUCTION

A young woman is in shock following a sports injury and needs oxygen. A man is having an anaphylactic reaction to a bee sting and needs assistance using his epinephrine auto-injector. Responders are often called upon to help give or administer medications. These medications come in several types and forms and are administered by different routes and in different doses, depending on the circumstance (Figure 11–1). Responders must understand how these drugs work, when to use them, how to use them, and what side effects they may cause.

INTRODUCTION TO BASIC PHARMACOLOGY

Pharmacology is the study of drugs and how they interact with the body. Drugs do not confer any new properties on cells. They can be given locally or be systemic. They tend to have actions at multiple sites, so they need to be thought of systemically even if administered locally.

Generally, all medications have indications, contraindications, and side effects to their administration. Indications are conditions that make administration of the drug appropriate. Contraindications are conditions that make administration of the drug inappropriate due to potential harmful effects. Side effects are any reactions to the drug other than the contraindication. Indicated drugs may have side effects, but the benefit of administering the drug is greater than the potential complications of the side effects.

The following protocols have been developed for use by responders in applicable provinces and territories. This set of assessment models, treatment principles, and protocols reflects the accepted medical practice for responders in applicable provinces and territories. Each protocol follows the current direction of the medical community, taking into consideration the limitations and special circumstances that may exist in pre-hospital care environments.

Protocols allow the responder to perform medical procedures that are normally in the domain of a physician. This allows for the initiation of care that patients would otherwise not receive until they arrived at a medical facility.

Figure 11–1 Medications come in several forms including tablets, capsules, powders, liquids, creams, and aerosol sprays.

QUALIFICATIONS REQUIRED TO ADMINISTER SPECIFIC MEDICATIONS

Medications can be beneficial but can also be dangerous if used incorrectly. Specialized training is required for those assigned to administer medications. This is particularly important for medications that are administered through an intravenous line (IV) or injection. Under certain circumstances and/or under medical direction, you may be able to provide a health product to a patient or to assist a patient with her own prescription medication. Medications require medical direction before they are administered to a patient.

> **NOTE:**
>
> *Administering medications through an intravenous (IV) line is an advanced skill and is performed at a higher level of care (i.e., a paramedic) than at the responder level.*

GUIDELINES FOR MEDICATION ADMINISTRATION

When administering or assisting a patient with medication, the responder has a responsibility to know the medication's potential effects and side effects as well as the actions with which the patient should be assisted. (Responders are responsible for ensuring that they have knowledge of the drug, what it can do, and the appropriate circumstances in which it can be administered.)

General Guidelines for Assisting with Medications

When administering or assisting a patient with medication, the responder should use proper technique, know how to observe drug effects, and take careful drug histories for the patient. Prior to having the patient take any medication, it is the responder's responsibility to ensure that the Six Rights of Medication administration have been met:

1. **Right person.** Make sure the person getting the medication is the one whose name is on the label of the medicine container.

2. **Right medication.** Read the label of the medication.

3. **Right dosage.** Use an accurately marked measuring container (if applicable).

4. **Right time.** Give the medication at the right time.

5. **Right route.** Read the directions carefully and administer with the correct method.

6. **Right documentation.** Completely document all of your care, including:

   • Time

   • Dose

   • Route

   • Effect

Also check the medication's colour, clarity (no particles), and concentration and that it hasn't expired. Observe carefully and document any side effects other than those indicated for the drug administered, if any. Always follow local protocol.

DRUG TERMINOLOGY

Addiction: A strong dependence on a drug; it may be physiological, psychological, or both, and it may be due to a decreased response to a drug with repeated use.

Antagonists: Drugs that combine with a receptor to prevent a response.

Contraindication: A medical or physiological factor that makes it harmful to administer a medication that would otherwise have therapeutic value.

Depressant: A substance that decreases a body function or activity.

Drug allergy: A systemic reaction to a drug resulting from previous sensitizing exposure and the development of an immunological mechanism.

Drug interaction: A modification, which can be beneficial or detrimental, of the effects of one drug by the prior or concurrent administration of another drug, thereby increasing or decreasing the pharmacological or physiological action of one or both drugs.

DRUG NAMES

Each drug has several names. The two most important are the generic name and the trade name.

Chemical name: A precise description of the drug's chemical composition and molecular structure (e.g., acetylsalicylic acid [Aspirin®]).

Generic name (also known as **non-proprietary name**): An abbreviated form of the chemical name of the drug. Generic medications usually have the same therapeutic efficacy as the non-generic medication and are generally less expensive (e.g., meperidine hydrochloride [Demerol]).

Trade name (also known as **brand name** or **proprietary name**): A copyrighted name designated by the drug company that owns the license to the medication. Trade names of drugs are considered to be proper nouns and therefore the first letter is capitalized (e.g., Demerol).

Official name: Followed by the initials "USP" or "NF," this name denotes the medication's listing in one of the official publications; it is usually the same as the generic name (e.g., meperidine hydrochloride USP).

Indications: The conditions that make administration of a drug appropriate.

Potentiation: The enhancing effect of one drug on another drug when administered together.

Side effect: An often unavoidable effect of using a drug; an action or effect other than those for which the drug was originally given.

Synergism: The combined action of two drugs such that the total effect exceeds the sum of the individual effects of each agent (e.g., 1 + 1 = 3).

Therapeutic action: The desired, intended action of a drug.

NOTE:

Information provided in these drug profiles is generic. In any conflict in data between your protocols and the drug profile, your protocol will take precedence. For example, those items currently listed as precautions in the nitrous oxide protocol are not reflected as precautions in the drug profile.

SPECIFIC DRUG PROFILES

Ipratropium Bromide (Atrovent®)

Classification: Anticholinergic, bronchodilator.

Mechanism: Anticholinergic (parasympatholytic) agent that inhibits vagally mediated reflexes by blocking the action of acetylcholine, the transmitter released from the vagus nerve.

Indications: Bronchospasm associated with COPD. To be used either alone or in combination with other bronchodilators, especially beta-adrenergics (e.g., albuterol).

Contraindications: Ipratropium bromide is contraindicated in known or suspected cases of hypersensitivity to ipratropium bromide or to atropine and its derivatives.

Precautions: Should be used with caution in people with narrow-angle glaucoma.

Adverse Effects: Respiratory: coughing, sputum increased; Nervous: dizziness, insomnia, tremor, nervousness; Gastrointestinal: nausea.

Doses and Routes of Administration: Nebulizer: Give 0.25–0.5 mg in 2.5 mL normal saline (one-unit dose vial) via small volume nebulizer (SVN) with a mouthpiece. Repeat according to medical control preference. Many medical protocols mix one-unit dose vial of ipratropium with one-unit dose vial of albuterol. MDI: The "puffer" supplies 0.02 mg per puff; used with a spacer; dosage is typically two puffs.

Onset: 5 to 15 minutes.

Peak Effects: 60 to 120 minutes.

Duration: 240 to 480 minutes.

Dosage Forms/Packaging: Inhalation solution unit dose vial is supplied as a 0.02% clear, colourless solution containing 2.5 mL with 25 vials per foil pouch.

Notes: Anticholinergics produce preferential dilatation of the larger central airways, in contrast to beta agonists, which affect the peripheral airways. May be more effective used in combination with beta agonists. Should be kept out of light in a foil pouch; avoid excessive humidity. Ipratropium bromide is an assist medication for people with shortness of breath due to asthma. Responders are to assist patients in taking their metered-dose inhaler.

Epinephrine Hydrochloride (Adrenaline "EPI", EpiPen®)

Classification: Sympathomimetic; natural catecholamine with alpha and beta effects.

Mechanism: Stimulates alpha- and beta-adrenergic receptors within the sympathetic nervous system.

Beta effects include:

- Increased heart rate
- Increased cardiac output
- Increased AV conduction
- Increased irritability
- Bronchodilation

Alpha effects include peripheral vasoconstriction at higher doses.

Indications: Bronchospasm, anaphylaxis, severe cardiac dysrhythmias as in asystole or ventricular fibrillation to increase the success of defibrillation.

Contraindications: None in cardiac arrest, known allergies.

Precautions: Extreme caution when treating someone for bronchospasm if patient has concurrent cardiovascular disease, narrow-angle glaucoma, caution in pregnancy (may decrease placental blood flow and can induce labour), caution with pre-existing tachycardias.

Adverse Effects: Respiratory: pulmonary edema (rare), dyspnea (rare); Nervous: nervousness, tremor, anxiety, headache, cerebral hemorrhage, agitation; Circulatory: tachycardia, ventricular fibrillation, palpitations, widened pulse pressure, hypertension, stroke, anginal pain; Integumentary: pallor, sweating, necrosis due to vascoconstriction.

Doses and Routes of Administration:

Cardiac arrest: 1.0 mg bolus IV 1:10,000 q 3 minutes.

Bronchospasm: 0.005 mg/kg SC 1:1,000 q 3 minutes to effect.

Anaphylaxis: 0.005 mg/kg SC 1:1,000 one dose; call medical director for repeat doses.

Severe, life-threatening bronchospasm, anaphylaxis: 0.2 mg IV 1:10,000; maximum total dosage IV is 0.5 mg.

ET 1:10,000 solution via ET tube (follow ET drug administration guidelines).

Onset: IV: 1 to 2 minutes; SC: 5 to 10 minutes.

Duration: 5 to 10 minutes.

Note: Epinephrine is an assist medication for patients with anaphylaxis (Figure 11–2).

Nitroglycerin

Classification: Antianginal, vasodilator.

Mechanism: Reduces cardiac oxygen demand primarily by dilating blood vessels, resulting in decreased blood flow (preload) to the heart from the body and decreased resistance to the heart's pumping (after load). Dilation of coronary arteries results in increased blood flow to cardiac tissue.

Figure 11–2 EpiPen®.

Indications: For cardiac chest pain when patient has his own nitroglycerin and a systolic pressure of above 100. (Must take baseline set of vital signs.)

Contraindications: Systolic BP less than or equal to 100 mmHg, known allergy or sensitivity to nitrates, if person has used Viagra® or Levitra® in the past 24 hours or Cialis® in the past 48 hours.

Precautions: Hypotension frequently occurs, especially in older adults, and must be expected. Therefore, ensure that the patient is not at risk of falling; administer while patient is sitting or lying down. Repeat check of vital signs and dosing of drug until pain is relieved, to a maximum of three doses (provided the systolic BP remains above 100, irrespective of any nitroglycerin taken by the patient prior to your arrival), or follow local protocol. If the patient has used Viagra® at any time in the past (beyond the 24-hour contraindication limit), there may be some cause for very careful monitoring of the patient's blood pressure.

Adverse Effects: Induces hypotension, dizziness, weakness, headache, nausea, vomiting, syncope, tachycardia, and tingling or burning under the tongue.

Onset, Doses, and Routes of Administration: Rapid onset via sublingual route (60 seconds) with 30-minute duration. Dose depends on strength of patient's prescription. Sublingual tablets are typically 0.3 or 0.6 mg with 0.3 mg being more common. In Canada, the spray is 0.4 mg/spray. Responders are to give one dose (q 5 min) to a maximum of three doses in any 30-minute period, based on local medical protocol.

Nitroglycerin comes in forms other than spray and/or tablet (Figure 11–3), none of which are approved for responder use. If the patient in your care has a nitroglycerin patch applied, it does not change the nitroglycerin protocol.

Metabolism: Rapidly metabolized in the body by the liver and excreted by the kidneys.

Notes: Nitroglycerin is an assist medication for patients suffering from ischemic chest pain. Responders are to assist patients in taking their nitro spray. If pain is completely relieved for more than five minutes, you may initiate the chest pain protocol again if the pain returns. This is considered a new episode, and a total of three additional doses of nitroglycerin can be given. This is applicable even if three nitroglycerin doses were already administered during the initial episode.

Acetylsalicylic Acid (ASA) (Novasen®, Aspirin®, Bufferin®)

Classification: Salicylate, antiplatelet, antipyretic, anti-inflammatory, non-opioid analgesic.

Mechanism: At low doses, it acts as an anticoagulant and impedes clotting by blocking prostaglandin synthesis, which prevents formation of platelet-aggregating substance thromboxane A2 (this is irreversible and can prolong bleeding time). As an analgesia/anti-inflammatory, it inhibits the synthesis of prostaglandin, preventing or reducing pain. As an antipyretic, it acts on the hypothalamus to produce peripheral vasodilation, causing sweating, which leads to heat loss and cooling by evaporation.

Indications: Acute coronary syndromes suggestive of an acute myocardial infarction.

Contraindications: Hypersensitivity, such as known severe allergy; in patient with a bleeding disorder (hemophilia, von Willebrand disease), if patient is unconsciousness.

Precautions: Use caution in patient with an active ulcer disease or asthma; impaired renal and hepatic function; may produce bronchoconstriction in asthmatics; in children and adolescents with influenza or chickenpox infections (may increase the risk of Reye's syndrome, which is a rare but serious childhood illness that has a mortality rate of 20–30%).

Doses and Routes of Administration: For an adult, 160–325 mg orally, chewed as soon as possible.

Figure 11–3 Nitroglycerin.

Note: ASA should be given even if patient has already taken ASA (however, doses higher than 1,000 mg may limit beneficial effect).

Nitrous Oxide (Entonox®)

Classification: Analgesic.

Mechanism: Inhalation of a 50% mixture of nitrous oxide and oxygen produces central nervous system depression and rapid pain relief. Analgesic works specifically on the central nervous system.

Indications: Relief of moderate to severe pain from any cause, such as acute myocardial infarction, musculoskeletal trauma, burns, other indications (e.g., urethral colic, labour).

Contraindications: Any altered level of consciousness such as head injury (masks neurological signs you need to monitor), chronic obstructive pulmonary disease, acute pulmonary edema (these patients require 100% oxygen), known pneumothorax or chest injury (nitrous oxide collects and expands in dead air spaces), abdominal distension (absent bowel sounds), major facial trauma (impairs ability to use mouthpiece), shock, decompression sickness, air embolism, ingestion of a depressant drug, cyanosis develops during administration, air transportation, usage in an enclosed area with no ventilation, patient has taken nitroglycerin within the last five minutes, inhalation injury with O_2 saturation of less than 100%.

Precautions: Improper Storage: Separation of N_2O_2 and O_2 where N_2O_2 rises to the top of the cylinder; always tip the cylinder back and forth prior to using. Separation occurs when the tank is stored below –6°C (21.2°F), gas is stagnant over a long period of time, or the tank has been stored in a vertical position. Combustible: Supports combustion. Inhalation by responder: Affects responder's competency in caring for people and driving ability. Dependence: Nitrous oxide is addictive.

Adverse Effects: There are nine common adverse effects in the use of nitrous oxide: aggravation of middle ear (increases pressure), drowsiness, nausea, vomiting, giddiness, dizziness, amnesia, decreased level of consciousness, and decreased cardiac output.

Dose: Self-administered. As the patient becomes drowsy, the mask or mouthpiece will drop away from the patient's face. Patient controls pain until pain is relieved.

Oral Glucose

Classification: Carbohydrate caloric.

Mechanism: Absorbed into the bloodstream, resulting in increased blood glucose levels, thereby providing an increased level of glucose for use by cells.

Indications: For some jurisdictions, oral glucose gel is indicated for someone with a known diabetic history and altered level of consciousness.

Contraindications: If airway management cannot be maintained, oral glucose is contraindicated.

Precautions: Patient must be placed semi-prone prior to administration; if this position cannot be achieved due to other complications, administration is contraindicated due to the possibility of causing aspiration.

Adverse Effects: May increase airway management problems.

Onset, Doses, and Routes of Administration: Via the buccal/sublingual route, glucose is absorbed slowly into the bloodstream. Responders administer approximately 12 g prior to transport. In approximately three to five minutes, responder should administer another dosage of approximately 12 g of oral glucose inside the lower cheek, again being cautious of the patient's airway. The effects of oral glucose are not immediate.

Figure 11–4 Oral glucose.

Notes: Place gel into a dependent buccal pouch (lower cheek). Administer half a tube of oral glucose at a time. A number of different brands of oral glucose containing 25 g of 40% dextrose are available on the market (Figure 11–4). Using a tongue depressor may help with administration. Document the time, route (oral), dose, and result. Oral glucose can be given by the responder to patients with hypoglycemia who are alert and able to follow commands.

Oxygen

Classification: Oxidizing agent (gas).

Description: Oxygen is an odourless, colourless, tasteless gas and is essential for life (Figure 11–5).

Indications: Hypoxia or anticipated hypoxia or in any patient with a medical problem or in a trauma situation to improve respiratory efficiency.

Contraindications: There are no contraindications to oxygen administration.

Precautions: In patients with COPD and very prolonged administration of high concentrations in a newborn.

Doses and Routes of Administration: Varies with route used.

Figure 11–5 Oxygen.

Calculating How Long an Oxygen Cylinder Will Last

Oxygen cylinder size is designated with a letter. If you know the size of your oxygen cylinder and the reading on the pressure gauge, you can calculate how long the supply will last. There are various protocols as to when to change your tank; however, in all cases, 200 psi is known as the safe residual pressure, and the tank should always be changed around this point.

The calculation is as follows:

$$\text{Duration of flow} = \frac{(\text{gauge pressure} - 200\ \text{psi}) \times C}{\text{Flow rate (L/min)}}$$

Where C = the cylinder constant

The constants for each size of cylinder are:

D cylinder = 0.16 L/psi

E cylinder = 0.28 L/psi

M cylinder = 1.56 L/psi

Salbutamol, Albuterol (Ventolin®)

Classification: Bronchodilator, sympathomimetic.

Mechanism: Relaxes the smooth muscles of the bronchial tree and the peripheral vasculature by stimulating beta-adrenergic receptors of the sympathetic nervous system. The action of this medication is relatively selective, affecting primarily the beta^2 receptors, however, beta^1-adrenergic receptors are also stimulated. As the dose of the drug is increased, the more beta^1 effects are produced.

Indications: Respiratory distress with bronchospasm; bronchospasm in anaphylaxis.

Contraindications: Known sensitivity or allergy.

Precautions: Caution in children; caution in patients sensitive to sympathomimetic amines; caution in patients with myocardial insufficiency, dysrhythmia, hypertension, diabetes mellitus, or thyrotoxicosis; should not be used concurrently with other beta-adrenergic drugs, such as isoproterenol; safety in pregnancy not firmly established.

Adverse Effects: Respiratory: coughing, bronchospasm; Nervous: restlessness, apprehension, tremor, dizziness, headache; Circulatory: palpitations, blood pressure changes, tachycardia, dysrhythmias—cardiac arrest, chest discomfort; Gastrointestinal: nausea; Skin: pallor, flushing, sweating.

Doses and Routes of Administration: Nebulizer: Give 2.5–5.0 mg in 2.5 mL normal saline (one-unit dose vial) via small volume nebulizer (SVN) with a mouthpiece.

Repeat according to medical control preference. Many medical protocols mix a one-unit dose vial of ipratropium with a one-unit dose vial of albuterol. MDI: 4–6 puffs of 0.1 mg per puff.

Onset: 5 to 10 minutes for maximum effect.

Duration: 3 to 4 hours (half-life of 2.7 to 5 hours).

Metabolism: Metabolized in liver into inactive metabolites.

Notes: Careful charting of air entry, lung sounds, degree of respiratory distress, and use of accessory muscles should be done pre- and post-treatment. Salbutamol is an assist medication for patients with shortness of breath due to asthma. Responders are to assist patients in taking their metered-dose inhaler (Figure 11–6).

Figure 11–6 Salbutamol, albuterol (Ventolin®).

ROUTES OF DRUG ADMINISTRATION

Enteral Administration

Enteral administration of drugs includes the following routes (Figure 11–7):

- Oral:
  - Easiest, safest, and most common form
  - Solid drugs must first dissolve before absorption
  - Patient must be able to control his own airway
- Sublingual:
  - Medications are delivered under the tongue and are rapidly absorbed into the blood
  - Are not to be swallowed or inhaled
- Buccal:
  - Drug is placed between the cheek and the gum and is absorbed across mucous membranes
  - Not common in a pre-hospital setting
- Rectal:
  - Not common but can be beneficial
  - Suppositories are solid at room temperature and dissolve with body heat
  - Liquids can be instilled with a syringe

Parenteral Administration

Parenteral administration of drugs includes the following routes:

- Intravenous:
  - Drug administered directly into the vein
  - Requires an IV line to be started (aseptic technique)
- Endotracheal:
  - Common in a pre-hospital setting for specific medications
  - Restricted to advanced life support (ALS) practitioners
- Intramuscular:
  - Good absorption due to rich blood supply of muscle tissue

Figure 11–7 Routes of drug administration.

  - Volume given must be carefully assessed based on patient's size and site of administration
- Subcutaneous:
  - Administered above the muscle, below the skin
  - Small volumes and slower onset than intramuscular (IM)
- Inhalation:
  - Rapid onset if drug reaches lower airways and passes into general circulation

PHARMACOKINETICS

Pharmacokinetics is the study of how the body handles a drug over a period of time, including:

- Drug absorption
- Drug distribution
- Biotransformation
- Excretion

Drug Absorption

Absorption involves the movement of drug molecules from the site of entry to the general circulation. Variables that affect drug absorption include:

- Blood flow to the site of administration
- Solubility of the drug
- pH
- Drug concentration
- Dosage form
- Route of drug administration

Drug Distribution

Distribution is the transport of a drug through the bloodstream to various tissues of the body and ultimately to its site of action. The rate of distribution depends on the permeability of the capillaries to the drug molecules. Cardiac output and regional blood flow also affect the rate and extent of distribution.

Biotransformation

Biotransformation is the process by which a drug is chemically converted to a metabolite. Its purpose is to "detoxify" a drug and render it less active. The liver is the primary site of drug metabolism. If drug metabolism is delayed, drug accumulation and cumulative drug effects may occur.

Excretion

Excretion is the elimination of toxic or inactive metabolites. The organs of excretion include the kidneys, intestines, lungs, sweat and salivary glands, and mammary glands.

PHARMACODYNAMICS

Pharmacodynamics is the theory of drugs and the mechanism of their actions. Most drugs produce their effects in one of the following ways:

- Drug-receptor interaction (lock-and-key mechanism)
- Agonists
- Antagonists
- Affinity
- Efficacy
- Types of receptors
- Drug-enzyme interaction
- Non-specific drug interaction

Drug-Receptor Interaction

Most drug actions result from a chemical interaction between the drug and various receptors throughout the body. The most common form of drug action is the drug-receptor interaction. Most drugs are thought to bind to drug receptors to produce their desired effect.

Many drugs used in the pre-hospital setting directly or indirectly affect the nervous system, often the autonomic nervous system (ANS). The sympathetic division of the ANS prepares the body for stress and emergencies. Epinephrine is one of the chemical messengers released by the sympathetic division. It can act on three different receptor types:

Factors That Influence the Actions of Drugs

The following factors can influence the actions of drugs:

- Age
- Body mass
- Sex
- Environment
- Time of administration
- Pathological state
- Genetic factors
- Psychological factors

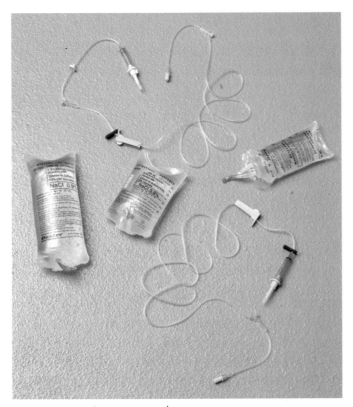

Figure 11–8 Intravenous therapy.

1. Alpha[1] receptors: When stimulated, they cause peripheral vasoconstriction.

2. Beta[1] receptors: When stimulated, they cause increased heart rate and increased force of cardiac contraction.

3. Beta[2] receptors: When stimulated, they cause bronchodilation.

The parasympathetic division of the ANS is designed to rest and restore the body to normal conditions. Parasympathetic receptors are called cholinergic receptors; when stimulated, they cause decreased heart rate and bronchodilation.

INTRAVENOUS (IV) THERAPY

- Intravenous administration is an advanced skill.

- As a responder, you are expected to maintain IV therapy in specific cases, such as patient transport.

- At times you may be asked to either set up a peripheral IV line, replace a solution bag, or to prepare an IV line (Figure 11–8).

To Set Up a Peripheral Intravenous Line

- Inspect the solution and packaging prior to assembling the drip set.

- Confirm and assemble the appropriate drip set and "lock off" the line.

- Hold the solution bag inverted and remove the protective cap on the port using the aseptic technique.

- Support the inverted solution bag and insert the spiked end of the IV drip chamber into the port with a straight push.

- Place the solution bag in the proper vertical position, and squeeze the drip chamber to fill it ½ to ⅔ full.

- Release the line lock, and purge air from the line.

- Confirm the indicated solution is flowing, then lock off the line.

- Once IV therapy has been initiated, adjust until the correct flow rate is achieved.

Crystalloid Solution Types:

- Normal saline: a 0.9% sodium chloride solution, an isotonic volume expander

- Dextrose: 3.3 % and sodium chloride 0.3 % (⅔ and ⅓)

- Ringer's lactate: A solution containing sodium chloride, potassium chloride, calcium chloride, and sodium lactate in distilled water

- D5W: 5% dextrose in water

Indications: Where an intravenous (IV) has already been established, the responder may be required to monitor it as per medical direction or oversight.

Calculating Flow Rates: To calculate flow rates for infusion of IV fluids, use the following formula:

$$\text{gtt*/min} = \frac{\text{volume to be infused} \times \text{gtt/mL of administration set}}{\text{Total time of infusion (in minutes)}}$$

*gtt = drops

NOTE:
There are two different drip chambers used in IV therapy: a micro-drip and a macro-drip. Ensure that you consider which chamber is being used when calculating the flow rate of IV fluids. In the flow rate calculation, a macro-drip has a constant of 10–15 gtt/mL and a micro-drip has a constant of 60 gtt/mL.

Changing an IV bag is indicated in the following circumstances:

- The bag is empty or has less than approximately 50 mL remaining.

- You are given instructions from the medical staff that the IV is to be changed en route during a transfer. In this circumstance, you can request that the nursing staff change the bag prior to the transfer or obtain a replacement bag from the hospital so you can change the bag en route.

- Glass solution bottles are exceptionally rare, but if a glass bottle is hanging and the patient is going on an air evacuation, you will need to change to a plastic bag so that the IV will run at high altitudes. Remember that gas expands at higher altitudes.

Follow this procedure when changing an IV bag:

1. Wash your hands and ensure aseptic technique.

2. Remove a new bag of solution from the outer wrappings and inspect it for leaks, discoloration, and the expiry date. Ensure that it has the correct contents and concentration as per hospital instructions and in accordance with the established protocols.

3. Close the flow clamp or line lock on the tubing.

4. Note how much solution remains in the old bag and invert the bag.

5. Remove the spike on the administration set from the old bag. Taking care not to contaminate the spike, remove the protective cap from the IV port on the new bag. Insert the spike into the IV port on the new bag.

6. Unlock the line and confirm the flow rate. Adjust the flow rate if necessary.

7. Document the procedure by noting the time you changed the IV bag and the amount and type of solution hung as well as the amount of solution that was discarded with the old bag. Example: 0930 (time) to 1,000 mL N/S started at 500 mL/hr/50 mL solution discarded [your signature].

Discontinuing an IV

An IV-endorsed paramedic will decide to remove an IV in the event of:

- Interstitial

- Thrombophlebitis

- Catheter embolism

- Infection at the venipuncture site (most likely will be seen on an inter-hospital transport); do not remove an IV catheter if a "do not remove" order has been given.

The procedure for discontinuing an IV is as follows:

1. Wash your hands, put on gloves, and ensure aseptic technique.

2. Gather and prepare your supplies (gauze, tape, disposable biohazard bag).

3. Turn off the flow-control clamp.

4. Remove the transparent dressing and the tape from the site when minimizing IV and catheter movement. It helps if you stabilize the hub of the catheter with one hand while removing the tape with the other.

5. Hold sterile gauze over the puncture site. Grasping the catheter by the hub, pull straight back. Do not use an alcohol swab for this procedure, as this may interfere with blood clotting and be painful for the patient.

6. Immediately apply firm pressure to the site using gauze and continue this for at least three to five minutes to stop the bleeding.

7. Once the bleeding has stopped, cover the puncture site with an adhesive bandage.

8. Inspect the catheter for completeness.

9. Document the time the IV was discontinued, the amount of solution infused, and the condition of the catheter.

Complications

In the course of monitoring an IV, several complications may arise that require intervention. Seven complications of IV administration include the following:

1. Interstitial

2. Circulatory overload

3. Thrombosis and thrombophlebitis

4. Catheter embolism

5. Infection of site

6. Allergic reaction

7. Air embolism

Interstitial

This means that the IV fluid is flowing into the surrounding tissues instead of into the vein due to complete or partial perforation of the vein through the opposite wall. This is identified by swelling around the injection site, and the skin will be cool to the touch. Flow rate may be diminished and pain may or may not be present.

Interventions:

- Once you have identified that the IV is interstitial, discontinue the IV.

- Record the time at which the IV was discontinued and the amount infused.

- If the swollen area is small, apply a cold pack.

- If the swollen area is large, apply warm, wet compresses to promote reabsorption of the fluid.

Circulatory Overload

This occurs when the patient's system is unable to manage the extra fluids administered, leading to cardiac and pulmonary complications similar to congestive heart failure or pulmonary edema. This can be caused by excessive fluid administration or rapid fluid delivery. Ensure careful monitoring of vital signs and IV flow line.

Interventions:

- Should the patient develop signs of fluid overload, immediately slow the IV rate to keep the vein open (TKVO).

- Place the patient in a semi-sitting position and apply oxygen if indicated.

- Transport the patient as quickly as possible and give the hospital notification of your arrival.

- Closely monitor the patient's vital signs en route and make sure you keep the patient warm to promote peripheral circulation.

- Document your findings, including slowing the IV rate. Someone with circulatory overload should be treated as a patient with congestive heart failure.

Thrombosis and Thrombophlebitis

Thrombosis is the formation of a clot and usually occurs at the tip of the catheter. Thrombophlebitis is inflammation of a vein due to the formation of a blood clot (thrombus = blood clot; phlebitis = inflammation of a vein).

A clot may form if:

- The IV is running too slowly.

- There is injury to the vein wall, either from the insertion or from mechanical irritation (e.g., excessive movement of the patient).

- The catheter is too large for the lumen (hollow) of the vein.

- The vein is too small to handle the amount or type of solution being administered.

- There is irritation to the vein by medications (e.g., drug infusions).

Thrombosis and thrombophlebitis can be prevented by choosing the appropriately sized vein for the gauge of catheter you are using and by ensuring that any potentially irritating medications are given through large veins with good blood flow. Keeping the infusion flowing at the established rate helps prevent the formation of a thrombus at the end of the needle. Stabilizing the IV site with an arm board or splint will prevent mechanical irritation.

Interventions:

- If thrombophlebitis develops, discontinue the IV.

- Record the time at which the IV was discontinued and the amount of fluid infused.

- Apply warm, wet compresses to decrease the pain and promote healing.

- Do not massage or rub the affected arm as this may dislodge the clot that has formed.

Catheter Embolism

This means that the catheter or a portion of it has broken off and been carried away in the bloodstream. Although rare, it can be caused by attempting to rethread the needle during insertion.

Interventions:

- Discontinue the IV but do not discard the catheter. Give the catheter to the hospital personnel for examination and follow-up.

- Record the time at which the IV was discontinued and the amount of solution infused.
- Be careful not to obstruct the arterial flow; check the distal pulse to ensure its presence.
- Apply high-flow oxygen to the patient if necessary.
- Notify the hospital and transport the patient as an emergency.

Infection of Site

You are more likely to recognize an infection when transporting a patient who already has an IV in place. The majority of infections are due to skin flora (microorganisms such as bacteria) entering the wound when the IV is started because of poor aseptic techniques. Infection is usually recognized by redness at the area, swelling of the site, or possible discharge.

Interventions:

- If possible, notify the sending facility before transporting the patient.
- Discontinue the IV and record the time.
- Document the amount of solution infused.
- Dispose of the catheter in a sterile container and give it to hospital personnel for testing.
- Dress the site with a sterile dressing and apply a warm pack.

Allergic Reaction

Caused by a hypersensitivity to an IV solution or an additive resulting in generalized rash, shortness of breath, rapid heart rate, and a drop in blood pressure.

Interventions:

- Decrease the IV rate to keep the vein open (or discontinue the IV).
- Record the time the IV rate was changed.
- Notify the hospital.
- Administer oxygen if necessary.

> **NOTE:**
>
> *Search for other substances that may have caused the reaction. If unable to find another cause for the reaction, discontinue the IV.*

Air Embolism

This can be caused by allowing an IV bag to run dry, significant air in the tubing, or loose connections between the IV tubing and the catheter or at the piggybacking sites. When setting up an IV, make sure you clear the tubing of all air bubbles. Change the IV bags before they are empty and make sure all connections are secured.

Interventions:

- Turn the patient on his left side with the head down 30°. If air has entered the heart chambers, this position may keep the air bubbles on the right side of the heart, where they can then enter the pulmonary circulation and be absorbed.
- Check the IV system for leaks.
- Administer oxygen if indicated.
- Notify the hospital and transport immediately.

> **NOTE:**
>
> *The skills noted below require specialized training and are intended only for people who provide advanced medical care.*

GUIDELINES FOR INJECTIONS

Safe administration of medications through injection requires following specific steps before, during, and after administration of the medication.

SYRINGES AND NEEDLES MUST BE USED ONLY ONCE—if disposable syringes are not available, sterilize glass syringes and needles by boiling.

The steps for safe administration of injections are:

- Medicines for injection are supplied either in rubber-capped vials or in glass ampoules.
- The use of multi-dose vials carries a risk of contamination; a new needle and syringe must always be used when drawing medicines from a multi-dose vial.
- Check that the name and strength of the medicine are marked on the vial or ampoule.
- If you cannot see or decipher the name of the medicine, discard the vial or ampoule.

- Glass ampoules may have a coloured band around the neck, indicating the level at which the top of the ampoule will break off cleanly.

- The rubber cap of a vial is held on by a metal cap with a small tear-off seal; do not remove this seal until the drug is required.

How to Give a Subcutaneous Injection

- Assemble the following items:

  - A disposable syringe

  - A 19- or 21-gauge needle for drawing the medicine into the syringe

  - A disposable 23- or 25-gauge needle for injecting the medicine

  - Alcohol swabs

  - The medicine

- If the medicine is in a multiple-dose vial, clean the rubber diaphragm on the vial with alcohol. If the medicine is in an ampoule, tap the ampoule gently with a finger to ensure that all the liquid is below the neck of the ampoule; then break off the top with a sharp snap:

  - If you are not experienced in this procedure, hold the top of the ampoule with a cloth or swab to avoid being cut by the edge of the glass.

- Remove the guard from the needle without touching the needle. If the medicine is in a vial, inject into the vial an amount of air equal to the amount of medicine to be withdrawn; this will make it easier to withdraw the medicine. Withdraw the correct amount of medicine. Change the needle to the appropriate gauge for the injection. Point the needle upward and push the plunger to expel any air in the syringe. Select a site for the injection and disinfect the skin with an alcohol swab.

- Between your thumb and forefinger, grasp a fold of skin large enough to offer plenty of space between the site of injection and your fingers. Insert the needle firmly and quickly at a 30 to 45° angle to a depth of about 2 cm (3/4 in.). Once the needle is under the skin, draw back the syringe plunger.

If no blood appears in the syringe, inject the medicine and withdraw the needle. If blood appears, repeat the procedure at a new site, using new sterile equipment. Place the needle, together with the syringe, directly into a proper sharps disposal bin.

How to Give an Intradermal Injection

- Assemble the following items:

  - A disposable syringe

  - A 19- or 21-gauge needle for drawing the medicine into the syringe

  - A disposable 25- or 27-gauge needle, only 1 to 1.6 cm (3/8 to 5/8 in.), for injecting the medicine

  - Alcohol swabs

  - The medicine

- This type of injection is usually performed on the inside of the forearm.

- If the medicine is in a multiple-dose vial, clean the rubber diaphragm on the vial with alcohol. If the medicine is in an ampoule, tap the ampoule gently with a finger to ensure that all of the liquid is below the neck of the ampoule; then break off the top with a sharp snap:

  - If you are not experienced in this procedure, hold the top of the ampoule with a cloth or swab to avoid being cut by the edge of the glass.

- Remove the guard from the needle without touching the needle. If the medicine is in a vial, inject into the vial an amount of air equal to the amount of medicine to be withdrawn; this will make it easier to withdraw the medicine. Withdraw the correct amount of medicine. Change the needle to one that is the appropriate gauge for the injection. Point the needle upward and push the plunger to expel any air in the syringe. Select a site for the injection and disinfect the skin with an alcohol swab.

- Grasp the forearm firmly in one hand, with the syringe in the other hand. With the bevel of the needle facing away from the skin, insert the needle into the skin, almost parallel with the arm (at an approximately 5 to 7° angle). Once the needle is inserted, inject the medicine and withdraw the needle. Place the needle, together with the syringe, directly into a proper sharps disposal bin.

How to Give an Intramuscular Injection

- Assemble the following items:
  - A disposable syringe
  - A disposable 19- or 21-gauge needle
  - Alcohol swabs
  - The medicine

- If the medicine is in a multi-dose vial, clean the rubber diaphragm on the vial with an alcohol swab. If the medicine is in an ampoule, tap the ampoule gently with a finger to ensure that all the liquid is below the neck of the ampoule; then break off the top with a sharp snap. Remove the guard from the needle without touching the needle. If the medicine is in a vial, inject into the vial an amount of air equal to the amount of medicine to be withdrawn in order to make withdrawal easy. Withdraw the correct amount of medicine. Expel any air from the syringe.

- Select a site for the injection: the preferred sites are the outer upper quadrant of either buttock or outer thigh muscle; do not use other parts of the buttock. In babies, use only the outer thigh muscle. Swab the skin at the injection site with alcohol swabs.

- Stretch the skin with your thumb and forefinger and, after finding the landmark, insert the needle at a right angle to the skin to a depth of about 2 cm ($^3/4$ in.), so as to penetrate the subcutaneous fat and enter the muscle (Figure 11–9).

- Draw back the syringe plunger. If no blood appears, inject the medicine and withdraw the needle. If blood appears, repeat the procedure at another site, using new sterile equipment. Place the needle, together with the syringe, directly into a proper sharps disposal bin.

Figure 11–9 Giving an intramuscular injection.

After You Have Given an Injection

- Place the needle together with the syringe directly into a proper sharps disposal bin.

- Never, under any circumstances, replace the needle guard on the needle or attempt to break the needle and syringe.

DISINFECTION

Instruments used in emergency care that pass through the skin of a patient pose an increased risk of infection for the patient. For this reason, there are certain standards to follow when disinfecting surgical instruments. Disinfectants are solutions used to inactivate any infectious agents that may be present in the blood or other bodily fluids. This will decrease the number of bacteria and viruses on an object but not sterilize it, reducing the risk to people who will be handling the objects during further cleaning and sterilization. There are various types of disinfectant solutions, which also have varying degrees of effectiveness. Sodium hypochlorite, or bleach, is one of the most common worldwide disinfectant solutions.

- Disinfectant solutions must always be available for:
  - Disinfecting working surfaces
  - Disinfecting equipment that cannot be sterilized further (such as in an autoclave, a steam-sterilization device)
  - Cleaning non-disposable items
  - Dealing with any spills involving bodily fluids or other known infectious material

- All needles and instruments should be soaked in a disinfectant solution for 30 minutes before cleaning.

- If reusable needles are to be cleaned, they must be handled very carefully and should be placed in a disinfectant before being cleaned and sterilized.

- Gloves should always be used when disinfecting equipment, especially when working with soiled materials, such as linen. Soiled linen should be put in leak-proof bags for transport. Thick gloves should be worn when needles and sharp instruments are being cleaned.

- To further clean soiled linen, wash it in cool water first; then disinfect with a diluted chlorine solution. After this, wash the linen with detergent at a temperature of at least 71°C (160°F) for 25 minutes.

- Some situations, such as a large spill of infected bodily fluid, may require higher concentrations of disinfectant, as lower concentrations of solution will actually be inactivated by the large amount of organic matter. Not only should a higher concentration be used, but the solution should stay in contact with the infected material for a longer period of time. This is known as "contact time," and it is the time the infectious material requires to become completely inactivated by the disinfectant solution.

- No matter what disinfectant solution is used, ensure it is used before its expiry date and always follow the manufacturer's or other specific guidelines for that particular solution.

SUMMARY

Administering medications requires specialized training. However, under certain circumstances and under medical direction, you may be able to provide a health product to a patient or to assist someone with taking their prescribed medication. To do so safely and effectively, it is important for you to use the proper technique, know how to observe drug effects, and take careful drug histories of the patient. It is your responsibility to ensure that the Six Rights of Medication administration have been met and to be familiar with the protocols that allow you to perform certain medical procedures. Knowing what drugs can do and the appropriate circumstances in which to use them can make the difference when attempting to save someone's life.

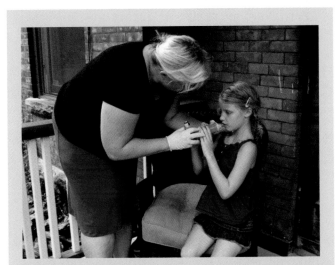

As you try to help the girl take her Ventolin®, she pushes away the spacer and resists the medication. What do you do?

Part *3*

Traumatic Injuries

INTRODUCTION

Several pairs of figure-skating partners are on the ice, practising for the championships. Pairs perform all types of spins, step sequences, and jumps. One of the men performs a throw jump, in which he throws his partner into a jump, and she bumps into another skater, slashing his leg with her blade. The injured skater cries out and falls to the ice, gripping his leg, which is bleeding badly. All the skaters skate to his side, horrified, and look around for help.

You go out onto the ice to help him. As you do, thoughts and questions rush through your mind: "Will I be able to control the bleeding? I'll need to obtain advanced medical care. Who can help? How will I make sure bystanders don't slow my care? I must act quickly to avoid complications."

Injury is a leading cause of death and disability in people aged 1 to 44 years. It greatly surpasses all major disease groups (cancer, heart disease, stroke) as a cause of death and disability in this age group. Injury is the leading reason for people to contact physicians and the most common cause of hospitalization among people under 45 years old. Statistics indicate that most people will have a significant injury at some time in their life. Some, because of their chosen professions, are more likely to be injured than others.

INJURIES

How Injuries Occur

The body has a natural resistance to injury. However, when certain external forms of energy produce forces that the body cannot tolerate, injuries occur. Mechanical forms of energy and the energy from heat, electricity, chemicals, and radiation can damage body tissues and disrupt normal body function. Superficial injuries include minor wounds or burns. Deep injuries include wounds caused by penetrating objects.

Some tissues, such as the soft tissues of the skin, have less resistance and are at greater risk of injury if exposed to trauma than the deeper, stronger tissues of muscle and bone. Some organs, such as the brain, heart, and lungs, are better protected by bones than other organs, such as those in the abdominal cavity. Understanding the forces that cause injury and the kinds of injury that each force can cause will help you recognize certain injuries someone may have.

Mechanical Energy

Mechanical energy produces the following forces: direct, indirect, twisting, and contracting. A direct force is the force of an object striking the body and causing injury at the point of impact. Direct forces can be either blunt or penetrating. For example, a fist striking the chin can break the jaw, or penetrating objects, such as bullets and knives, can injure structures beneath the skin at the point where they penetrate. Direct force can cause internal and external bleeding, head and spinal injuries, fractures, and other problems, such as crushing injuries.

An indirect force is the force of a blunt object striking the body in one body part and causing injury to another. For example, a fall on an outstretched hand may result in an injury to the arm, shoulder, or collarbone.

In twisting, one part of the body remains stationary while another part of the body turns. A sudden or severe twisting action can force body parts beyond their normal range of motion, causing injury to bones, tendons, ligaments, and muscles. For example, if a ski and its binding keep the lower leg in one position while the body falls in another, the knee may be forced beyond its normal range of motion. Twisting injuries are not always this complex. They more often occur as a result of simple actions such as stepping off a curb or turning to reach for an out-of-the-way object.

Sudden or powerful muscle contractions often result in injuries to muscles and tendons. These commonly occur in sports activities, such as throwing a ball far or hard without properly warming up or preparing your muscles. Although it happens rarely, sudden, powerful muscle contractions can even pull a piece of bone away from the point at which it is normally attached. Figure P3–1 shows how these forces can result in injuries. These four forces, products of mechanical energy, cause the majority of injuries. Soft tissue injuries and injuries to muscle and bone (musculoskeletal injuries) are most often the result.

Direct

Indirect

Twisting

Contracting

Figure P3–1 Four forces—direct, indirect, twisting, and contracting—cause the majority of all injuries.

Energy from Heat, Electricity, Chemicals, and Radiation

Together, the energy from heat, electricity, chemicals, and radiation accounts for a significant proportion of all injuries in Canada. Exposure to any of these can result in burns. Thermal burns, burns caused by heat, are the most common. Sources of electricity, such as common household current or lightning, can penetrate the body, causing external and internal damage. Electrical current can also affect the part of the brain that controls breathing and heartbeat. When certain chemicals contact the skin, they cause burns. Solar radiation from the sun's rays causes sunburn. The average person is rarely exposed to other forms of radiation.

Factors Affecting Injury

A number of factors affect the likelihood of injury—among them age, sex, geographic location, economic status, and alcohol use and abuse. The type and frequency of injuries can also be affected by fads and seasonal activities. As certain activities gain and lose popularity or as activities such as softball or skiing change with the seasons, the injury statistics reflect these changes.

Injury statistics consistently show that:

• Injury rates are higher among people under age 45.

• Males are at greater risk than females for most types of injury.

• Motor vehicle crashes are the leading cause of deaths from injuries in Canada.

Many factors influence injury statistics. Whether people live in a rural or an urban area, whether a home is built of wood or brick, the type of heat used in the home, and the climate all affect the degree of risk. Death rates from injury are typically higher in rural areas. The death rate from injuries is higher in low-income areas than in high-income areas.

The use and abuse of alcohol is a significant factor in many injuries and fatalities, even in young teenagers. The deaths of almost half of all fatally injured drivers involve alcohol, as do those of many adult passengers and pedestrians. Alcohol use also contributes to other injuries. It is estimated that a significant number of people who die as a result of falls, motor vehicle collisions,

TABLE P3–1: LEADING CAUSES OF DEATH FROM INJURIES IN CANADA (2003–2004)

Cause	Percentage
Motor vehicle collisions	38.6
Falls	34.8
Assault and purposely inflicted injury	8.2
Suicide and self-inflicted injury	5.6
Miscellaneous	4.8
Fire and flames	3.1
Motor vehicles (non-traffic)	2.1
Other road vehicles	1.1
Drowning	0.7
Natural and environmental factors	0.6
Air and water transport	0.2
Choking/suffocation	0.1
Railway	0.1

Note: Poisoning is not included in these data.

drownings, fires, assaults, and suicides have high blood alcohol concentrations.

Table P3–1 shows the leading causes of death from injuries.

Injury Prevention

Many people believe that injuries just happen—their targets are unfortunate results of circumstance. However, overwhelming evidence shows that injury, like disease, does not occur at random. Rather, many injuries are predictable, preventable events resulting from the interaction of people and hazards, whether at home, at work, or during recreation.

Preventing injuries is everyone's responsibility. As a responder, injury prevention may be part of your job.

As an athletic therapist, you are responsible for preventing athletic injuries. As an emergency team member, you may be responsible for ensuring that safety codes and regulations are met. A firefighter or police officer who supervises or instructs others may be responsible for their safety. In any event, responders should take all precautions to ensure their personal safety and to be role models of safe behaviour.

There are three general strategies for preventing injuries:

1. Persuade people to alter risky behaviour.

2. Require behaviour change by law and regulation.

3. Provide automatic protection through product and environmental design.

Laws and regulations that require you to conform to safety measures, such as wearing safety belts when driving and wearing protective clothing when on the job, are only moderately effective. The most successful injury prevention strategy is the built-in protection of product design. For instance, automatic protection, such as airbags in motor vehicles, does not require people to make choices.

Typically, people who engage in risky behaviours are the hardest to influence, regardless of whether safer behaviours are required. For example, despite the overwhelming evidence of alcohol-related injuries and fatalities, people still drink when driving and when operating equipment.

It has been estimated that if everyone worked to prevent injuries, about half of all injuries would not occur. Everyone has a personal responsibility to promote safety, both in their own life and in the lives of others. Taking the following steps could significantly reduce the risk of injury:

1. Know your injury risk.

2. Take measures that can make a difference. Adopt behaviours that decrease your risk of injury and the risk of others, both on and off the job.

3. Think safety. Be alert for and avoid potentially harmful conditions or activities that increase your injury risk or that of co-workers. Take precautions, such as wearing appropriate protective clothing—helmets, outer garments, and effective barriers—to prevent disease transmission and buckle up when driving or riding in motor vehicles.

4. Encourage others to take a Red Cross first aid course. This can decrease their risk of injury significantly.

Chapter *12*

Soft Tissue Injuries

You are dispatched to a factory workshop. A worker is screaming and gripping his right hand, which is bleeding heavily. The drill press he was using is still on. The man is red faced and begins to stagger around, leaving a trail of blood. What do you do?

INTRODUCTION

A baby falls off a couch and gets jabbed in the abdomen on the sharp corner of a glass table; a toddler grabs a knife off the counter and cuts her finger; a child gets a black eye when he's banged in the head by a swing; an adolescent gets stabbed in the chest during a gang fight; and an adult cuts her hand while working in a tool and die shop. What do these injuries have in common? They are all soft tissue injuries.

In the course of growing up and in our daily lives, soft tissue injuries occur often and in many different ways. Fortunately, most soft tissue injuries are minor, requiring little attention. Often only an adhesive bandage or ice and rest are needed. Some injuries, however, are more severe and require immediate medical attention. In this chapter, you will learn how to recognize and care for the most common type of injuries: soft tissue injuries.

Types of Soft Tissue Injuries

An injury to the soft tissues is called a wound. Soft tissue injuries are typically classified as either closed or open wounds. A wound is closed when the soft tissue damage occurs beneath the surface of the skin, leaving the outer layer intact. A wound is open if there is a break in the skin's outer layer. Open wounds usually result in external bleeding.

Burns are a special kind of soft tissue injury. A burn occurs when intense heat, caustic chemicals, electricity, or radiation contacts the skin or other body tissues. Burns are classified as either superficial, partial-thickness, or full-thickness. Superficial burns affect only the outer layer of skin. Partial-thickness burns damage both skin layers. Full-thickness burns penetrate the layers of skin and can affect other soft tissues and even bone. Burns are discussed in more detail later in this chapter.

Closed Wounds

The simplest closed wound is a bruise, also called a contusion (Figure 12–1, a-b). Contusions result when the body is subjected to a blunt force, such as when you bump your leg on a table or chair. This usually results in damage to soft tissue layers and blood vessels beneath the skin, causing internal bleeding. When blood and other fluids seep into the surrounding tissues, the area discolours and swells. The amount of discoloration and swelling varies depending on the severity of the injury. At first, the area may only appear red. Over time, more blood may leak into the area, making it appear dark red or purple. Violent forces can cause more severe soft tissue injuries involving larger blood vessels, the deeper layers of muscle tissue, and even organs deep within the body. These injuries can result in profuse internal bleeding. With deeper injuries, a responder may or may not immediately see bruising.

Crush Injury

A crush injury can occur when a crushing force is applied to any part of the body. These injuries can be severe and cause internal bleeding, fractures, and organ

a

b

Figure 12–1, a-b A bruise.

damage with the skin still intact. This type of injury may occur from force that has been applied over a short or relatively long period of time. The latter is seen most often when the injured person has been trapped with his limbs compressed for a long period of time. When the crushing object has been removed from a person, toxins that may have built up in the crushed area can be released into the bloodstream, causing further damage. Unless the object is hindering the ABCs or you are trained to remove it, leave the object in place. Allow more advanced medical personnel to remove the object or extricate the person.

NOTE:

In a remote workplace environment, leaving the object in place may not be an option. Contact advanced medical care for directives on what to do in this situation.

Compartment Syndrome

When pressure builds up to dangerous levels within the muscles, this is called compartment syndrome. The pressure blocks circulation to the cells. This can affect muscle groups in the arms, hands, legs, feet, and buttocks because they are covered by tough membranes that do not readily expand. Within the muscle compartment, swelling and/or bleeding creates pressure on capillaries and nerves. The capillaries collapse when the pressure in the compartment becomes greater than the blood pressure within the capillaries, disrupting blood flow to muscle and nerve cells. Without a steady supply of oxygen and nutrients, nerve and muscle cells begin to die within hours. Unless the pressure is relieved quickly, this syndrome can cause permanent disability or death.

Compartment syndrome can be caused by a traumatic injury, such as a fracture of one of the long bones in the body, or other conditions, such as a badly bruised muscle, complication after surgery, blockage of circulation, a crush injury, or anabolic steroid use.

Signs and Symptoms

The classic sign of compartment syndrome is pain, especially when the muscle is stretched. Other signs and symptoms may be present:

- The pain may be intensely out of proportion to the injury, especially if no bone is broken.
- There may also be a tingling or burning sensation in the muscle.
- The muscle may feel tight or full.
- If the area becomes numb or paralysis sets in, this means that cell death has begun; in this case, efforts to lower the pressure in the compartment may not be successful in restoring function to the muscle.

Acute compartment syndrome is a medical emergency requiring immediate treatment. Obtain more advanced medical care.

Blast Injuries

Blast injuries occur when pressure waves generated by an explosion strike the body surfaces. Blast injuries can occur from bombing, underwater blasts, natural gas explosions, or explosions in a mine, shipyard, or chemical plant. Blasts release large amounts of energy in the form of pressure and heat. Injuries due to the blast are almost exclusively confined to the ear, the respiratory system, and the gastrointestinal tract. As a result, injuries can include loss of hearing, pulmonary hemorrhage, pulmonary edema, pneumothorax, pulmonary embolism, abdominal hemorrhage, and bowel perforation. Thermal burns may also occur from the release of energy in the form of heat. Blast injuries may be difficult to identify because sometimes there are no visible external injuries, whereas internal injuries may be severe.

There are four mechanisms of injury resulting from blasts:

1. Injuries from the blast itself
2. Injuries from flying debris (shrapnel) from the blast
3. Trauma from being thrown by the blast
4. Injuries or illnesses caused by hazardous material being dispersed by the blast

Myocardial Contusion

The heart muscle may be bruised after blunt force to the chest (motor vehicle collision, CPR, a fall, etc.). The person may have some pain in the chest (from the blunt force) and may feel the heart racing. More advanced medical care should be obtained as the person may require monitoring over a period of time.

> ### NOTE:
> *Blood may be splashed when you are caring for a subungual hematoma. For this reason you should use PPE, such as a mask, gown, and protective eyewear, in addition to gloves.*

Subungual Hematoma

When there is a blow to a finger or toe, it frequently causes a collection of blood to form under the nail bed, and this is called a subungual hematoma. A subungual hematoma throbs and can be very painful. If the blood is released, the patient will feel some relief.

To care for a subungual hematoma:

1. Clean the area.

2. Ensure that the patient's hand is on a firm surface.

3. Use a nail drill to create a small hole in the middle of the blood pocket. If there is no nail drill available, heat the end of a paperclip until it is red hot and use it to create the hole. Because there are no nerve endings in this area, the procedure should be painless.

4. If releasing the blood does not stop the pain, you should suspect a fracture of the bones.

5. If pressure builds after a time, the hole may require reopening.

6. Clean the injured area and apply a dressing.

Open Wounds

Open wounds are injuries that break the skin. These breaks can be as minor as a scrape of the surface layers or as severe as a deep penetration. The amount of bleeding depends on the severity of the injury. Any break in the skin provides an entry point for disease-producing micro-organisms. There are four main types of open wounds:

1. Abrasions

2. Lacerations

3. Avulsions

4. Punctures

An abrasion is the most common type of open wound. It is characterized by skin that has been rubbed or scraped away (Figure 12–2, a-b). This often occurs when a person falls and scrapes his hands or knees. An abrasion is sometimes called a rug burn, or road rash. Because the scraping of the outer skin layers exposes sensitive nerve endings, an abrasion is usually painful.

a

b

Figure 12–2, a-b An abrasion.

Bleeding is easily controlled and not severe since only the capillaries are affected. Because of the way the injury occurs, dirt and other matter can easily become embedded in the skin, making it especially important to clean the wound.

A laceration is a cut, usually from a sharp object. The cut may have either jagged or smooth edges (Figure 12–3, a-b). Lacerations are commonly caused by sharp-edged objects, such as knives, scissors, or broken glass. A laceration can also result when a blunt force splits the skin. This often occurs in areas where bone lies directly under the skin's surface, such as the eyebrow. Deep lacerations can also affect the layers of fat and muscle, damaging both nerves and blood vessels. Lacerations usually bleed freely and, depending on the structures involved, can bleed profusely. Because the nerves may also be injured, lacerations are not always immediately painful.

An avulsion is an injury in which a portion of the skin and sometimes other soft tissue is partially or completely torn away (Figure 12–4, a-b). A partially avulsed piece of skin may remain attached but hangs like a flap. Bleeding is usually significant because avulsions often involve deeper soft tissue layers. Sometimes a force is so violent that a body part, such as a finger, may be severed.

A complete severing of a part is called an amputation (Figure 12–5). Although damage to the tissue is severe,

bleeding is usually not as bad as you might expect. The blood vessels usually constrict and pull in (retract) at the point of injury, slowing bleeding and making it relatively easy to control with direct pressure. With today's technology, reattachment is often successful, making it important to send the severed part to the hospital with the patient.

A puncture wound results when the skin is pierced with a pointed object such as a nail, a piece of glass, a splinter, or a knife (Figure 12–6, a-b). A bullet wound is also a puncture wound. Because the skin usually closes around the penetrating object, external bleeding is generally not severe. However, internal bleeding can be severe if the penetrating object damages major blood vessels or internal organs. An object that remains in the open wound is called an impaled object (Figure 12–7, a-b). An object may also pass completely through a body part, making two open wounds: one at the entry point and one at the exit point.

Although puncture wounds generally do not bleed profusely, they are potentially more dangerous than wounds that do because they are more likely to become infected. Objects penetrating the soft tissues carry micro-organisms that cause infections. Of particular danger is the micro-organism that causes tetanus, a severe infection.

a

b

Figure 12–3, a-b A laceration.

Figure 12–4, a-b An avulsion.

Figure 12–5 An amputation.

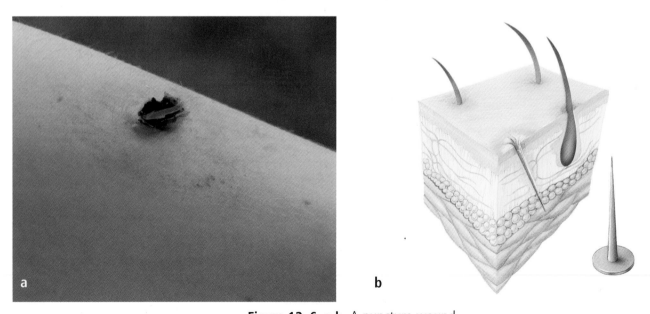

Figure 12–6, a-b A puncture wound.

a

b

Figure 12–7, a-b An impaled object.

Abscesses

An abscess is a localized collection of pus within tissues, usually in hair-bearing areas (Figure 12–8). It is also known as a boil. To care for an abscess:

1. Drain the abscess (this will occur naturally if it is left alone); draining can be hastened by local application of hot/warm compresses until the skin bursts.

2. Once the skin has burst, clean it and then apply dry dressings.

3. Continue to cleanse intermittently with antibacterial solution as necessary.

4. Do not squeeze the abscess as this will likely spread the infection deeper.

5. If the abscess involves the face, neck, groin, or buttocks or if it is very painful, seek further medical attention.

Infection

Injuries causing breaks in the skin carry great risk of infection. Since the skin tends to collect micro-organisms, injuries involving breaks in the skin can become infected unless properly cared for.

The best initial defence against infection is to cleanse the area thoroughly. For minor wounds—those that are small and do not bleed severely—wash the area with soap and water. Most soaps are effective in removing harmful bacteria. Do not use alcohol because it can damage tissues. Once washed, rinse the wound under running water for five minutes (if possible); then apply an antibiotic ointment (as long as the injured person has no allergy or sensitivities to antibiotics). Wounds that require medical attention because of more extensive tissue damage or bleeding need not be washed immediately. These wounds will be cleaned thoroughly in the medical facility as a routine part of the care. It is more important for you to control bleeding. Some

Figure 12–8 An abscess.

Tetanus

- A serious infection can cause severe medical problems. One such infection is tetanus, caused by the organism *Clostridium tetani*. This organism, commonly found in soil and the feces of cows and horses, can infect many kinds of wounds. Worldwide, tetanus kills thousands of people annually.

- Tetanus is introduced into the body through a puncture wound, abrasion, laceration, or burn. Because the organism multiplies in an environment that is low in oxygen, puncture wounds and other deep wounds are at particular risk for tetanus infection. It produces a powerful toxin, one of the most lethal poisons known, that affects the central nervous system and specific muscles. People at risk for tetanus include drug addicts, people with burns, and people recovering from surgery. Newborn babies can be infected through the stump of the umbilical cord.

- Signs and symptoms of tetanus include difficulty swallowing, irritability, headache, fever, and muscle spasms near the infected area. Later, as the infection progresses, it can affect other muscles, such as those in the jaw, causing the condition called "lockjaw." Once tetanus gets into the nervous system, its effects are irreversible.

- The best way to prevent tetanus is to be immunized against it and then receive periodic booster shots. Immunizations assist the natural function of the immune system by building up antibodies, disease-fighting proteins that help protect the body against specific bacteria. Because the effects of immunization do not last a lifetime, booster shots help maintain the antibodies that protect against tetanus. Booster shots are recommended every 5 to 10 years, whenever a wound has been contaminated by dirt, or whenever an object, such as a rusty nail, causes a puncture wound. Most children in Canada receive an immunization known as DPT, which includes the tetanus toxoid. Always contact your physician if you are unsure how long it has been since you received a tetanus immunization or booster.

- If an injury occurs, the best defence against tetanus is to thoroughly clean an open wound. Major wounds should be cleaned and treated at a medical facility. Clean a minor wound with soap and water and apply a clean or sterile dressing. If signs of wound infection develop, seek medical attention immediately. Infected wounds of the face, neck, and head should receive immediate medical care since the tetanus toxin can travel rapidly to the brain. A physician will determine whether a tetanus shot or a booster shot is needed, depending on the person's immunization status.

Gangrene

Like tetanus, gangrene is caused by bacteria that thrive in the absence of oxygen. Gangrene causes a sudden onset of pain and swelling, with local tissue discoloration and a brownish, foul-smelling watery discharge. Note that the discharge is highly infectious. The person may also have a low-grade fever or experience shock. Rapidly progressive and very painful infections may be necrotizing fasciitis (i.e., "flesh eating disease") and need urgent medical care. The most definitive characteristic is the presence of crackling (crepitus) beneath the skin due to tiny air bubbles.

To care for gangrene:

- Perform first aid.

- Provide rapid transport to advanced medical care.

- Treat the patient for shock and administer oxygen if indicated.

Gangrene.

Figure 12–9, a-b An infected wound.

soft tissue injuries warrant having a tetanus shot, such as if the person was injured with a rusty piece of metal. In these cases, the person should seek more advanced medical care.

Signs of Infection

Sometimes even the best care for a soft tissue injury is not enough to prevent infection. When a wound becomes infected, the area around the wound becomes swollen and red. The area may feel warm or throb with pain. Some wounds have a pus discharge (Figure 12–9, a-b). Red streaks may develop that progress from the wound toward the heart. More serious infections may cause the injured person to develop a fever and feel ill. Infections require a physician's care.

Dermatitis

Dermatitis is an inflammation of the skin and it is a very common condition in a workplace setting. Most cases of dermatitis result from direct contact with a chemical irritant or from an allergy.

The signs and symptoms include:

- A history of reaction to an irritant
- Redness, irritation, swelling (Figure 12–10)
- Itchiness or pain
- Blisters (in some cases)

- Thickening and cracking of the skin (in some cases)

Dermatitis is not contagious, but it can spread if left untreated. It is essential that the correct care be started early.

Prevention of dermatitis is important. Follow these general guidelines:

- Whenever harmful material is used, take the correct precautions, including the use of proper equipment.
- Maintain personal cleanliness.
- Use barrier creams:
  - When clothing does not provide protection, creams may do so. It is important to choose the correct barrier cream for the situation.

Figure 12–10 Dermatitis.

Figure 12–11 Dressings come in various sizes.

Figure 12–12 Different types of bandages are used to hold dressings in place, apply pressure to control bleeding, help protect a wound from dirt and infection, and provide support to an injured body part.

■ Use the cream correctly and remove it after you have finished handling the materials.

To care for dermatitis:

• For serious cases, see Absorbed Poisons in Chapter 17.

• Avoid the irritant.

• Protect skin with a suitable size of dressing.

• Seek further medical attention if the signs of irritation persist for 3–4 days.

• Early recognition and care can prevent minor cases from becoming major ones.

Dressings and Bandages

All open wounds need some type of covering to help control bleeding and prevent infection. These coverings are commonly referred to as dressings and bandages. There are many different types of both.

Dressings

Dressings are pads placed directly on the wound to absorb blood and other fluids and to prevent infection. To minimize the chance of infection, dressings should be sterile. Most dressings are porous, allowing air to circulate to the wound to promote healing. Standard dressings include varying sizes of cotton gauze, commonly ranging from 5 to 10 cm (2 to 4 in.) square (Figure 12–11). Much larger dressings called universal dressings are used to cover very large wounds and multiple wounds in one body area. Some dressings have non-stick surfaces to prevent the dressing from sticking to the wound.

A special type of dressing, called an occlusive dressing, does not allow air to pass through. Aluminum foil, plastic wrap, and petroleum jelly–soaked gauze are examples of this type of dressing. These dressings are used for certain chest and abdominal injuries that are discussed in Chapter 15.

Bandages

A bandage is any material used to wrap or cover any part of the body. Bandages are used to hold dressings in place, to apply pressure to control bleeding, to help protect a wound from dirt and infection, and to provide support to an injured limb or body part. Many different types of bandages are available commercially (Figure 12–12). A bandage applied snugly to create pressure on a wound or injury is called a pressure bandage.

A common type of bandage is a commercially made adhesive compress. Available in assorted sizes, it consists of a small pad of non-stick gauze (the dressing) on a strip of adhesive tape (the bandage) that is applied directly to small injuries. Also available is the bandage compress, a thick gauze dressing attached to a gauze bandage. This bandage can be tied in place. Because it is specially designed to help control severe bleeding, the bandage compress usually comes in a sterile package.

Figure 12–13 Roller bandages are wrapped around a body part, over a dressing, using overlapping turns until the dressing is completely covered.

a

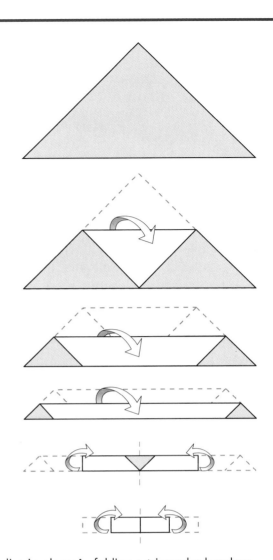

b

Figure 12–14, a-b a, Triangular bandages can be used to hold a splint in place; **b**, folding a triangular bandage.

Figure 12–15 Triangular bandages can be used to support an injured shoulder, arm, or hand.

A roller bandage is usually made of gauze or gauze-like material. Some gauze bandages are made of a self-adhering material that easily conforms to different body parts. Roller bandages are available in assorted widths from 1 to 30 cm (1/2 to 12 in.) and lengths from 5 to 10 metres (16 to 33 feet). A roller bandage is generally wrapped around the body part, over a dressing, using overlapping turns until the dressing is completely covered (Figure 12–13). It can be tied or taped in place. A folded strip of roller bandage may also be used as a dressing or compress. In the next chapter, you will learn to use roller bandages to hold splints in place.

Another commonly used bandage is the triangular bandage. Folded, it can hold a dressing or splint in place on most parts of the body (Figure 12–14, a-b). Used as a sling, the triangular bandage can support an injured shoulder, arm, or hand (Figure 12–15).

Figure 12–16, a-d When applying a bandage: **a**, secure the end of the bandage in place; **b**, wrap the bandage around the body part until the dressing is completely covered; **c**, tie or tape the bandage in place; and **d**, ensure the bandage is not too tight by checking distal circulation.

Applying a Bandage

To apply a roller bandage, follow these general guidelines:

- Secure the end of the bandage in place (Figure 12–16, a). Wrap the bandage around the body part until the dressing is completely covered and the bandage extends several centimetres beyond the dressing (Figure 12–16, b). Tie or tape the bandage in place (Figure 12–16, c).

- Do not cover the fingers or toes, if possible. By keeping these parts uncovered, you will be able to

Stitches

It can be difficult to judge when a wound should be seen by a doctor for stitches. A quick rule of thumb is that stitches are needed when the edges of skin do not fall together or when the wound is more than 2.5 cm (1 in.) long. Stitches speed the healing process, lessen the chances of infection, and improve the look of scars. The wound should be stitched within the first few hours after the injury. The following major injuries may require stitches:

- Bleeding from an artery or uncontrollable bleeding

- Deep cut or avulsion that shows the muscle or bone, involves joints near the hands or feet, gapes widely, or involves the thumb or the palm of the hand

- Large or deep puncture

- Large or deeply embedded object

- Human or animal bite

- Wound that, if left unattended, could leave a conspicuous scar, such as one that involves the lip or eyebrow

If you are caring for a wound and think it may need stitches, it probably does.

tell if the bandage is too tight (Figure 12–16, d). If the fingers or toes become cold or begin to turn pale or blue, the bandage is too tight and should be loosened slightly.

- If blood soaks through the bandage, apply additional dressings and another bandage. Leave the blood-soaked ones in place.

Care for Wounds

Closed Wounds

Most closed wounds do not require special medical care. Cold can be effective in helping control both pain and swelling. When applying ice or a chemical cold pack, place a gauze pad, towel, or other cloth between the ice and the skin to protect the skin (Figure 12–17). Apply the cold for 20 minutes every hour until pain is relieved.

Figure 12–17 Ice can reduce pain and swelling. Ensure it is not placed directly on the skin.

Figure 12–18 Use a figure-eight pattern to apply a pressure bandage to a shoulder.

Do not dismiss a closed wound as "just a bruise." Be aware of possible serious injuries to internal organs or other underlying structures, such as the muscles or bones. Take the time to evaluate how the injury happened and whether more serious injuries could be present. If a patient complains of severe pain or cannot move a body part without pain, or if you think the force that caused the injury was great enough to cause serious damage, obtain more advanced medical care immediately. Care for these injuries is described in later chapters.

Major Open Wounds

A major open wound is one with severe bleeding, deep destruction of tissue, or a deeply impaled object. To care for a major open wound, follow these general guidelines:

- Quickly control bleeding using direct pressure. Apply direct pressure by placing a sterile dressing over the wound with your gloved hand. If nothing sterile is available, use any clean covering, such as a towel or a handkerchief. If you do not have a glove and a cloth is not available, have the patient use his hand.

- Continue direct pressure by applying a pressure bandage. Apply a pressure bandage using a figure-eight pattern for a shoulder injury (Figure 12–18), elbow injury (Figure 12–19), forearm, wrist, and hand injury (Figure 12–20), or a knee injury (Figure 12–21).

- Obtain more advanced medical care.

- Wash your hands immediately after completing care, even though you wore gloves.

Figure 12–19 Use a figure-eight pattern to apply a pressure bandage to the elbow.

Figure 12–20 A pressure bandage for the palm of the hand.

Figure 12–21 Use a figure-eight pattern to apply a pressure bandage to a knee.

Figure 12–22 Wrap a severed body part in sterile gauze, put it in a plastic bag, and put the bag on ice.

If the patient has an injury in which a body part has been amputated, try to retrieve the severed body part. Wrap the part in sterile gauze, if any is available, or in any clean material, such as a washcloth. Place the wrapped part in a plastic bag. If possible, keep the part cool by placing the bag on ice (Figure 12–22). Be careful to keep the ice from directly contacting the amputated part so that it does not freeze. Make sure the part is transported to the medical facility with the patient.

If the patient has an impaled object in the wound:

- Leave the object in place unless it involves the cheek or interferes with breathing.

- Use bulky dressings to stabilize the object (Figure 12–23, a). Any movement of the object can result in further tissue damage.

- Control bleeding by bandaging the dressings in place around the object (Figure 12–23, b).

Minor Open Wounds

A minor wound, such as an abrasion, is one in which damage is only superficial and bleeding is minimal. To care for a minor wound, follow these general guidelines:

- Cleanse the wound with soap and water.

- Rinse the wound with running water for five minutes (if possible).

Figure 12–23, a-b **a**, Use bulky dressings to support an impaled object; **b**, control bleeding and hold the dressing in place by applying a bandage.

- Apply an antibiotic ointment to the wound (as long as the patient has no allergy or sensitivity to antibiotics).

- Place a sterile dressing over the wound.

- Hold the dressing in place with a bandage or tape.

Removing Slivers

A sliver is a sharp, thin piece of some material that has broken off and penetrated the skin. There are typically three types of slivers:

1. Wood: These are likely flesh-coloured and difficult to see. To find a wood sliver, wet the area with a coloured antiseptic solution (e.g., iodine) and soak for 30 seconds. Gently wipe away the remaining liquid; the sliver will have likely soaked up some of the liquid, making it easier to see.

2. Metal: These are generally easy to see and remove; treat as a wood sliver (although you can use a clear antiseptic solution if you wish).

3. Glass: These are usually invisible and difficult to remove. Soak in warm, diluted antibacterial detergent for 20 minutes.

To remove a sliver (when it is appropriate to do so):

1. Determine the angle at which the sliver entered the skin (Figure 12–24, a).

2. Grasp the sliver with disinfected forceps and withdraw it at the same angle (Figure 12–24, b).

3. Treat as a puncture or laceration.

Removing Fish Hooks

If there is a chance that removing an impaled fish hook might injure vital structures (e.g., muscles or nerves around the eye), do not remove it. Immobilize the fish hook and seek medical attention. If removing the fish hook won't create any risks, take it out using one of the following methods.

Method 1

1. With one hand, press down on the back of the hook shank by the eye of the hook to push the barb away from any tissue.

2. With the other hand, quickly jerk out the hook. This causes less damage than the second method.

3. Wash the injured area with soap and water.

4. Dress the wounds.

Method 2

1. Move the hook in a curve so that the barbed tip exits through the skin.

2. Clip off the barbed tip and remove the remainder of the hook by pulling it back the way it entered.

Figure 12–24, a-b To remove a sliver: **a**, determine the angle at which it entered the skin; and **b**, with disinfected forceps, grasp and withdraw it at the same angle.

Figure 12–25, a-b A superficial burn.

This avoids forcing the eye of the hook through tissue.

3. Wash the injured area with soap and water.

4. Dress the wounds.

Burns

Burns are another type of soft tissue injury, caused primarily by heat. Burns can also occur when the body is exposed to caustic chemicals, electricity, or solar or other forms of radiation.

When burns occur, they first affect the top layer of skin. If the burn progresses, the dermis can also be affected. Deep burns can damage underlying tissues. Burns that break the skin can cause infection, fluid loss, and loss of temperature control. Burns can also damage the respiratory system and the eyes.

The severity of a burn depends on the:

• Temperature of the source of the burn

• Length of exposure to the source

• Location of the burn

• Extent of the burn

• Person's age and medical condition

In general, people under age 5 and over age 60 have thinner skin and often burn more severely. People with acute trauma or chronic medical problems such as fractures, heart or kidney problems, or diabetes tend to have more complications resulting from burns; the effects of burns in these people may be more severe.

Severity of Burns

Burns are classified by their cause, such as heat, chemicals, electricity, or radiation. They are also classified by depth. The deeper the burn, the more severe it is. Generally, three depth classifications are used: superficial, partial-thickness, and full-thickness.

Superficial Burns

A superficial burn involves only the top layer of skin (Figure 12–25, a-b). The skin is red and dry, and the burn is usually painful. The area may swell. Most sunburns are superficial burns. Superficial burns generally heal in five to six days without permanent scarring.

Partial-Thickness Burns

A partial-thickness burn involves both the epidermis and the dermis (Figure 12–26, a-b). These injuries are also red and have blisters that may open and weep clear fluid, making the skin appear wet. The burned skin may look blotched. These burns are usually painful, and the area often swells. Although the burn usually heals in three or four weeks, a skin graft may still be necessary. Extensive partial-thickness burns can be serious, requiring more advanced medical care. Scarring may occur from partial-thickness burns.

Figure 12–26, a-b A partial-thickness burn.

Full-Thickness Burns

A full-thickness burn destroys both layers of skin, as well as any or all of the underlying structures—fat, muscles, bones, and nerves (Figure 12–27, a-b). These burns may look brown or charred, with the tissues underneath sometimes appearing white. They can be either extremely painful or relatively painless if the burn destroys nerve endings in the skin. Full-thickness burns are often surrounded by painful partial-thickness burns.

Full-thickness burns can be life-threatening. Because the burns are open, the body loses fluid, and shock is likely to occur. These burns also make the body highly prone to infection. Scarring occurs and may be severe. Skin grafts are usually required.

Identifying Critical Burns

It is important that you be able to identify a critical burn. A critical burn is one that requires immediate, more advanced medical care. Critical burns are potentially life-threatening, disfiguring, or disabling. Knowing whether you should obtain more advanced medical care for a burn injury can sometimes be difficult. It is not always easy or possible to assess the severity of a

Figure 12–27, a-b A full-thickness burn.

burn immediately after injury. Even superficial burns to large areas of the body or to certain body parts can be critical. You cannot judge severity by the pain the patient feels because nerve endings may have been destroyed. More advanced medical care must be obtained for the following burns:

- Inhalation injuries causing breathing difficulty or signs of burns around the mouth and nose

- Flame burns that occurred in a confined space

- Burns covering more than one body part

- Burns to the head, neck, hands, feet, or genitals

- Any partial-thickness or full-thickness burns to a child or an older adult

- Burns resulting from chemicals, explosions, or electricity

- Burns that result in a great deal of pain or unconsciousness in the patient

Expect that burns caused by flames or hot grease will require medical attention, especially if the patient is under 5 or over 60 years of age. Hot grease is slow to cool and difficult to remove from the skin. Burns that involve hot liquid or flames contacting clothing will also be serious since the clothing keeps the heat in contact

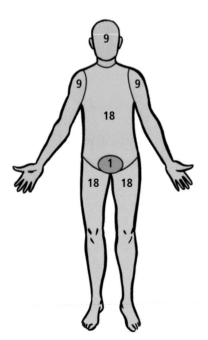

Figure 12–28 The Rule of Nines is one method to help determine how much of the body is burned.

NOTE:
If the eyes have been burned due to a flash burn, rinse them with saline or water; then have the patient close the eyes and cover them with moist, sterile dressings.

with the skin. Some synthetic fabrics melt and stick to the body. They may take longer to cool than the soft tissues. Although these burns may appear minor at first, they can continue to worsen over a period of time.

Estimating the Extent of Burns

When communicating with more advanced medical personnel about a burned patient, you may be asked how much of the body is burned. The Rule of Nines is a common method for estimating what percentage of the body is affected by burns (Figure 12–28).

In an adult, the head equals 9% of the total body surface. Likewise, each arm also equals 9% of the body. Each leg equals 18%, as does the front or back of the trunk. For example, if the front of the trunk (18%) and one entire arm (9%) are burned, you would estimate that 27% of the body's surface area has been burned.

If you do not remember the Rule of Nines, simply communicate how the burn occurred, the body parts involved, and the approximate degree of burn. For example, "The patient was injured when an overheated car radiator exploded. The patient has partial-thickness burns on his face, neck, chest, and arms." The Rule of Nines is most useful when determining body surface area for large burns.

If someone has small burns on his body, you may want to use the Rule of Palms. The Rule of Palms is another method for estimating what percentage of the body is affected by burns. The palm of the patient's hand is roughly equivalent to 1% of his body surface area.

Estimating the Extent of Burns for Babies

The Rule of Nines is modified when determining the extent of body surface area for a baby. For a baby, the head and neck equal 18% of the total body surface. Additionally, each upper extremity equals 9%, each lower extremity equals 14%, and each surface of the trunk equals 18% (Figure 12–29).

Figure 12–29 The Rule of Nines is modified when determining the percent of body burned on a baby.

Care for Thermal Burns

Look for fire, smoke, downed electrical wires, and warning signs for chemicals or radiation. If the scene is unsafe and you have not been trained to manage the situation, summon other specially trained personnel.

If the scene is safe, approach the person cautiously. If the source of heat is still in contact with the person, take steps to remove and extinguish it. This may require you to smother the flames or extinguish them with water or to remove smoldering clothing. If the burn is caused by hot tar, cool the area with water but do not attempt to remove the tar.

If the burn is superficial, you may not need to obtain more advanced medical care unless the patient is in a great deal of pain or becomes unconscious. More advanced medical care should be obtained if a partial-thickness burn covers more than 10% of the body or the patient is in a great deal of pain, becomes unconscious, or has a full-thickness burn.

Do a primary survey. Make sure ABCs are present. Pay close attention to the patient's airway.

As you do a secondary survey, look for additional signs of burn injuries. Look also for other injuries, especially if there was an explosion or electric shock. Treat any non-life-threatening injuries.

If thermal burns are present, follow these three basic care steps:

1. Cool the burned area.

2. Cover the burned area.

3. Minimize shock.

Cool the Burned Area

Even after the source of heat has been removed, soft tissue will continue to burn for minutes afterward, causing more damage. Therefore, it is essential to cool burned areas immediately with large amounts of cool water (Figure 12–30, a). If a partial- or full-thickness burn covers more than 10% of the body, cool only a small area at a time. Cooling the patient too quickly may cause the patient to go into shock. Do not use ice or ice water as ice can cause critical body heat loss. Instead, flush or immerse the area using whatever resources are available—a tub, shower, or garden hose. You can apply soaked cloths to any area that cannot be immersed or is too painful to be immersed. Be sure to keep these compresses cool by adding more water until the site has returned to body temperature.

Figure 12–30, a-b **a**, It is important to cool a burn with large amounts of cool water; **b**, cover the burned area.

Allow adequate time for the burned area to cool. If pain continues or if the edges of the burned area are still warm to the touch when the area is removed from the water, continue cooling. When the burn is cool, remove any remaining clothing from the area by carefully removing or cutting material away. Do not try to remove any clothing that is sticking to skin.

In some regions, you may be provided with more specific directions for when and how to cool burns.

Cover the Burned Area

Burns often expose sensitive nerve endings. Cover the burned area to keep out air and help reduce pain (Figure 12–30, b). Use non-stick, sterile dressings and loosely bandage them in place. The bandage should not put pressure on the burn surface. If the burn covers a large area of the body, cover it with clean, dry sheets or other cloth. Small burns (under 10% of the body) may be covered with a moist dressing.

Covering the burn helps prevent infection. For a small, superficial burn, you can put an antibiotic ointment on after it is cooled (if the patient has no allergy or sensitivity to it). Do not put other ointments, butter, oil, or other commercial or home remedies on any burn. Oils and ointments seal in heat and do not relieve pain or can contaminate open skin areas, causing infection. Do not break blisters. Intact skin helps prevent infection.

For small superficial burns or small burns with open blisters that are not sufficiently severe or extensive to require medical attention, care for the burned area as an open wound. Wash the area with soap and water. Immerse the burn in water if possible, instead of using running water, as running water can damage tissues. Ensure that the water you are immersing the burn in is clean and stays cool. Cover the burn with a non-stick dressing and bandage. Tell the patient to watch for signs of infection.

For a large partial-thickness burn, after cooling the skin, cover it loosely with a dry, sterile dressing, preferably non-stick gauze. If the patient has full-thickness burns, cover the burn with a dry sterile dressing and obtain more advanced medical care if necessary.

Minimize Shock

Pain and loss of body fluids from full-thickness and large partial-thickness burns can cause shock. Lay the patient down unless he is having difficulty breathing (dyspnea). People with burns tend to chill. Help the patient maintain normal body temperature by protecting him from drafts. Administer oxygen if it is available and it is safe to do so.

Special Situations

Chemical Burns

Chemical burns are common in industrial settings but also occur in the home. Cleaning solutions, such as household bleach, oven or drain cleaners, toilet bowl cleaners, paint strippers, and lawn or garden chemicals, are common sources of caustic chemicals. Caustic chemicals destroy tissues and cause chemical burns. Typically, burns result from chemicals that are strong acids or alkalis. These substances can quickly injure the skin. As with heat burns, the stronger the chemical and the longer the contact, the more severe the burn. The chemical will continue to burn as long as it is on the skin. You must remove the chemical from the skin as quickly as possible and then obtain more advanced medical care immediately.

With a chemical powder or granules, brush the chemical from the skin before flushing. Whether the substance is liquid, granular, or powder, flush the burn continuously with large amounts of cool, running water. A continuous flow of water will remove a dry substance before the water can activate it. Continue flushing until you can obtain more advanced medical care. Have the patient remove contaminated clothing if possible. Take steps to minimize shock.

Chemical burns to the eyes can be exceptionally traumatic. If an eye is burned by a chemical, flush the affected eye until you can obtain more advanced medical care (or for at least 20 minutes) (Figure 12–31). Flush the affected eye from the nose outward to prevent washing the chemical into the unaffected eye.

With all chemicals, ensure that you protect yourself from the chemicals and avoid contaminating any unaffected areas of the patient.

Figure 12–31 Flush a chemical burn to the eye for at least 20 minutes.

Figure 12–32 An electrical burn.

Electrical Burns

The human body is a good conductor of electricity. When someone comes in contact with an electrical source, such as a power line, a malfunctioning household appliance, or lightning, he conducts the electricity through his body. Some body parts, such as the skin, resist the electrical current. Resistance produces heat, which can cause electrical burns along the flow of the current (Figure 12–32). The severity of an electrical burn depends on the type and amount of contact, the current's path through the body, and how long the contact lasted. Electrical burns are often deep. Although these wounds may look superficial, the tissues beneath may be severely damaged. Some electrical burns will be marked by characteristic entry and exit wounds indicating where the current has passed through the body (Figure 12–33). In the secondary survey, look for two burn sites. Cover any burn injuries with a non-stick sterile dressing and give care to minimize shock.

With someone who was hit by lightning, look and care for life-threatening conditions, such as respiratory or cardiac arrest. The patient may also have fractures, including spinal fracture, so do not move him unless necessary.

Inhalation Injuries

Note soot or burns around the mouth or nose or the rest of the face and singed hair and/or eyebrows, which may signal that air passages or lungs have been burned

(Figure 12–34). Burns that resulted from a fire in an enclosed, confined space are likely to be associated with inhalation injuries of the airway and lungs. When possible, move the patient to a well-ventilated place out of the confined area. If you suspect a burned airway or burned lungs, continually monitor breathing and obtain advanced medical care immediately. Air passages may swell, impairing or stopping breathing. Oxygen should be administered if available.

Radiation Burns

Solar radiation from both the sun and other sources can cause radiation burns. Radiation burns are often caused by the sun and are similar to thermal burns. Usually, they are mild, but they can be painful (Figure 12–35). They may blister, involving more than one skin layer. Care for sunburns as you would any other burn. Cool the burn and protect the burned area from further damage by keeping it out of the sun.

Figure 12–33 An exit wound of an electrical burn.

Lightning

Lightning causes more deaths than most other weather hazards. Lightning occurs when particles of water, ice, and air moving inside storm clouds lose electrons. Eventually, the cloud becomes divided into layers of positive and negative particles. Most electrical currents run between the layers inside the cloud. Occasionally, the negative charge flashes toward the ground. An electrical current snakes back and forth between the ground and the cloud many times in the seconds that we see a flash crackle down from the sky. Anything tall—a tower, a tree, or a person—becomes a path for the electrical current.

Travelling at speeds up to 500 kilometres per second, a lightning strike can hurl a person through the air, burn his clothes off, and sometimes cause the heart to stop beating. The most powerful lightning strikes carry up to 50 million volts of electricity, enough to keep 13,000 homes running. Lightning can "flash" over a person's body, or, in its more dangerous path, it can travel through blood vessels and nerves to reach the ground.

Besides burns, lightning can also cause brain and spinal damage, cardiac arrest, fractures, and ruptured ear drums.

If you see or hear a storm approaching in the distance:

- Go inside a large building or home.
- Get inside a car and roll up the windows.
- Stop swimming or boating as soon as you see or hear a storm; water conducts electricity.
- Stay away from land-line telephones, except in an emergency.
- Stay away from telephone poles and tall trees if you are caught outside.
- Stay off hilltops; try to crouch down in a ravine or valley.

- Stay away from farm equipment and small metal vehicles such as motorcycles, bicycles, and golf carts.
- Avoid wire fences, clotheslines, metal pipes, rails, and other conductors.
- Stay several metres apart if you are in a group.

You can also reduce the chances of being struck by lightning by assuming the "lightning position" in situations of risk. This position requires you to squat down and ball yourself up so you are as low to the ground as possible without lying down. Wrap your arms around your legs. This provides a safer path for electrons to flow from the ground rather than through your torso. It is also comfortable enough that you can hold this position for a bit of time. Close your eyes. Although this position doesn't guarantee your safety from lightning, it does reduce your risk.[16]

© iStockphoto.com/Linda Blair

Figure 12–34 Burns to the face may indicate an inhalation injury.

Figure 12–35 Radiation burns can be painful.

People working in special settings, such as certain medical, industrial, or research sites, may be exposed to other types of radiation. If this type of radiation causes a burn, treat it as you would any other burn.

SUMMARY

Caring for wounds is not difficult. You need only follow the basic guidelines to control bleeding and minimize the risk of infection. Remember that with minor wounds your primary concern is to cleanse the wound to prevent infection. With major wounds, control the bleeding quickly using direct pressure and obtain more advanced medical care. Dressings and bandages, when correctly applied, help control bleeding, reduce pain, and minimize the danger of infection.

Burns damage the layers of the skin and sometimes the internal structures as well. Heat, smoke inhalation, chemicals, electricity, and radiation all cause burn injuries. When caring for a patient with burns, always ensure your safety first. When the scene is safe, approach the patient and do a primary survey and a secondary survey if necessary.

Once the patient has been removed from the burn source and is in a well-ventilated area, follow the steps of burn care:

- Cool the burned area to minimize additional tissue destruction.

- Keep air away from the burned area by covering it with non-stick sterile dressings.

- To minimize shock, maintain the patient's normal body temperature.

- Obtain more advanced medical care for any critical burn.

- If inhalation injury is possible, provide supplemental oxygen.

In addition, always check for inhalation injury if the patient has a heat or chemical burn involving the face. With electrical burns, check carefully for additional problems such as breathing difficulty, cardiac problems, and fractures.

You notice that the man is starting to breathe rapidly and he tells you he is feeling nauseous. What do you do?

Musculoskeletal Injuries

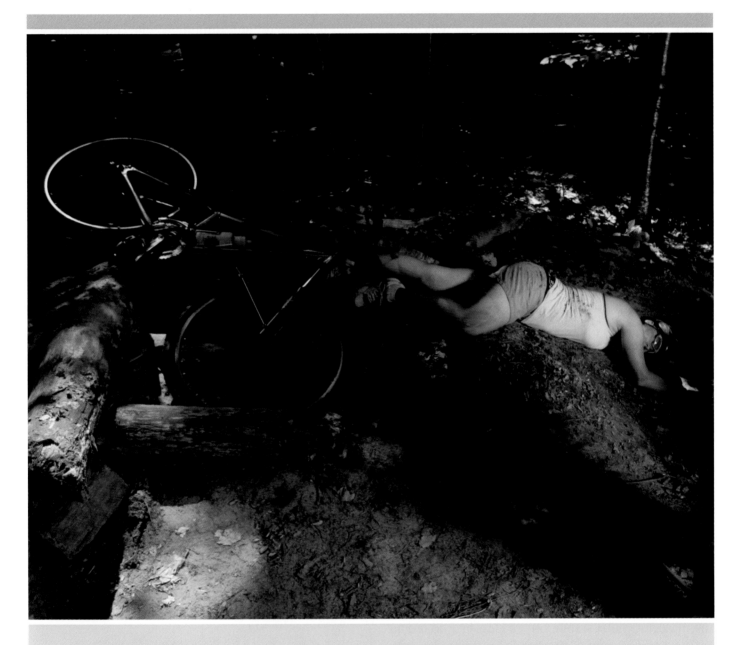

A mountain biker goes over the handle bars. She hits the ground and screams in pain. Her leg is deformed and she cannot stand up. What do you do?

INTRODUCTION

Injuries to the musculoskeletal system are common. Millions of people at home, at work, or at play injure their muscles, bones, or joints. No age group is immune. An athlete may fall and bruise the muscles of the thigh, making walking painful. Heavy machinery may fall on a worker and break ribs, making breathing difficult. A person who braces a hand against a dashboard in a car crash may injure the bones at the shoulder, disabling the arm. A person who falls while snowboarding may fall and injure her wrist, tear the supportive ligaments, and make it impossible to use her hand.

Injuries to the extremities, the arms and legs, hands and feet, are quite common. They range from simple bruises to open fractures, where bone protrudes through the skin. With any injury to the extremities, the prompt care you give can help prevent further pain and damage.

Although musculoskeletal injuries are almost always painful, they are rarely life-threatening. However, when not recognized and taken care of properly, they can have serious consequences and even result in permanent disability or death. Developing a better understanding of the structure and function of the body's framework will help you assess musculoskeletal injuries and give appropriate care.

Injuries to the Musculoskeletal System

Injuries to the musculoskeletal system occur in a variety of ways. They are more commonly caused by forces generated by mechanical forms of energy but can result from heat, chemical, or electrical forms of energy.

Types of Musculoskeletal Injuries

The four basic types of musculoskeletal injuries are fractures, dislocations, sprains, and strains. Injuries to the musculoskeletal system can be classified according to the body structures damaged. Some injuries may involve more than one type of injury. For example, a direct blow to the knee may injure both ligaments and bones. Injuries are also classified by the nature and extent of the damage.

Fracture

A fracture is a partial or complete break in bone tissue. Fractures include chipped or cracked bones, as well as bones that are broken all the way through (Figure 13–1). Fractures are commonly caused by direct and indirect bending forces. However, if strong enough, twisting forces and strong muscle contractions can cause a fracture, for example, a femur fracture.

Fractures are classified as open or closed. An open fracture involves an open wound. Open fractures often occur when the limb is severely angulated or bent, causing bone ends to tear the skin and surrounding soft tissues, or when an object, such as a bullet, penetrates the skin and breaks the bone. Closed fractures leave the skin unbroken and are more common than open fractures. Open fractures are more serious than closed fractures because of the risks of infection and severe blood loss. Although fractures are rarely an immediate threat to life, any fracture involving a large bone can cause hypovolemic shock because bones and soft tissue may bleed heavily.

Cracked bone

Broken bone

Chipped bone

Figure 13–1 Fractures include chipped or cracked bones, as well as bones that are broken all the way through.

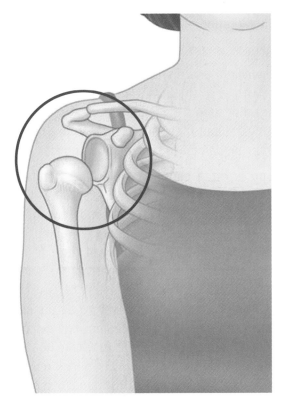

Figure 13–2 A dislocation is a displacement or separation of a bone from its normal position at a joint.

Fractures are not always obvious unless there is a telltale sign, such as an open wound with protruding bone ends or a severely deformed body part. You must always consider the way in which the injury occurred, which is often enough to suggest a possible fracture.

Dislocation

A dislocation is a displacement or separation of a bone from its normal position at a joint (Figure 13–2). Dislocations are usually caused by severe forces such as twisting or falls. After repeated injury, joints may dislocate easily because their bones and ligaments do not provide adequate protection. Others, such as the elbow or the joints of the spine, are well protected and therefore dislocate less easily.

When bone ends are forced far enough beyond their normal position, ligaments stretch and tear. Subsequent dislocations are then more likely to occur. A force violent enough to cause a dislocation can also cause a fracture and can damage nearby nerves and blood vessels.

Dislocations are generally more obvious than fractures because the joint appears to be deformed. The displaced

bone end often causes an abnormal lump, ridge, or depression, sometimes making dislocations easier to identify than other musculoskeletal injuries. An injured person is also unable to move a joint that is dislocated because the bones are out of place.

Sprain

A sprain is the stretching or tearing of ligaments and other tissues at a joint. A sprain usually results when the bones that form a joint are forced beyond their normal range of motion (Figure 13–3). The more ligaments that are torn, the more severe the injury. The sudden, violent forcing of a joint beyond its limit can completely rupture ligaments and dislocate the bones. Severe sprains may also involve a fracture of the bones that form the joint.

Mild sprains, which only stretch ligament fibres, generally heal quickly. The person may have only a brief period of pain or discomfort (7–10 days) and quickly return to activity with little or no soreness. For this reason, people often neglect sprains, and the joint is often reinjured. Severe sprains, or sprains that involve a fracture, usually cause pain when the joint is moved or used. It is important to take care of a sprain to aid in healing.

Often a sprain is more disabling than a fracture. When fractures heal, they usually leave the bone as strong as it was before; it is unlikely that a repeat break would occur at the same spot. On the other hand, once

Figure 13–3 A sprain usually results when the bones that form a joint are forced beyond their normal range of motion.

ligaments become stretched or torn, the joint may become less stable if the injury does not receive proper care. A less stable joint makes the injured area more susceptible to reinjury.

Strain

A strain is the excessive stretching and tearing of muscle or tendon fibres. It is sometimes called a "muscle pull" or "tear." Because tendons are tougher and stronger than muscles, tears usually occur in the muscle itself or where the muscle attaches to the tendon. Strains are often the result of overexertion, such as lifting something too heavy or overworking a muscle. They can also result from sudden or uncoordinated movement. Strains commonly involve the muscles in the neck or back, the front or back of the thigh, or the back of the lower leg. Strains of the neck and lower back can be particularly painful and therefore disabling.

Like sprains, strains are often neglected, which commonly leads to reinjury. Strains sometimes recur chronically, especially to the muscles of the neck, lower back, and back of the thigh. Neck and back problems are two of the leading causes of absenteeism from work, accounting for millions of dollars in lost productivity annually. Using proper body mechanics and ergonomics, these injuries can often be prevented.

Signs and Symptoms of Musculoskeletal Injuries

Common Signs and Symptoms of Musculoskeletal Injuries

Five common signs and symptoms associated with musculoskeletal injuries are:

1. Pain
2. Swelling
3. Deformity

> Tendonitis is an inflammation of a tendon due to overuse or systemic inflammatory diseases. It can present with pain and stiffness in the tendon area or a burning sensation around the whole joint.

4. Discoloration of the skin
5. Inability to use the affected part normally

Pain, swelling, and discoloration of the skin commonly occur with any significant injury. Irritation to nerve endings that supply the injured area causes pain. Pain is the body's signal that something is wrong. The injured area may be painful to touch and to move.

Swelling is often caused by bleeding from damaged blood vessels and tissues in the injured area. It may also be due to excessive fluid production by the capsule surrounding the joint. However, swelling is often deceiving. It may appear rapidly at the site of injury, develop gradually, or not appear at all. Swelling by itself, therefore, is not a reliable sign of the severity of an injury. Nor is it a reliable way to determine which structures are involved as bleeding may discolour the skin in surrounding tissues (this may take hours or days to appear). At first, the skin may only look red. As blood seeps to the skin's surface, the area begins to look bruised.

Deformity may also be a sign of significant injury (Figure 13–4). Abnormal lumps, ridges, depressions, or unusual bends or angles in body parts are types of deformities.

Figure 13–4 Deformity may be a sign of significant injury.

Marked deformity is often a sign of fracture or dislocation. Comparing the injured part with the uninjured side may help you detect deformity.

An injured person's inability or unwillingness to move or use an injured part may also indicate a significant injury. The person may tell you she is unable to move or that it is simply too painful to move. Moving or using injured parts can disturb tissues, further irritating nerve endings, which causes or increases pain. Often the muscles of an affected area will spasm in an attempt to keep the injured part from moving.

Similarly, an injured person often supports the injury in the most comfortable position. To care for musculoskeletal injuries, try to avoid causing additional pain.

Specific Signs and Symptoms of Serious Musculoskeletal Injuries

In the secondary survey, you may notice certain telltale signs and symptoms that help you determine the type of injury. Often what the patient feels or can recall about the moment of injury provides important clues.

Sprains or strains are fairly easy to tell apart. Because a sprain involves the soft tissues at a joint, pain, swelling, and deformity are usually confined to the joint area. Strains involve the soft tissue structures that, for the most part, stretch between joints. In most strains, pain,

Figure 13–5 Strains generally involve an area between the joints.

swelling, and any deformity are generally in the areas between the joints (Figure 13–5).

However, it is not always easy to determine if a musculoskeletal injury is serious, requiring more advanced medical care. Always suspect a serious injury when the following signs and symptoms are present:

• Significant deformity

• Moderate or severe swelling and discoloration

• Inability to move or use the affected body part

• Bone fragments protruding from a wound

• Patient feels bones grating or felt or heard a snap or pop at the time of injury

• Patient reports a feeling of the affected joint "giving way"

• Loss of circulation or feeling in an extremity

• Cause of the injury suggests that the injury may be severe

Care for Musculoskeletal Injuries

Some musculoskeletal injuries are obvious because they involve severe deformities, such as protruding bones or bleeding. The patient may also be in severe pain, although such injuries are rarely life-threatening. Complete the primary survey and care for any life-threatening conditions. Then do the secondary survey and care for any other injuries. When you find a musculoskeletal injury, immediately obtain more advanced medical care if:

• The injury involves severe bleeding

• The injury involves the head, neck, or back

• The injury impairs walking or breathing

• There is severe angulation with reduction or loss in sensation and/or circulation

• You see or suspect multiple musculoskeletal injuries

General Care

You identify and care for injuries to the musculoskeletal system during the secondary survey. Because they often appear similar, it may be difficult for you to determine exactly what type of injury has occurred. As you do the secondary survey, think about how the body normally looks and feels. Compare the injured side with the uninjured side.

During the interview, ask how the injury happened. The cause of injury is often enough to make you suspect a serious musculoskeletal injury. As the patient or bystanders explain how the injury occurred, listen for clues, such as a fall from a height or another significant impact to the body that would have the potential to cause a serious injury. Also ask the patient if any areas are painful.

Then do a head-to-toe examination of the entire body, beginning with the head. Check each body part. Start with the neck, followed by the shoulders, the chest, and so on. As you conduct the secondary survey, look and listen for clues that may indicate a musculoskeletal injury.

The general care for all musculoskeletal injuries is similar. Just remember the acronym RICE for rest, immobilize, cold, and elevate (Figure 13–6).

> R – rest
>
> I – immobilize
>
> C – cold
>
> E – elevate

Rest

Avoid any movements or activities that cause pain. Help the patient find the most comfortable position. If you suspect head and/or spine injuries, leave the patient lying flat and move him only if absolutely necessary.

Immobilize

If you suspect a serious musculoskeletal injury, you must immobilize the injured part before giving additional care, such as applying ice or elevating the injured part. To immobilize, use a splint or another method to keep the injured part from moving.

The purpose of immobilizing an injury is to:

- Lessen pain

- Prevent further damage to soft tissues

- Reduce the risk of serious bleeding

- Reduce the possibility of loss of circulation to the injured part

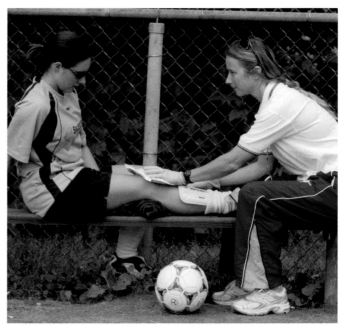

Figure 13–6 General care for all musculoskeletal injuries is similar—rest, immobilize, cold, elevate.

- Prevent closed fractures from becoming open fractures

If you are not able to transport the patient and more advanced medical care is on the way, the ground can temporarily immobilize an injured area effectively. However, if necessary, you can further immobilize an injured part by applying a splint, sling, or bandages to keep the injured body part from moving. A splint is a device that maintains an injured part in place. To effectively immobilize an injured part, a splint must extend above and below the injury site (Figure 13–7).

When using a splint, follow these basic principles:

- Have the appropriate, effective equipment.

- Splint only if you can do it without causing further injury.

- Splint the injured area and the joints above and below the injury site.

- Check for proper circulation and sensation before and after splinting.

If splinting a part causes circulation or sensation to become impaired, loosen the splint and wait for advanced medical care.

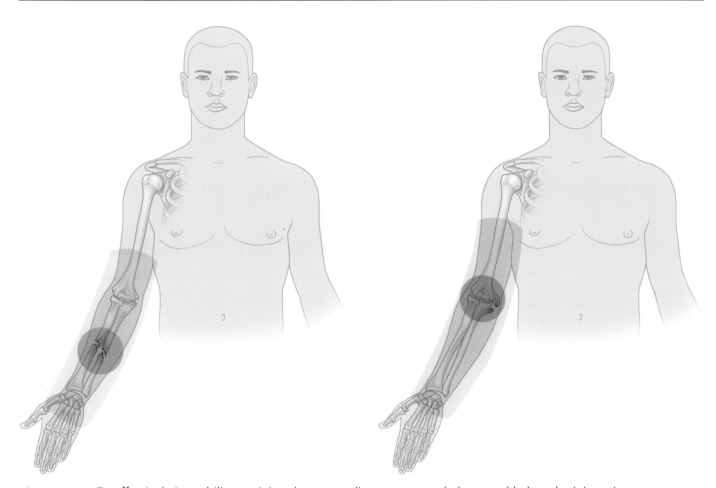

Figure 13–7 To effectively immobilize an injured part, a splint must extend above and below the injury site.

Types of Splints

Splints are of four general types: soft, rigid, anatomical, and traction. Soft splints include folded blankets, towels, pillows, slings, or triangular bandages (Figure 13–8). A blanket can be used to splint an injured ankle (Figure 13–9). A sling, which can be made from a triangular bandage, is tied to support an arm, a wrist, or a hand (Figure 13–10). A folded triangular bandage is used to hold dressings or splints in place.

Rigid splints include boards, metal strips, and folded newspaper or cardboard (Figure 13–11). For example, a padded rigid splint can be applied to an injured arm (Figure 13–12). Anatomical splints refer to the use of the body as a splint. You may not ordinarily think of the body as a splint, but it works very well and requires no special equipment. For example, an arm can be splinted to the chest. An injured leg can be splinted to the uninjured leg (Figure 13–13).

A traction splint is a special type of splinting device used primarily to immobilize fractures of the femur. One end attaches to the hip and the other at the ankle. When traction is engaged, a constant, steady pull is applied against opposite ends of the leg, stabilizing the fractured bone ends and keeping them from causing any further damage (Figure 13–14). Each commercial brand of traction splint has its own unique method of application, and responders must be thoroughly familiar with and proficient in the technique of applying the splint being used.

As a responder, you are likely to have commercially made splints immediately available to you. Commercial splints include padded board splints, air splints, specially designed flexible splints, vacuum splints, and traction splints (Figure 13–15). You should become familiar with the splinting devices you are likely to have before you use them.

Figure 13–8 Soft splints include folded blankets, towels, and triangular bandages.

Figure 13–9 A blanket can be used to splint an injured ankle.

Figure 13–10 A triangular bandage can be tied to support an arm, wrist, or hand.

Figure 13–11 Rigid splints can include boards, folded newspaper, or cardboard.

Figure 13–12 A rigid splint can be used to support an injured arm.

Figure 13–13 An injured leg can be splinted to the uninjured leg.

Figure 13–14 A traction splint is primarily used to immobilize femur fractures.

Figure 13–15 Commercial splints.

Rule of Thirds in Splinting

To determine if the injury is a joint or mid-shaft injury, use the Rule of Thirds. Each long bone (see Chapter 4) is divided into thirds; if the injury is located in the upper third, in the lower third, or in the joint, assume the injury is a joint injury. If the injury is in the middle third of the bone, assume it is a mid-shaft injury.

How to Splint

Follow these guidelines when splinting an injured body part:

1. Support the injured part. If necessary, have the patient or a bystander help you.

2. Cover any open wounds with a dressing and bandage to help control bleeding and prevent infection.

3. If the injury involves an extremity, check for circulation and sensation at a site below (distal to) the injury. Expose the foot or hand if possible to check for distal circulation, check the colour of the digits below the injury, feel the hand or foot for warmth, or check for capillary refill in the fingers or toes. Ensure that the patient has feeling in the fingers or toes; compare the injured side with the non-injured side in terms of pulse, skin colour, capillary refill, mobility, and sensation.

4. If using a rigid or anatomical splint, pad the splint so that it is shaped to the injured part; this can be done using the uninjured limb as a guide. This will help prevent further injury and provide comfort to the patient.

5. Secure the splint in place with folded triangular bandages (cravats) or straps provided with the splint.

6. Recheck circulation below the injury site to ensure that circulation has not been restricted due to the splint being applied too tightly. Loosen the splint if the patient complains of numbness or if the fingers or toes turn blue (discolour) or become cold.

7. Elevate the splinted part, if possible.

After the injury has been immobilized, recheck the ABCs and vital signs and take steps to care for shock. Shock is likely to develop as a result of a serious musculoskeletal injury. Help the patient rest in the most comfortable position, apply ice or a cold pack, maintain normal body temperature, and reassure her. Determine what additional care is needed and whether to obtain more advanced medical care if it has not already been done. Provide ongoing survey and care.

If more advanced medical care is not available within 30 minutes, and there is decreased or absent distal circulation, sensation, and/or mobility; gross angulation of the limb; tenting of the skin; or great discomfort, a single attempt may be made to straighten the limb, with the patient's willingness.

To do this, gently straighten the limb, using gentle traction, into anatomical position. Grasp the limb above and below the site of injury and pull gently. Do not

Osteoporosis

Osteoporosis, a degenerative bone disorder, affects one in four women over the age of 50 and one in eight men. Fair-skinned women with ancestors from northern Europe, the British Isles, Japan, or China are genetically predisposed to osteoporosis. Inactive people are also more susceptible to osteoporosis.

Osteoporosis occurs when there is a decrease in the calcium content of bones. Normally, bones are hard, dense tissues that endure tremendous stresses. Bone-building cells constantly repair damage that occurs as a result of everyday stresses, keeping bones strong. Calcium is a key to bone growth, development, and repair. When the calcium content of bones decreases, bones become frail, less dense, and less able to repair the normal damage they incur.

This loss of density and strength leaves bones more susceptible to fractures. Where once tremendous force was necessary to cause fractures, they may now occur with little or no aggravation, especially to hips, vertebrae, and wrists. Spontaneous fractures are those that occur without trauma. The person may be taking a walk or washing dishes when the fracture occurs. Some hip fractures thought to be caused by falls are actually spontaneous fractures that caused the person's fall.

Osteoporosis can begin at any age. The amount of calcium absorbed from the diet naturally declines with age, making calcium intake increasingly important. When calcium in the diet is inadequate,

calcium in bones is withdrawn and used by the body to meet its other needs, leaving bones weakened.

Building strong bones at an early age is the key to preventing osteoporosis. Calcium and exercise are necessary to bone building. Many physicians recommend more than 1,000 milligrams of calcium per day for women age 19 and over. Three to four daily servings of low-fat dairy products should provide adequate calcium. Magnesium and vitamin D are also necessary because they aid in calcium absorption. Exposure to sunshine enables the body to make vitamin D. Fifteen minutes of sunshine on the hands and face of a young, light-skinned individual is enough to supply the recommended dietary allowance of 5 to 10 micrograms of vitamin D per day. Dark-skinned and older adults need more sun exposure. People who do not receive adequate sun exposure need to consume vitamin D. The best sources are vitamin-fortified milk and fatty fish, such as tuna and salmon.

Calcium and magnesium supplements combined with vitamin D are available for those who do not take in adequate calcium and/or magnesium. However, before taking a supplement, consult a physician. Many highly advertised supplements are ineffective because they do not dissolve in the body.

Exercise seems to increase bone density and the activity of bone-building cells. Regular exercise may reduce the rate of bone loss by promoting new bone formation and may also stimulate the skeletal system to repair itself.

attempt this if a joint injury, such as a dislocation, is suspected or you observe firm resistance to movement, a significant increase in pain, or the sound or feeling of bone fragments grating.

Cold

Regardless of whether the injury is a closed fracture, dislocation, sprain, or strain, apply ice or a cold pack. Cold helps ease pain and discomfort. Commercial cold

packs can be stored in a kit until ready to use, or you can make an ice pack by placing ice in a plastic bag and wrapping it with a towel or cloth. Place a layer of moistened gauze or cloth between the source of cold and the skin to prevent skin damage. Do not apply an ice or cold pack directly over the fracture because doing so would require you to put pressure on the fracture site and could cause discomfort to the patient. Instead, place cold packs around the site. In general, cold should be applied for 20 minutes every hour for the first 24 to 48 hours after the injury.

Elevate

Elevating the injured area above the level of the heart helps slow the flow of blood, reducing swelling. Elevation is particularly effective in controlling swelling in extremity injuries. However, never attempt to elevate a seriously injured limb area unless it has been adequately immobilized.

Considerations for Transporting a Patient

Some musculoskeletal injuries are obviously minor, and the patient may choose not to get emergency medical care. Others are more serious, requiring more advanced medical care. Obtain more advanced medical care immediately if you suspect an injury involving severe bleeding, injuries to the head or spine, or an injury that impairs breathing, or if you see or suspect multiple musculoskeletal injuries. Fractures of large bones, or multiple fractures, can cause severe internal bleeding and may lead to shock.

Some situations may require you to move the patient before an ambulance arrives. If possible, always splint the injury before moving the patient. If you are in a position in which you must transport the patient to a medical facility, one person should monitor the patient at all times.

UPPER EXTREMITY INJURIES

The upper extremities are the arms and hands. Upper extremity bones include the clavicle, scapula, humerus, radius and ulna, carpals and metacarpals, and phalanges. Figure 13–16 shows the major structures of the upper extremities.

The upper extremities are commonly the most injured area of the body. Injuries to the upper extremities occur in many different ways. The most frequent cause is falling on the hand of an outstretched arm. Since the hands are rarely protected, abrasions occur easily. A falling person instinctively tries to break the fall by extending the arms and hands, so these areas receive the force of the body's weight. This can cause a serious injury to the hand, forearm, upper arm, or shoulder, such as a severe sprain, fracture, or dislocation (Figure 13–17).

When caring for serious upper extremity injuries, minimize any movement of the injured part. If a patient is holding the arm securely against the chest, do not change the position. Holding the arm against the chest is an effective method of immobilization, keeping an injured body part from moving. Allow the patient to

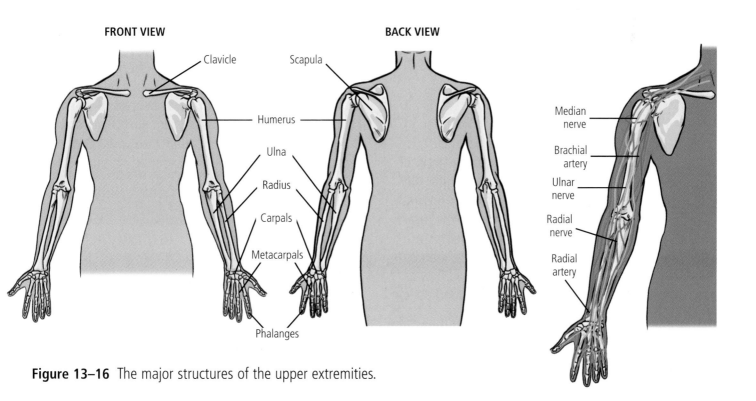

Figure 13–16 The major structures of the upper extremities.

continue to support the arm in this manner. You can further assist her by binding the injured arm to the chest. This eliminates the need for special splinting equipment and still provides an effective method of immobilization.

Injuries to the upper extremities may also damage blood vessels, nerves, and other soft tissues. It is particularly important to ensure that blood flow and nerve function have not been impaired. Always check for circulation and sensation below the injury site, both before and after splinting. Sometimes when a splint is applied too tightly, blood flow may be impaired. If this occurs, loosen the splint. If you suspect that either the blood vessels or the nerves have been damaged, minimize movement of the area and obtain more advanced medical care immediately.

Shoulder Injuries

The shoulder consists of three bones that meet to form the shoulder joint. These bones are the clavicle, scapula, and humerus. The most common shoulder injuries are sprains. However, injuries of the shoulder may also involve a fracture of one or more of these bones or dislocation of the shoulder joint.

The most frequently injured bone of the shoulder is the clavicle, injured more commonly in children than in adults. Typically, the clavicle is fractured as a result of a fall. The person usually feels pain in the shoulder area.

Figure 13–17 A fall can cause a serious injury to the hand, arm, or shoulder.

The pain may radiate down the arm. A person with a fractured clavicle usually attempts to ease the pain by holding the arm against the chest. Since the clavicle lies directly over major blood vessels and nerves to the arm, it is important to immobilize the injured area to prevent injury to these structures.

Scapular fractures are not common. A fracture of the scapula typically results from violent force. The signs

One technique for checking how the body is reacting to illness or injury is to check the capillaries' ability to refill with blood. Capillary refill is an estimate of the amount of blood flowing through the capillary beds, such as those in the fingertips. The capillary beds in the fingertips are normally rich with blood, which causes the pink colour under the fingernails. When a serious illness or injury occurs, the body attempts to conserve blood in the vital organs. As a result, capillaries in the fingertips are among the first blood vessels to constrict, thereby limiting their blood supply. Also, when blood flow to an extremity is disrupted, due to injury, blood does not circulate to the capillaries appropriately.

To check capillary refill, squeeze the patient's nail bed and then release. In a healthy person, the normal response is for the area beneath the nail to turn pale as you press it and turn pink again as you release and it refills with blood. If the area does not return to pink within two seconds, this indicates insufficient circulation.

and symptoms of a fractured scapula are the same as for any other extremity fracture, although you are less likely to see deformity of the scapula. The most significant signs and symptoms are extreme pain and the inability to move the arm.

It takes great force to break the scapula, so you must consider that the force may have been great enough to injure the ribs or internal organs in the chest. If this is the case, the person may have difficulty breathing (dyspnea).

A dislocation is another common type of shoulder injury. Like fractures, dislocations often result from falls. This happens frequently in contact sports, such as football and rugby. A player may attempt to break a fall with an outstretched arm or may land on the tip of the shoulder, forcing the arm against the joint formed by the scapula and clavicle (this is commonly referred to as a separation). This can result in ligaments tearing, causing the end of the clavicle to displace. Dislocations also occur at the joint where the humerus meets the socket formed by the scapula. For example, when an arm in a throwing position is hit, it forces the arm to rotate backward. Ligaments tear, causing the upper end of the arm to dislocate from its normal position in the shoulder socket.

Shoulder dislocations are painful and can often be identified by the deformity present. As with other shoulder injuries, the person often tries to minimize the pain by holding the arm in the most comfortable position.

Care for Shoulder Injuries

To care for shoulder injuries, first control any external bleeding with direct pressure. Apply a pressure bandage using a figure-eight pattern. Allow the patient to continue to support the arm in the position in which she is holding it (usually the most comfortable position) and, if possible, splint it in that position. If the patient is holding the arm away from the body, use a pillow, rolled blanket, or similar object to fill the gap between the arm and chest to provide support for the injured area. Check for circulation and sensation in the hand and fingers. Then splint the arm in place. This can be done by merely binding the arm to the chest or by placing the arm in a sling and binding the arm to the chest

with a cravat (Figure 13–18, a-c). Recheck for circulation and sensation. Apply cold to the injured area to help minimize pain. Take steps to minimize shock.

Upper Arm Injuries

The humerus can be fractured at any point, although it is usually fractured at the upper end near the shoulder or in the middle of the bone. The upper end of the

a

b

c

Figure 13–18, a-c Splint the arm against the chest in the position the patient was holding it.

humerus often fractures in older adults and in young children as a result of a fall. Breaks in the middle of the bone occur mostly in young adults.

When the humerus is fractured, there is danger of damage to the blood vessels and nerves supplying the entire arm. Most humerus fractures are very painful and prevent the person from using the arm. A fracture can cause considerable arm deformity.

Care for Upper Arm Injuries

To care for a serious upper arm injury, immobilize the upper arm, from the shoulder to the elbow. This can be done in the same way as for shoulder injuries. Control any external bleeding with direct pressure. Place the arm in a sling and bind it to the chest with triangular bandages. You can use a short splint, if one is available, to give more support to the upper arm (Figure 13–19). Apply cold in the best way possible. Always check for circulation and sensation in the hand and fingers before and after immobilizing the injured area.

Elbow Injuries

Like other joints, the elbow can be sprained, fractured, or dislocated. Injuries to the elbow can cause permanent disability since all the nerves and blood vessels to the forearm and hand go through the elbow. Therefore, take elbow injuries seriously. Injuries to a joint such as the elbow can be made worse by movement.

Figure 13–19 A short splint can provide additional support for an injury to the upper arm.

Care for Elbow Injuries

If the patient says that she cannot move the elbow, do not try to move it. Control any external bleeding with direct pressure and a pressure bandage using a figure-eight pattern. Check for circulation and sensation. Support the arm and immobilize it from the shoulder to the wrist.

Immobilize the elbow in the position in which you find it. Place the arm in a sling and secure it to the chest, as shown in Figure 13–18, a-c. If this is not possible, immobilize the elbow with a splint and two triangular bandages. If the elbow is bent, apply the splint diagonally across the underside of the arm (Figure 13–20, a). The splint should extend beyond both the upper arm and

Figure 13–20, a-b a, If the elbow is bent, apply a splint diagonally across the underside of the arm; **b**, if the arm is straight, apply a splint along the underside of the arm.

Figure 13–21 Fractures of both bones of the forearm may lead to an S-shaped deformity.

Figure 13–22 If the forearm is fractured, place a splint under the forearm and secure it.

the wrist. If the elbow is straight, apply the splint along the arm. Secure the splint at the wrist and upper arm with triangular bandages or roller bandages (Figure 13–20, b). Recheck for circulation and sensation. Obtain more advanced medical care. Apply ice or a cold pack and take steps to care for shock. Provide ongoing survey and care.

Forearm, Wrist, and Hand Injuries

The forearm is the upper extremity from the elbow to the wrist. Fractures of the two forearm bones, the radius and ulna, are most common in children and older adults. If a person falls on the palmar surface of an outstretched arm, both bones of the lower arm may break, but not always in the same place. With forearm fractures, the arm may look S-shaped (Figure 13–21). Because the radial artery and nerve are near these bones, a fracture may cause severe bleeding or a loss of movement in the wrist and hand. The wrist is also a common site of sprains.

Because the hands are used in so many daily activities, they are very susceptible to injury. Most injuries to the hands and fingers involve only minor soft tissue damage. However, a serious injury may damage nerves, blood vessels, and bones. Home, recreational, and industrial mishaps often produce lacerations, avulsions, burns, and fractures of the hands. Because the hand structures are delicate, deep lacerations can cause permanently disabling injuries.

Care for Forearm, Wrist, and Hand Injuries

Begin by controlling any external bleeding with direct pressure. To bandage the hand, apply a pressure bandage using a figure-eight pattern. Check for circulation and sensation and then care for the injured forearm, wrist, or hand by immobilizing the injured part. When using a rigid splint, support the injured part by placing a splint underneath the forearm. Extend the splint beyond both the hand and elbow. Place a roll of gauze or a similar object in the palm to keep the palm and fingers in a normal position. Then secure the splint with triangular bandages or roller gauze (Figure 13–22). Recheck circulation and sensation. Then put the arm in a sling and secure it to the chest.

You can immobilize injured hands and fingers using a soft splint made of a roll of gauze or rolled up cloth and bandages (Figure 13–23, a-b). You can splint an injured finger to an adjacent finger with tape (Figure 13–24). Do not attempt to put displaced finger or thumb bones back into place. Always apply ice or a cold pack to forearm, wrist, and hand injuries; elevate the injured area; and seek medical attention.

LOWER EXTREMITY INJURIES

Injuries to the leg, the entire lower extremity, can involve both soft tissue and musculoskeletal damage. The major bones of the thigh and lower leg are large and strong enough to carry the body's weight. Bones of the leg include the femur, patella, tibia, and fibula, as

Figure 13–23, a-b A roll of gauze can be used to immobilize a hand: **a**, start wrapping at the wrist; **b**, cover the hand with the gauze.

well as the tarsals, metatarsals, and phalanges. Because of the size and strength of the bones in the thigh and lower leg, a significant amount of force is required to cause a fracture.

The femoral artery is the major supplier of blood to the legs and feet. If it is damaged, which may happen with a fracture of the femur, the blood loss can be life-threatening. If there is a very weak pulse or no pulse at all below the injury, this is a sign of damage to the femoral artery.

Serious injury to the lower extremities can result in their inability to bear weight. Since the patient may be unable to walk, you should obtain more advanced medical care.

Figure 13–24 An injured finger can be splinted to an adjacent finger.

Thigh and Lower Leg Injuries

The femur is the largest bone in the body. Because it bears most of the weight of the body, it is most important in walking and running. Thigh injuries range from bruises and torn muscles to severe injuries such as fractures. The upper end of the femur meets the pelvis at the hip joint (Figure 13–25). Most femur fractures involve the upper end of the bone. Even though the hip joint itself is not involved, such injuries are often called hip fractures.

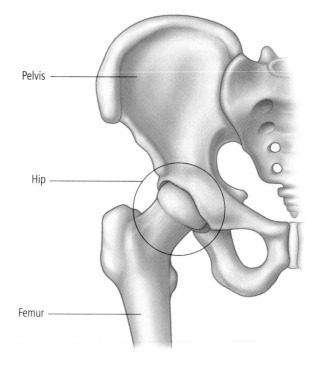

Figure 13–25 The upper end of the femur meets the pelvis at the hip joint.

Figure 13–26 A fractured femur often produces a characteristic deformity. The injured leg is shorter than the uninjured leg and may be turned outward.

Figure 13–27 It is important to stop any external bleeding and help the patient rest in the most comfortable position.

A fracture of the femur usually produces a characteristic deformity. When the fracture occurs, the thigh muscles contract. Because the thigh muscles are so strong, they pull the broken bone ends together, causing them to overlap. This may cause the injured leg to be noticeably shorter than the other leg. The injured leg may also be turned outward (Figure 13–26). Other signs and symptoms of a fractured femur may include severe pain and swelling and the inability to move the leg.

A fracture in the lower leg may involve one or both bones (fibula and tibia). Often both are fractured simultaneously. However, a blow to the outside of the lower leg can cause an isolated fracture of the fibula. Because the fibula and tibia lie just beneath the skin, open fractures are common. Lower leg fractures may cause a severe deformity in which the lower leg is bent at an unusual angle (angulated). These injuries are painful and result in an inability to move the leg. However, fractures of the fibula, and some very small fractures of the tibia, may not cause any deformity, and the person may be able to continue to use the leg.

Care for Thigh and Lower Leg Injuries

Initial care for the patient with a serious injury to the thigh or lower leg is to stop any external bleeding, immobilize the injured area, and help the patient rest in the most comfortable position (Figure 13–27). Obtain more advanced medical care immediately. They are much better equipped to care for and transport a patient with a serious leg injury. Consider that the ground can adequately immobilize the legs, if the surface is relatively flat and firm, until you are able to obtain more advanced medical care.

Figure 13–28 To splint an injured leg, secure the injured leg to the uninjured leg with triangular bandages. A pillow or rolled blanket can be placed between the legs.

Figure 13–29 Rigid splints can also be used to splint an injured leg.

Figure 13–30, a-b Two types of traction splints.

However, there may be situations, such as moving the patient, in which you will need to splint an injured leg. Securing the injured leg to the uninjured leg with several wide triangular bandages is one simple method. If available, place a pillow or rolled blanket between the legs and bind the legs together in several places above and below the site of the injury (Figure 13–28). If rigid splints are available, apply one long splint to the outside of the injured leg, extending above the hip and beyond the foot. Place a shorter padded splint to the inside of the leg, also extending beyond the foot (Figure 13–29). Secure the splints to the leg with triangular bandages. Other commercial splints, such as air splints or vacuum splints, can also be used if available. Regardless of the type of splint applied, always check and recheck the circulation and sensation of the foot. Apply ice or a cold pack to reduce pain.

A fractured femur can injure the femoral artery, and serious bleeding can result. The likelihood of shock is great. Therefore, take steps to minimize shock. Keep the patient lying down and try to keep her calm. Maintain normal body temperature, administer oxygen if it is available, and obtain more advanced medical care. Provide ongoing survey and care.

Some fractures of the femur may require traction splinting. Traction helps prevent broken bone ends from causing further injury and helps reduce pain and minimize shock. However, not all responders are trained to use traction splints. If you are not trained or if you need assistance, immobilize the injured leg in the best way possible and provide ongoing survey and care until you can obtain advanced medical care. Figure 13–30, a-b, shows two types of traction splints.

Knee Injuries

The knee joint is very vulnerable to injury. The knee includes the lower end of the femur, the upper ends of the tibia and fibula, and the patella (kneecap). The kneecap is a bone that moves on the lower front surface of the thigh bone. Knee injuries range from cuts and bruises to sprains, fractures, and dislocations. Deep lacerations in the area of the knee can later cause severe joint infections. Sprains, fractures, and dislocations of the knee are common in athletic activities that involve quick movements or exert unusual force on the knee.

The most agile of joints, the knee is also the most vulnerable. It joins the two longest bones of the body. Four ligaments attach to the bones and hold the knee together. Two cartilage discs serve to increase joint stability, facilitate joint lubrication, and spread out the weight-bearing forces. The cartilage can be torn due to a torsion injury. Repeated and excessive shocks to the knee can also splinter the cartilage pads and stretch or fray ligaments.

The kneecap is unprotected in that it lies directly beneath the skin. This part of the knee is very vulnerable to bruises and lacerations, as well as dislocations. Violent forces to the front of the knee, such as those caused by hitting the dashboard of a motor vehicle or by falling and landing on bent knees, can fracture the kneecap.

Care for Knee Injuries

To care for an injured knee, first control any external bleeding. Apply a pressure bandage using a figure-eight pattern. If the knee is bent and cannot be straightened without pain, support it in the bent position (Figure 13–31). If the knee is straight or can be straightened

Figure 13–31 Support a knee injury in the bent position if the patient cannot straighten the knee.

without pain, splint the leg as you would an injury of the thigh or lower leg or apply a long rigid splint to the leg. Other commercial splints can also be used if available. Apply ice or a cold pack. Help the patient rest in a comfortable position. Obtain more advanced medical care. Provide ongoing survey and care.

Ankle and Foot Injuries

Ankle and foot injuries are commonly caused by twisting forces. Injuries range from minor sprains with little swelling and pain that heal with a few days' rest to fractures and dislocations. As with other joint injuries,

Arthroscopy

In 1994, *Sports Illustrated* magazine marked its 40th anniversary by selecting the 40 people who "most significantly altered or elevated the world of sports in the last four decades." One of those honoured was Canadian doctor Robert W. Jackson, an athlete in his own right but selected for this honour because he extended the careers of numerous professional athletes through a process known as arthroscopic surgery.

The train-track scars that once criss-crossed the injured knees of many athletes have almost disappeared. Both the scars and the trauma of knee surgery have been diminished with the advent of arthroscopy.

The recovery after arthroscopy is remarkable considering that about 25 years ago knee surgery meant a five-day hospital stay, a cast, and months of rehabilitation. With arthroscopic surgery, many athletes can have day surgery in a hospital or clinic setting and begin athletic therapy or physiotherapy within days of the procedure.

The arthroscope, a thin, flexible fibre-optic scope, allows physicians to perform delicate joint surgery without cutting muscles and ligaments and without lifting the kneecap to get to the injured area. After injecting a saline solution to distend the knee joint, the surgeon inserts the arthroscope through small puncture wounds into the space of the knee joint. By projecting magnified images inside the knee onto a screen, the arthroscope allows orthopedic surgeons to use microsurgical instruments to smooth arthritic surfaces, remove chipped bones and cartilage, and sew up torn ligaments.

Thousands of people undergo arthroscopic surgery each year. Arthroscopes, some less than 1.7 millimetres in diameter, are being used to repair shoulders, ankles, wrists, and even jaws. Not all joint problems can be repaired with arthroscopy, but most surgeons would agree that advances in arthroscopy have had a profound impact on the lives of people who might otherwise be incapacitated.

you cannot always distinguish between minor and severe injuries. You should initially care for all ankle and foot injuries as if they are serious. As with other lower extremity injuries, if the ankle or foot is painful to move, if it cannot bear weight, or if the foot or ankle is swollen, a physician should evaluate the injury. Foot injuries may also involve the toes. Although these injuries are painful, they are rarely serious.

Fractures of the feet and ankles can occur when a person forcefully lands on the heel. With any great force, such as falling from a height and landing on the feet, fractures are possible. The force of the impact may also be transmitted up the legs. This can result in an injury elsewhere in the body, such as the thigh, pelvis, or spine.

Care for Ankle and Foot Injuries

Care for ankle and foot injuries by controlling external bleeding and immobilizing the ankle and foot in the best way possible. Some commercial splints are specifically designed for ankle and foot injuries. Secure the splint to the injured area with two or three triangular bandages or a roller bandage. Once it is splinted, elevate the injured ankle or foot to help reduce the swelling. Apply ice or a cold pack. Suspect that anyone who has fallen or jumped from a height may have additional injuries. Obtain more advanced medical care. Keep the patient from moving until this care has been obtained. Provide ongoing survey and care.

SUMMARY

Injuries are a leading health problem in Canada. When the body experiences violent forces, many kinds of injuries can occur. Injuries may affect soft tissues, nerves, muscles, bones, ligaments, and tendons. These injuries can have permanent, disabling effects on the body and can even be life-threatening.

The musculoskeletal system is a complex group of structures that provide protection, support, and movement for the body. The musculoskeletal system has four main structures: bones, muscles, tendons, and ligaments. Sometimes it is difficult to tell whether an injury is a fracture, dislocation, sprain, or strain. Since you cannot be sure which injury someone might have, always care

for the injury as if it were serious. If you're awaiting more advanced medical care, do not move the patient. Control any bleeding first and take steps to minimize shock. Provide ongoing survey and care. If you are going to transport the patient to a medical facility, be sure to first immobilize the injury before moving her.

You can care for serious musculoskeletal and soft tissue injuries to the extremities by focusing on minimizing pain, shock, and further damage to the injured area. You can do this by:

- Managing airway or breathing problems
- Controlling any external bleeding
- Checking circulation and sensation below the site of injury before and after immobilizing
- Immobilizing the injured area of the body
- Applying ice or a cold pack to the injured area
- Limiting movement of, or by, the patient
- Calming and reassuring the patient
- Maintaining normal body temperature
- Administering oxygen
- Obtaining more advanced medical care
- Providing ongoing survey and care

As you examine the biker, you find that her injured leg appears to be noticeably shorter than her other leg and her pulse is weak. What do you do?

Head and Spine Injuries

You respond to an industrial incident involving someone who has fallen from a height of approximately three metres (10 feet). You arrive to find a man lying on the ground. He is unconscious. Looking at the scene, it is difficult to determine exactly what has happened and what his injuries might be. What do you do?

INTRODUCTION

It's summer vacation at the lake. A group of teenage boys are swimming around in the lake when one of them says he's going to dive off the edge of a cliff about 12 metres (39 feet) up. The water is normally a safe depth, about 5 metres (16 feet) deep, but it's been a drier season than usual and the lake is only about 3½ metres (11 feet) deep. He dives straight down and strikes his head on the sandy bottom. His friends rush to pull him out and find him unconscious, having broken his neck.

Each year, tens of thousands of Canadians suffer a head and/or spine injury serious enough to require medical care. Most of these people are males between the ages of 15 and 30. Motor vehicle collisions account for about half of all head and spine injuries. Other causes include falls, sports and recreational activities, and violent acts such as assault.

Besides those who die each year from head and spine injury, thousands become permanently disabled. Today there are many thousands of people in Canada permanently disabled from head or spine injuries. These survivors have a wide range of physical and cognitive impairments, including paralysis, behavioural disorders, and speech and memory problems.

Fortunately, prompt, appropriate care can help minimize the damage from most head and spine injuries. In this chapter, you will learn how to recognize when a head and/or spine injury may be serious. You will also learn how to provide the appropriate care to minimize injuries to the head and spine.

PREVENTING HEAD AND/OR SPINE INJURIES

Injuries to the head and/or spine are a major cause of death, disability, and disfigurement. However, many such injuries can be prevented by managing the risks in all parts of your life:

- Wear a seat belt
- When appropriate, wear approved helmets, eyewear, faceguards, and mouthguards
- Prevent falls
- Obey rules in sports and during recreational activities
- Avoid inappropriate use of drugs
- Inspect work and recreational equipment periodically
- Think and talk about safety and managing risks

Wearing Seat Belts

Always wear seat belts, including shoulder restraints, when driving or riding in a car. Be sure, also, that all passengers wear them. Airbags provide additional protection. All small children riding in a car must be in approved safety seats correct for their age, height, and weight.

Wearing Helmets and Eyewear

Helmets can prevent many needless injuries to the head. They are designed for different purposes, have varying degrees of protection, and offer protection only for their intended use (Figure 14–1). For example, the industrial work helmet, called a hard hat, provides adequate protection against falling debris but does not offer the proper protection for riding a motorcycle.

Any open form of transportation, such as a motorcycle, moped, or all-terrain vehicle, exposes the head and spine to injury. Wearing a helmet can help reduce such injuries. The ideal helmet, sometimes called a full-face helmet, protects the lower face and jaw and has a large clear or

Figure 14–1 Helmets are designed for multiple purposes, and offer protection only for their intended use.

tinted face shield. In all cases, the helmet should be the correct size and fit comfortably and securely.

Eyewear can help prevent many needless injuries that result in loss of sight. Anytime you operate machinery or perform an activity that may involve flying particles or splashing chemicals, you should wear protective eyewear such as goggles.

Safeguarding Against Falls

Although most falls occur at home and involve young children and older adults, falls can and do occur in the workplace. Take precautions to prevent falls. Floor surfaces should be made of non-slip material. Stairs should have non-slip treads and handrails and be well lit. Rugs should be secured to the floor with double-sided tape. All spills should be cleaned up promptly.

In the workplace:

- Use all appropriate safety equipment when working above ground level.

- When using ladders, make sure there are three points of contact on the ladder at all times (e.g., two hands and a foot or two feet and a hand).

- Keep floors and aisles free of clutter and ensure that nothing is blocking stairwells, work sites, or exits.

- Check equipment, such as warehouse forklifts, ladders, and scaffolding, regularly for worn or loose parts.

Extra prevention for children:

- If there are small children in the home, gates should be placed at the top of stairs.

- Babies and children should always ride in approved safety seats. Ensure that the seats are the right fit and are properly installed.

- Ensure that children and adults wear an approved, properly fitting helmet for any activity in which a blow to the head may occur.

Managing Risks in Sports and Recreation

Participants in sports or recreational activities should know their physical limitations. Proper protective equip-ment is necessary for any activity in which serious injury may occur. In all sports involving physical contact, participants should wear mouthguards. Most importantly, everyone must know and follow the rules. Rules not only make activities fair, they also help prevent injuries. The coach, athletic therapist, or more experienced participant may impose additional rules for the safety of newcomers. Participants should never engage in a new activity until they know the rules and risks involved.

Diving is one of the leading causes of head and/or spine injuries. Divers must always be careful around water:

- Ensure that the water is deep enough before diving.

- Enter unknown water and pools feet first.

- Check for objects below the surface, such as logs or piling, before diving.

Thinking and Talking About Managing Risks

People too often neglect to think about managing risks in their daily lives, yet we are most vulnerable to injury at work, during recreational activities, or while travelling. Take the time to inspect and think about your daily environment. You should consider the following five questions:

1. Are there things you could do in your workplace or at home to help prevent injuries to yourself or others?

2. Are you taking unnecessary risks in any activities?

3. Do you follow rules meant for your safety?

4. Do you maintain your vehicle appropriately?

5. Do you ever attempt an activity without being in the physical condition that would allow you to do it without injury?

Talk with others about preventing injuries at work, at home, and in recreation. Everyone needs to know about managing risks. Seek guidance to help prevent injuries that could permanently affect your life or the lives of others. Discuss safety when using mechanical devices or equipment or when approaching a potentially dangerous scene.

RECOGNIZING SERIOUS HEAD AND SPINE INJURIES

Injuries to the head and spine can damage both bone and soft tissue, including brain tissue and the spinal cord. It is usually difficult to determine the extent of damage in head and spine injuries. In most cases, the only way to assess the damage is by having an X-ray or scan done at a hospital. Since you have no way of knowing exactly how severe an injury is, always provide initial care as if the injury is serious. Remember your priorities of care to treat a head and/or spine injury before minor bleeding. There is a significant difference between a head injury and an injury to the head. An injury to the head is often a superficial injury, for example, a cut to the face or scalp, whereas a head injury often involves brain trauma. Focus on treating the most serious injuries during the initial assessment.

The Brain

Injuries to the head can affect the brain. Blood from a ruptured vessel in the brain can accumulate in the skull (Figure 14–2). Because there is very little empty space in the skull, bleeding can build up pressure that can cause further damage to brain tissue.

Bleeding in the skull can occur rapidly or slowly over a period of days. This bleeding will affect the brain, causing changes in consciousness. An altered level of consciousness is often the first and most important sign of a serious head injury.

Bleeding in the skull is divided into three general types:

Epidural Hematoma

An epidural hematoma is an arterial bleed occurring between the skull and dura mater, usually resulting from a low-velocity blow (Figure 14–3). The signs and symptoms appear quickly, and the person usually presents with a brief loss of consciousness, then regained consciousness, and then a rapid decline in consciousness. As this decline occurs, pupils may become sluggish, dilated, or non-reactive. Motor function may also be impaired on one side of the body (the side opposite the injury).

Subdural Hematoma

A subdural hematoma is venous bleeding in the subdural space, resulting from a violent blow to the head (Figure 14–4). Neurological deficits may present themselves immediately after the blow or days later. The signs and symptoms may not appear immediately after

Figure 14–2 Blood from a ruptured vessel in the brain can accumulate in the skull.

Figure 14–3 An epidural hematoma is an arterial bleed between the skull and the dura mater.

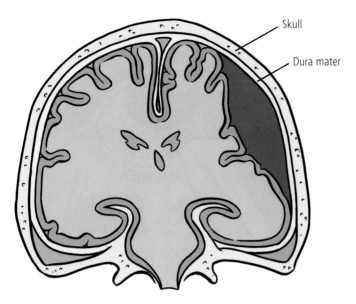

Figure 14–4 A subdural hematoma is a venous bleed in the subdural space.

the impact, although other signs of trauma can be seen. The signs and symptoms will appear as the pressure resulting from the bleed increases. Headaches, visual disturbances, personality changes, difficulty speaking, and deficits in motor function are all possible symptoms of someone with this type of bleeding.

Intracerebral Hematoma

An intracerebral hematoma is caused by damage to the blood vessels in the brain itself due to either blunt or penetrating trauma. There is often more than one contusion, and they can enlarge over time. Specific neurological findings depend on the location and size of the hematoma.

SPINE INJURIES

Injuries to the spine can fracture the vertebrae and sprain the ligaments. These injuries usually heal without problems. With severe injuries, however, the vertebrae may shift and compress or sever the spinal cord. This can cause temporary or permanent paralysis, even death. The extent of the paralysis depends on which area of the spinal cord is damaged.

Mechanism of Injury

Consider the mechanism of injury to help you determine whether someone has suffered a head and/or spine

injury (Figure 14–5). Survey the scene and think about the forces involved in the injury. Strong forces are likely to cause severe injury to the head and spine. For example, a driver whose head breaks a car windshield in a crash may have a serious head and/or spine injury. A diver who hits his head on the bottom of a swimming pool may also have a serious head and/or spine injury. Evaluate the scene for clues as to whether a serious head and/or spine injury has occurred.

You should consider the possibility of a head and/or spine injury in a number of situations. These include:

- Any motor vehicle crash
- Any ejection from a motor vehicle
- A fall from a height greater than the individual's height
- Any injury in which the person's helmet is broken
- Any injury involving a severe blunt force to the head or trunk
- Any injury, such as a gunshot wound, that penetrates the head or trunk
- Any diving mishap
- Unconsciousness of unknown cause
- Any incident involving a lightning strike

Signs and symptoms that indicate a head and/or spine injury may be obvious right away or may develop later (Table 14–1). These signs and symptoms alone do not always suggest a head and/or spine injury, but they may when combined with the cause of the injury. Regardless of the situation, always obtain more advanced medical care when you suspect a head and/or spine injury.

CARE FOR SERIOUS HEAD AND SPINE INJURIES

Head and spine injuries can become life-threatening emergencies. A serious injury can cause someone to stop breathing. Care for serious head and spine injuries also involves supporting the respiratory, circulatory, and nervous systems. Provide the following care while waiting to obtain more advanced medical care:

- Minimize movement of the head and spine.
- Maintain an open airway.

Compression

Distraction

Flexion

Rotation

Hyperextension

Penetration

Figure 14–5 The mechanism of injury may help you to determine if the patient has suffered a head and/or spine injury.

TABLE 14–1: SIGNS AND SYMPTOMS OF HEAD AND SPINE INJURIES

- Changes in the level of consciousness
- Severe pain or pressure in the head, neck, or back
- Swelling
- Tingling or loss of sensation in the extremities (arms and legs)
- Partial or complete loss of movement of any body part
- Unusual bumps or depressions on the head, neck, or back
- Blood or other fluids draining from the ears, nose, mouth, or open wounds
- Profuse external bleeding of the head, neck, or back
- Irregular breathing
- Open wounds to the scalp
- Seizures
- Sudden impaired breathing or vision
- Unusual or unequal pupil size
- Nausea or vomiting
- Persistent headache
- Loss of balance
- Incontinence
- Specific changes in blood pressure and pulse
- Bruising of the head, especially around the eyes ("raccoon eyes") or behind the ears ("Battle's signs")

- Control any external bleeding.
- Provide ongoing survey and care.
- Administer oxygen if available.

NOTE:

Remember to assess the patient using the Glasgow Coma Scale.

Minimize Movement

Caring for a head and/or spine injury is similar to caring for any other serious soft tissue or musculoskeletal injury. Immobilize the injured area and control any bleeding. Because movement of an injured head and/or spine can damage the spinal cord irreversibly, keep the patient as still as possible until you can obtain more advanced medical care. To minimize movement of the head and neck, use a technique called in-line stabilization:

1. Instruct the patient to remain still and minimize movement.

2. Place your hands on both sides of the patient's head.

3. Slowly rotate the head until the chin is in line with the middle of the chest.

4. Maintain manual stabilization and continue care.

Once you have manually stabilized the head and neck, do not remove your hands from the patient until the patient has been fully secured to the spinal immobilization device, unless advanced medical care has determined that there is no longer a need for spinal immobilization and has discontinued it.

The head in this anatomically correct, neutral position helps prevent further damage to the spinal column (Figure 14–6, a-b). If a second responder is available, that person can give care for any other conditions while

NOTE:

When applying in-line stabilization, the responder must ensure that his arms are completely stable before placing them on the patient's head.

you keep the head and neck stable. There are, however, some circumstances in which you would not move the patient's head in line with the body. These include:

- When the patient's head is severely angled to one side

- When the patient complains of pain, pressure, or muscle spasms in the neck when you begin to align the head with the body

- When the responder feels resistance when attempting to move the head in line with the body

In these circumstances, support the patient's head in the position in which you found it, except when the patient's airway cannot be maintained open in that position.

If the head is manually stabilized in anatomical position, a rigid cervical collar should be applied (Figure 14–7, a-b). This collar helps minimize movement of the head and neck and keeps the head in line with the body. It is important to note that these devices reduce movement and some range of motion but do not by themselves provide adequate immobilization of the spine. The collar must always be used in conjunction with manual in-line stabilization or a mechanical immobilization device.

Sizing a Hard Cervical Collar

Proper sizing of a hard cervical collar is very important. If the collar is too short, it will not provide enough support, whereas if it is too tall, it may hyperextend the neck. Hard collars come in a variety of sizes and are also available as a single collar that is adjustable for different sizes.

To size and apply the hard collar, the responder should carry out the following steps:

1. Ensure that the patient's head is placed in the neutral position. If this is not possible due to pain or resistance by the patient, do not apply the hard collar; immobilize in that position.

2. The first responder applies manual in-line stabilization from behind the patient and maintains this hold throughout the procedure. The first responder's fingertips should not extend beyond the patient's earlobe, as this would make applying the collar difficult.

Figure 14–6, a-b Support the patient's head in line with the body using in-line stabilization.

Figure 14–7, a-b **a,** An adjustable rigid cervical collar; **b,** non-adjustable rigid cervical collars.

3. The second responder measures the distance between the top of the patient's trapezius and an imaginary line from the bottom of the patient's chin to the floor using his fingers (Figure 14–8).

4. Match this measurement to the appropriate size of collar. (Familiarize yourself with the brand of hard collar you are using and the manufacturer's measurement marks.)

5. Assemble the chin piece, if required. For one type of collar, sliding the black fastener up and into the small hole does this. Press firmly to snap into place. You may also need to pre-form this type of collar to simplify its application.

6. The second responder properly angles the collar for placement.

7. The second responder positions the collar bottom.

8. The second responder positions the front of the collar underneath the patient's chin while maintaining the patient's head in the neutral position. The chin piece should rest snugly up against the patient's chin. The lower portion of the collar should be centred and resting on the patient's breastbone.

9. The second responder secures the collar with the Velcro® strap.

10. After the collar is applied, the second responder visually checks to make sure it is correctly placed and fitted properly. The first responder maintains in-line stabilization until the patient is secured to a spinal immobilization device and his head is secured to that device.

Immobilize the Patient

Once the cervical collar has been applied and in-line stabilization maintained, the patient's entire body should be immobilized. When a head and/or spine injury is suspected, spinal immobilization should be considered to move a patient out of a dangerous place, to rescue him, or to transport him. This can be done using the following equipment:

• Rigid splint, such as a backboard

• Large towel or blanket

• Straps or folded triangular bandage(s)

Local protocol may dictate what equipment is to be used.

Figure 14–8 To select the correct size cervical collar, measure the distance from the top of the shoulders to the bottom of the chin.

If you do not have a backboard available, support the patient in the position in which you found him until you can obtain more advanced medical care.

Once the cervical collar is in place, the patient is positioned on a backboard. This is done by "log-rolling" the patient onto the board. This technique keeps the head in line with the body. It requires a minimum of two responders: one to maintain in-line stabilization and another to position the backboard and roll the patient's body. However, it is highly preferable to have three responders available to perform this technique. With three responders, one can provide in-line stabilization and the second and third can log-roll the patient and position the backboard (Figure 14–9). When the patient is in a position in which the back is visible, check the

Babies and children have large heads and may require padding under the body when being put on a board. Collars and other equipment specifically designed for children should be used when possible.

Figure 14–9 Log-roll a patient onto a backboard while keeping the spine in as straight a line as possible.

Figure 14–10 Use several straps and/or triangular bandages to secure the patient to the backboard.

Figure 14–11 There are commercially available head immobilization devices.

Figure 14–12 Attaching the head straps on a Kendrick Extrication Device (K.E.D.®).

back quickly for signs of trauma such as bleeding, deformity, discoloration, or muscle spasms.

Before strapping the patient to the backboard, ensure that he is in the correct position. If the patient is too low, too high, or too far to one side of the board, you must move him.

Once the patient is on the board properly, use several straps and/or triangular bandages to secure her body to the backboard (Figure 14–10). There are several different configurations you can use to strap the patient onto the board. A common one is to secure the chest by criss-crossing the straps. Regardless of which method is used, the straps should be snug, but not so tight as to restrict movement of the chest during breathing. With the remaining straps, secure the patient's hips, thighs, and legs. If necessary, secure the hands in front of the body.

Once the patient's body is secured to the backboard, secure her head. If the patient's head does not appear to be resting in line with the body, you may need to place a small amount of padding, such as a small folded towel, under the head to fill any space left. Normally, approximately 2.5 cm (1 in.) of padding is all that is needed to keep the head in line with the body while at the same time providing comfort for the patient. Next, use tape to secure the forehead.

You may have a commercially made head immobilization device available (Figure 14–11). Many of these use Velcro® straps to secure the head. You should follow the manufacturer's directions when using these devices.

Use of an Upper Body Motion Restriction Device

You might be called upon to assist more advanced medical personnel to immobilize someone with an upper body motion restriction device, such as a Kendrick Extrication Device (K.E.D.®) (Figure 14–12). The steps are as follows:

1. After manual in-line stabilization and the application of a rigid cervical collar, the K.E.D.® or short backboard device can be placed behind the patient. If using a K.E.D.®, it should be positioned snugly beneath the patient's armpits to prevent it from moving up the torso.

HEAD GRIP PROCEDURES

Head Grip

1. Kneel behind the patient's head, keeping yourself aligned with the patient's body.

2. Place your elbows on the ground and then place your hands on either side of the patient's head. Your fingers should not extend past the patient's ears. Place your thumbs on the patient's forehead, your index and middle fingers on the cheekbone, and your ring and little fingers below the ears.

3. If you need to manipulate the patient's airway, move your index and middle fingers to the angle of the jaw and displace the mandible (the lower jaw) upward but maintain the head in the neutral position.

Trapezius Squeeze (Trap Stabilization)

1. Kneel behind the patient's head, keeping yourself aligned with the patient's body.

2. Place your elbows on the ground or on your knees and then extend your arms along either side of the patient's head.

3. Slide your hands under the patient's trapezius muscles, palms up, fingers pointing along the long axis of the body (parallel to the spine). Do not turn your hands to cradle the patient's neck.

4. Move your forearms in to support the patient's head.

5. Apply firm pressure to maintain the patient's head in position.

Modified Trap Stabilization

1. Kneel behind the patient's head, keeping yourself aligned with the patient's body.

2. Support your elbow on the ground or against your knee and then grip the patient's trapezius muscles.

3. Rest your elbow against the ground or your knee and support the patient's head as in the head grip. Apply firm pressure to stabilize the head between your hand and forearm.

Sternal Forehead Grip

This head grip is typically used for transferring a patient from one responder to another.

1. Kneel with one leg even with the patient's chest or shoulders and the other leg by the patient's head.

2. Place your elbow and forearm along the patient's sternum.

3. Place your hand on the patient's face, with your thumb on one cheekbone and your index and middle fingers on the other cheekbone. You can arch your hand upward to stay clear of the patient's nose and mouth. Do not restrict respiration.

4. Place your other elbow on your knee and then place your hand on the patient's forehead. Apply firm pressure to hold the head and neck in position. Avoid rotating the head or compressing the head and neck toward the body. Arch your hand to allow room for sandbags or other device to be placed or removed and for your partner to adjust his grip.

Sternal/Spinal Grip

1. Position yourself, kneeling beside the patient, next to his back.

2. Place your elbow and forearm along the patient's sternum.

3. Place that hand on the patient's face, with your thumb on one cheekbone or mandible and your index and middle fingers on the other cheekbone or mandible.

4. Position your other arm along the patient's spine and grip the occiput (the back of the head).

2. The middle torso is immobilized by fastening the middle and lower chest straps. The straps should be snug so that fingers cannot be slipped beneath the straps.

3. When using a K.E.D.®, each groin/leg strap is positioned and fastened separately, forming a loop. These straps prevent the device from moving up and the lower end from moving laterally.

4. The head is padded and secured to the device.

5. The upper torso is then immobilized by securing the chest strap.

6. The patient is carefully moved as a unit to a long backboard by rotating the person and K.E.D.® onto the board. The legs are held proximal to the knees and lifted during the transition.

7. The patient is centred on the backboard, any groin straps are loosened, and the legs are slowly lowered to an in-line position.

8. The patient is secured to the backboard, keeping the K.E.D.® in place.

If the patient is standing and you suspect a spinal injury, you can immobilize him while standing. This technique takes at least two responders (Figure 14–13).

1. Have one responder apply a cervical collar while the other maintains manual in-line stabilization.

2. Place the long backboard behind the patient. Check the placement of the board from in front of the patient to ensure that it is aligned correctly.

3. With one responder on each side of the patient, each should place his lower arm under the patient's armpit and grasp the next highest handhold on the backboard. The responder's free hand should hold the patient's elbows. If there is a third responder, that person is positioned behind the backboard with arms wrapped around the board, maintaining manual in-line stabilization. If there are only two responders, the free hand of the responders on each side of the patient can be used to hold the patient's head in position.

4. Lower the patient to the ground while holding the head stable.

5. After the patient is completely immobilized and secured to the board, you can release manual in-line stabilization.

Rapid Extrication

In some cases, it may be necessary to move a patient quickly using only manual in-line stabilization.

The circumstances in which this may be required are as follows:

- The scene is not safe.
- Life-saving care cannot be given due to the location or position of the patient.
- It is necessary to move the patient to gain access to another patient with life-threatening emergencies.

A rapid extrication should be performed by at least two responders in order to move a patient from a sitting position to a long backboard. As with using a short backboard, ensure that the patient's head is in a neutral position, apply a cervical collar, and use short, coordinated moves until the patient can be moved and secured onto a backboard.

If the patient must be removed quickly and there is no upper body motion restriction device available, you can do the following:

1. First responder maintains manual in-line stabilization of the patient's head.

2. Second responder places a cervical collar on the patient.

3. Second responder places a blanket, which is pre-rolled, around the patient, with the centre of the blanket placed at the anterior midline of the cervical collar.

4. Second responder wraps the ends of the blanket around the cervical collar and places them under the patient's arms from the front.

5. Second responder turns the patient using the ends of the blanket until the patient's back is toward the door opening.

6. First responder takes control of the blanket ends, which can be put under the patient's shoulders, along with the motion of the upper body, while second responder takes control of the patient's lower body.

Figure 14–13 You can immobilize a patient with a suspected spinal injury while they are standing.

If the situation requires immediate extrication due to dangers at the scene, just pull the patient out of the situation, taking precautions to stabilize the head and neck in the best way possible.

Maintain an Open Airway

You do not always have to roll the patient onto his back to check breathing. A cry of pain, regular chest movement, or the sound of breathing tells you the patient is breathing. If the patient is breathing, support him in the position in which you found him. If he begins to vomit, position him onto one side to keep the airway clear. Ask other responders to help move the patient's body while you maintain in-line stabilization.

Monitor Vital Signs

After immobilizing the patient, monitor the vital signs. Pay close attention to the patient's level of consciousness and breathing. A serious head injury will often cause changes in consciousness. The patient may give inappropriate responses when asked his name, the time, the place, or what happened or may speak incoherently. The patient may be drowsy, appear to fall asleep, and then suddenly awaken or lose consciousness completely. Breathing may become rapid or irregular. Because injury to the head and/or spine can paralyze chest nerves and muscles, breathing can stop. If this happens, perform rescue breathing. Patients with serious head and/or spine injuries need supplemental oxygen. Administer oxygen if it is available.

Control External Bleeding

Some head and neck injuries include soft tissue damage. Because there are many blood vessels in the head and two major arteries—the carotid arteries—in the neck, the patient with this type of injury can lose large amounts of blood quickly. If there is external bleeding, control it promptly. If applying a pressure dressing to the neck, be careful not to stop the carotid arteries from getting blood to the head.

Maintain Normal Body Temperature

A serious injury to the head and/or spine can disrupt the body's normal heating or cooling mechanism. When this happens, a person is more susceptible to shock. For example, a person suffering a serious head and/or spine injury while outside on a cold day will be more likely to suffer from hypothermia, a life-threatening cooling of the body. This is because the normal shivering response to rewarm the body may not work. It is always important to minimize shock by maintaining normal body temperature.

Removing Helmets and Other Equipment

If you determine that it is necessary to remove a helmet from a patient to provide care, you must do so correctly to avoid causing further harm to the patient.

Helmets fall into multiple categories, including sports helmets and motorcycle helmets. Sports helmets usually have an opening in front, which allows for easier access to the airway. You can usually remove the face mask on a football helmet by unsnapping the plastic clips that hold the face mask to the helmet or by cutting the plastic clips. It is more difficult to access the airway with a motorcycle helmet in place, as they usually cover the full face and the airway.

The steps for a *non-athletic* helmet removal require two responders and are as follows:

Figure 14–14, a-c a, one responder immobilizes the head by holding both sides of the helmet while the second responder loosens the strap; **b**, the second responder holds the patient's mandible and base of the skull; and **c**, the first responder removes the helmet while the second responder maintains manual stabilization

1. If the patient is wearing glasses, remove them before attempting to remove the helmet.

2. The first responder applies stabilization by holding both sides of the helmet, with the fingers on the patient's lower jaw. This will prevent the helmet from moving around if the strap is loose.

3. The second responder loosens the strap at the D-rings while the first responder maintains stabilization (Figure 14–14, a).

4. The second responder then places one hand on the patient's mandible at an angle, with the thumb on one side and the long and index fingers on the other. With the other hand, the second responder holds the back of the patient's head (occipital region) (Figure 14–14, b).

5. The first responder then removes the helmet halfway, making sure to clear the patient's ears, while the second responder readjusts his hand position under the patient's head. The first responder then removes the helmet the rest of the way, making sure to tilt it backward to avoid hitting the patient's nose (Figure 14–14, c).

6. The second responder maintains manual stabilization throughout, from below, preventing head tilt. After the helmet has been removed, the first responder replaces the hands over the ears, taking over responsibility for stabilization.

7. The first responder maintains manual stabilization from above until a cervical collar can be applied and complete immobilization is achieved with a backboard.

For a responder, the removal of athletic equipment, such as football helmets, is usually more challenging than the removal of a motorcycle helmet. Unlike a motorcycle helmet, removal of a football or hockey helmet alone, without removal of the athlete's shoulder pads, increases the risk of cervical movement and further spinal injury. If an athlete is suspected of having a head and/or spine injury, the helmet should only be removed when:

- The face mask does not allow easy access to the airway.

- The design of the helmet and chinstrap, even in the absence of the face mask, does not allow for a controlled airway or adequate ventilation.

- The design of the helmet and chinstraps do not hold the head securely in place (immobilization of the helmet does not also immobilize the head).

- The helmet prevents immobilization of the patient for transport in an appropriate position.

The face mask should be removed after an athlete is suspected of having a head and/or spine injury, even if the patient is still conscious. A football helmet face mask is held in place using four loop-straps, two on the top and one on either side. Each of these loop-straps must be removed by one responder while a second responder minimizes neck movement and maintains the neck in a neutral position. The loop-straps can be removed using a variety of tools, such as a screwdriver, pruning shears, and several other commercial devices designed specifically for this task. However, this is a skilled task, requiring practice. The two side loop-straps are removed first, followed by the two top loop-straps. Never use items such as razor blades or scalpels to remove the loop-straps, as these items increase the risk of injury to the athlete and the responder and may delay removal of the face mask.

To remove a helmet and shoulder pads, one responder must provide manual stabilization while a second responder cuts away the chinstrap, shoulder pad straps, and jersey. Then the internal cheek pads should be removed (using a tongue depressor) and the helmet's air bladder system deflated, if necessary (using a syringe or air pump), while another trained responder stabilizes the athlete's chin and back of the neck. Two to four other trained responders should be placed at strategic locations along the body to support the shoulders, upper torso, and other locations based on the size of the athlete. The responders then lift the athlete and one responder slides the helmet off the head by rotating the helmet in an anterior direction. Do not attempt to spread the helmet by the ear holes, as this will only tighten the helmet on the head, causing further spinal movement and possible injury. Once the helmet is off, a responder should immediately remove the shoulder pads by spreading apart the front panels and pulling them around the athlete's head. Remove any clothing or equipment under the shoulder pads. Lower the athlete back to the ground.

Removing protective equipment such as a football helmet and shoulder pads is a skilled technique, requiring hours of practice. It often requires five responders trained in this skill. If you encounter this type of situation during an athletic event, look to the certified athletic trainer to assist in removal of the face mask, helmet, and shoulder pads, as the necessary tools will be included in athletic emergency kits. Prior planning and interdisciplinary practice among the responder, certified athletic trainer, and emergency department personnel is recommended prior to the beginning of the athletic season, particularly for football.

CARE FOR SPECIFIC HEAD AND FACIAL INJURIES

The head is easily injured because it lacks the padding of muscle and fat that are in other areas of the body. You can feel bone just beneath the surface of the skin over most of the head, including the chin, cheekbones, and scalp (Figure 14–15).

Skull Fracture

A skull fracture accompanied by a brain injury is very serious. The signs and symptoms include:

- Visible damage to the scalp
- Deformity of the skull or face
- Pain or swelling
- Fluid (clear or pinkish) coming from the nose, ears, mouth, or a head wound

Figure 14–15 The head is easily injured because it lacks the padding of muscles and fat that are in other areas of the body.

- Unusual pupil size
- "Raccoon eyes" (bruising around the eyes)
- "Battle's signs" (behind-the-ear bruising)

With a skull fracture, it may be appropriate to take spinal precautions.

Injuries to the Brain

Brain damage can occur with an open or closed wound. The severity of the injury often depends on the mechanism of injury and the force involved. All head injuries should be considered serious. The signs and symptoms include:

- Changes in the level of consciousness
- Paralysis or flaccidity (limp, lacking tone) (usually on one side of the body)
- Unequal facial movements and/or disturbances in vision or pupils
- Ringing in the ears or disturbances in hearing
- Limb rigidity
- Loss of balance
- Pulse that becomes rapid and weak
- High blood pressure with slow pulse
- Breathing problems
- Vomiting
- Incontinence

When the brain sustains an acceleration (or moving) injury, there is usually damage at two points. The brain initially strikes the skull, called the "coup effect," and then there is a second point of damage when the brain strikes the skull on the opposite side, in what is called the "contre-coup effect."

Concussion

A concussion is a complex injury affecting the brain that usually does not result in permanent physical damage to the brain tissue. It can be caused by either a direct blow to the head, face, neck, or elsewhere, with an "impulse" force transmitted to the brain.

Concussions typically result in the rapid onset of short-lived symptoms such as memory loss, dizziness, balance problems, headache, or loss of consciousness. The patient may say he "saw stars" or even "blacked out." You can even have a concussion without loss of consciousness.

The signs and symptoms include:

- Confusion
- Inability to recall what happened just before and after the injury
- Repetitive questioning
- Irritability, uncooperativeness, combativeness
- Inability to answer questions or follow commands
- Persistent vomiting
- Headache
- Balance problems
- Dizziness
- Nausea and/or vomiting
- Ringing in the ears
- Fatigue
- Restlessness
- Seizures
- Brief loss of consciousness

In a sports situation, it is important that athletes showing any symptoms or signs of a concussion not be allowed to return to the current game or practice. The player should not be left alone and should be monitored. The player should be medically evaluated and follow a supervised return-to-play process that takes a minimum of a week to complete.[17] Anyone suspected of having a concussion should be examined by a physician.

Penetrating Wounds

If an object is impaled in the skull, leave it in place and stabilize it with bulky dressings. Dress the area around the wound with sterile gauze but allow blood to drain. Avoid putting direct pressure to a head injury that may involve a skull fracture.

Figure 14–16 To avoid putting pressure on a deep scalp wound, apply pressure around the wound.

NOTE:

If an object has penetrated but cannot be seen (e.g., a bullet), cover the wound lightly with sterile dressings.

Scalp Injury

Scalp bleeding can be minor or severe. The bleeding is usually easily controlled with direct pressure. Because the skull may be injured, be careful to press gently at first. If you feel a depression, a spongy area, or bone fragments, do not put direct pressure on the wound. Attempt to control bleeding with pressure on the area around the wound (Figure 14–16). Examine the injured area carefully because the patient's hair may hide part of the wound. If you are unsure about the extent of a scalp injury, obtain more advanced medical care.

If the patient has only an open wound, control the bleeding with direct pressure. Apply several dressings and hold them in place with your hand (Figure 14–17, a). Secure the dressings with a roller bandage (Figure 14–17, b).

Cheek Injury

Injury to the cheek often involves soft tissue only. Control bleeding from the cheek in the same way as

Figure 14–17, a-b a, Apply pressure to control bleeding from a scalp wound by holding several dressings against the wound; **b**, secure the dressings with a roller bandage.

other soft tissue bleeding. Begin by examining both the outside and inside of the cheek. Bleeding from inside may result from a blow that caused the teeth to cut the inside of the cheek or from a laceration or puncture wound outside. To control bleeding, place several folded dressings inside the mouth, against the cheek. If possible, have the patient hold them in place. If external bleeding is also present, place dressings on the outside of the cheek and apply direct pressure with your hand (Figure 14–18, a) or a pressure bandage (Figure 14–18, b).

An embedded object in the cheek cannot be easily stabilized, makes control of bleeding more difficult, and

may become dislodged and obstruct the airway. You can remove the object by pulling it out the same way it entered. If doing this is difficult or is painful to the patient, leave the object in place and stabilize it with bulky dressings and bandages.

If an object passes completely through the cheek and becomes embedded, you may have to remove it to control bleeding and keep the airway open. This circumstance is the only exception to the general rule of not removing embedded objects from the body.

If you remove the object, fold or roll several dressings and place them inside the mouth. Be sure not to

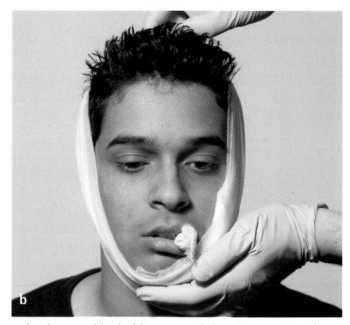

Figure 14–18, a-b a, Apply pressure to control bleeding from a cheek wound by holding several dressings against the wound; **b**, apply direct pressure with a pressure bandage.

obstruct the airway. Apply dressings to the outside of the cheek as well. The patient may not be able to hold these in place, so you may have to hold them. Bleeding inside the cheek can cause the patient to swallow blood. If the patient swallows enough blood, nausea or vomiting could result, which would complicate the situation. When possible, place the patient in a seated position, leaning forward slightly so that blood will not drain into the throat. As with any situation involving serious bleeding or an embedded object, obtain more advanced medical care.

Nose Injury

Nose injuries are often caused by a blow from a blunt object. The result is often a nosebleed (epistaxis). In most cases, you can control bleeding by having the patient sit with the head slightly forward while pinching the nostrils together (Figure 14–19). Other methods of controlling bleeding include applying an ice pack to the bridge of the nose or putting pressure on the upper lip just beneath the nose.

Once you have controlled the bleeding, tell the patient to avoid rubbing, blowing, or picking the nose since this could restart the bleeding. Later, the patient may apply a little petroleum jelly inside the nostril to help keep it moist.

If you think an object is in the nostril, look into the nostril. If you see the object and can easily grasp it with your fingers, then do so. However, do not probe the nostril with your finger. Doing so may push the object farther into the nose and cause bleeding or make it more difficult to remove later. If the object cannot be removed easily, the patient should seek medical attention.

High blood pressure or changes in altitude can also cause nosebleeds (epistaxis). You should obtain more advanced medical care if the bleeding cannot be controlled within 10 to 15 minutes, it stops and then recurs, or the patient says the bleeding is the result of high blood pressure. If the patient loses consciousness, place him on his side to allow blood to drain from his nose.

Eye Injury

Although rarely life-threatening, eye injuries can be scary as the person can lose vision. Eyes can be injured in any manner. Cuts, impaled objects, and burns are among the ways eyes can be injured. Loss of vision; bruising; swelling; burning, tingling, or scratching sensations; and fluid coming from the eyes are all indicators of eye injuries.

See Figure 14–20 for the anatomy of the eye. When you assess someone with an eye injury, you will need to obtain answers to a few questions: When did the injury occur? Were both eyes affected? What symptoms did the patient first notice? Next, carefully examine each eye separately and then together using a small penlight.

Figure 14–19 To control a nosebleed, have the patient lean forward while pinching the nostrils together.

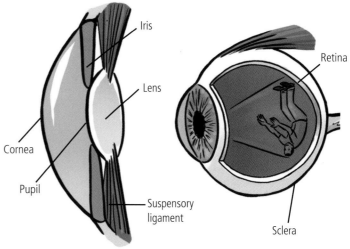

Figure 14–20 The anatomy of the eye.

Here is the procedure for the examination:

- Orbits (the bones in the skull surround and create the structure that holds the eyeballs): Check for bruising, swelling, lacerations, tenderness, depression, and deformity.

- Eyelids: Check for bruising, swelling, and lacerations.

- Mucous membranes: Check for redness, pus, and foreign objects.

- Eyeballs (globes): Check for abnormal colouring, laceration, and foreign objects.

- Pupils: Check for size, shape, and equality. Also check for reaction to light. The pupils should be black, round, and equal in size. They should react to light by constricting.

- Eye movement: Check to see that the eyes can move in all directions. Check for abnormal gaze or pain upon movement.

Here are the basic rules for emergency care of an injured eye:

- Many EMS systems do not allow flushing of an injured eye, except for a chemical injury. Flushing would cause irreversible damage if the eye has been perforated. Follow local protocol.

- Do not put salves or medicines in the injured eye. If this is necessary, a physician will do so.

- Do not remove blood or blood clots from the eye. However, you can sponge blood from the patient's face to help keep him comfortable.

- Only force the eyelid open if you have to flush out chemicals.

- If someone has an eye injury, do not allow the patient to walk without help, especially up or down stairs.

- Do not allow the patient to eat or drink.

- Never panic. It will upset the patient, and you may lose his trust.

- Reassure the patient constantly.

- Ideally, the patient should be transported in a supine position.

Foreign Objects

A foreign object can enter the eye usually by being blown or driven in. Examples of foreign objects may include particles of dirt, sand, cinders, coal dust, or fine pieces of metal. These must be removed or they may cause inflammation, scarring, or infection. They also may scratch the cornea. Signs and symptoms of foreign objects in the eye include pain, excessive tearing, and abnormal sensitivity to light.

Do not allow the patient with a foreign object in the eye to rub his eyes. Rubbing can force a particle with sharp edges into tissues, making removal difficult.

It is always safer for responders to allow EMS personnel with more training to remove a foreign object. However, if removal is necessary and local protocols allow it, there are several ways in which you might proceed. They are as follows:

- Hold the lids apart and flush the eye with clean water (Figure 14–21). Note that some EMS systems do not allow flushing except for chemical burns. Follow local protocol.

- If the object is under the upper eyelid, draw the upper lid down over the lower lid (only if there is no facial makeup, such as glitter or mascara, that will further aggravate the area). When you let it return to its normal position, its undersurface will be drawn over the lashes of the lower lid, which will sweep away the foreign object.

Figure 14–21 Flushing the eye with clean water.

Figure 14–22 Use the corner of a piece of sterile gauze to remove an object under the lower eyelid.

- Grasp the eyelashes of the upper lid. Turn up the lid over a cotton swab. The foreign object may then be carefully removed with the corner of a piece of sterile gauze.

- If the object is under the lower eyelid, pull down the lower lid to expose the inner surface. Then use the corner of a piece of sterile gauze to remove the object (Figure 14–22).

Should a foreign object become lodged in the eyeball, do not try to remove it. Doing so may force the object deeper into the eye, causing further damage. In this case, place a rigid eye shield over the injured eye. Obtain more advanced medical care.

Orbits

Trauma to the face may result in a fracture of the bones that form the orbits, or eye sockets (Figure 14–23). Someone with an orbit injury may complain of double or decreased vision, numbness above the eyebrow or over the cheek, or massive discharge from the nose.

Fractures of the lower part of the orbit are the most common. They can cause paralysis of the upward gaze, that is, the patient's eyes would not be able to follow your finger upward. Someone with an orbit fracture needs hospitalization and surgery.

If there is no injury to the eyeball, place cold packs over the injured orbit to help reduce the swelling. However, if the eyeball is injured or you are in doubt, do not apply cold packs. Obtain more advanced medical care.

Eyelids

Lid injuries include bruising, burns, swelling or drooping, and lacerations (Figure 14–24). Anything that damages the lid may also damage the eyeball. In general, there is not much that can be done for these injuries in the field, beyond gentle patching.

To control bleeding from the eyelid, apply light pressure. Don't use any pressure if the eyeball itself is injured.

Never attempt to remove embedded material, such as gravel. Use sterile gauze soaked in saline to keep the wound from drying. If the lid is avulsed, preserve it and send it with the patient for later grafting.

Figure 14–23 Facial trauma may result in a fracture of the eye sockets.

Figure 14–24 Eyelid injuries include bruising, burns, swelling or drooping, and lacerations.

> ### NOTE:
>
> *When caring for an eye injury, it is appropriate to just cover the injured eye, unless local protocol dictates otherwise. If the patient feels more comfortable having both eyes covered, then do so.*

Globes

Injuries to the globe include bruises, lacerations, foreign objects, and abrasions. It is generally best to treat these in the hospital, where specialized equipment is available. In the field, keep the patient with an injury to the globe supine.

Chemical Burns to the Eye

Chemical burns to the eye are quite common (Figure 14–25) and represent one of the most urgent emergencies related to the eyes. Permanent damage can occur within seconds of the injury. The first 10 minutes are crucial to the final outcome. Remember, burning and tissue damage will continue as long as the chemical remains in the eye, even if it is diluted.

Figure 14–25 Chemical burns to the eyes are quite common.

Figure 14–26, a-b For an impaled object in the eye: **a**, pack around the object with bulky dressings, without applying pressure; **b**, bandage over and around the dressings to secure them in place.

To provide emergency care, begin immediate, continuous irrigation with water. Do not use anything other than water. The water does not need to be sterile, but it must be clean. You must wear protective glasses when providing this care. Gently hold the patient's eyelid open so that all the chemical can be flushed away. You may have to force the eyelid open because of the patient's pain.

Pour water from the inside corner across the eyeball to the outside edge. This will help avoid contaminating the uninjured eye. Irrigate continuously for 10 to 15 minutes.

Remove any solid particles from the surface of the eye with a moistened cotton swab. Contact lenses must be removed or flushed out. If not, chemicals could be trapped between the lens and the cornea. Follow local protocol.

Following irrigation, wash your hands thoroughly to avoid contaminating your own eyes.

Impaled Objects

Only a physician should remove an object impaled in the eye. You must protect the patient from further injury until he can reach a doctor. Therefore, you must stabilize the object in place.

Begin by stabilizing the patient's head. Keep the patient supine. Pack around the object with bulky dressings, without applying pressure (Figure 14–26, a). Bandage over and around the dressings to keep them in place (Figure 14–26, b).

Once the object has been stabilized, cover both eyes with sterile gauze or eye pads while maintaining the patient's head in a neutral position.

After covering, stay with the patient and ensure he knows someone is there. It is common for the patient to panic.

Extruded Eyeball

During a serious injury, the eyeball may be knocked out of the socket, or extruded (Figure 14–27). Do not try to replace it. Instead, cover it with a moist dressing and protective cup. Do not apply any pressure.

Figure 14–27 The eyeball may be extruded during a serious injury.

Other Eye Injuries

For all other emergencies involving the eye, patch the eye and arrange for transportation. Such emergencies may include eye infections, a black eye, corneal abrasions, light burns, and heat burns. Follow local protocol.

Removing Contact Lenses

Millions of people in Canada wear contact lenses. Some may wear a lens in one eye only, so be sure to examine both eyes carefully. Other people, especially older adults, wear both contact lenses and eyeglasses. To detect lenses, shine a penlight into each eye. A soft lens will show up as a shadow on the outer portion of the eye. A hard lens will show up as a shadow over the iris. In general, remove contact lenses only when there has been a chemical burn to the eye. Always follow local protocols.

Ear Injury

Ear injuries are common. Either the soft tissue of the outer ear or the eardrum within the ear may be injured. Open wounds, such as lacerations or abrasions, can result from recreational injuries, for example, falling off a bike. An avulsion of the ear may occur when a pierced earring catches on something and tears the earlobe. You can control bleeding from the soft tissues of the ear by applying direct pressure to the affected area.

If the patient has a serious head and/or spine injury, blood or other fluid may be in the ear canal or draining from the ear. Cover the ear lightly with a sterile dressing without applying direct pressure, stabilize the head and spine, and obtain more advanced medical care.

The ear can also be injured internally. A direct blow to the head may rupture the eardrum. Sudden pressure changes, such as those caused by an explosion or a deep-water dive, can also injure the ear internally. The patient may lose hearing or balance or experience inner ear pain. These injuries require more advanced medical care.

A foreign object, such as dirt, an insect, or a piece of cotton, can easily become lodged in the ear canal. If you can easily see and grasp the object, remove it. Do not try to remove any object by using a pin, a toothpick, or any sharp item. You could force the object farther back or puncture the eardrum. Sometimes you can remove the object if you pull down on the earlobe, tilt the head to the side, and shake or gently strike the head on the affected side. If you cannot easily remove the object, the patient should be seen by a physician.

Mouth and Jaw Injuries

Your primary concern for any injury to the mouth or jaw is to ensure an open airway. Injuries in these areas may cause breathing problems if blood or loose teeth obstruct the airway. A swollen or fractured trachea may also obstruct breathing.

If the patient is bleeding from the mouth and you do not suspect a head and/or spine injury, place him in a seated position with the head tilted slightly forward. This will allow any blood to drain from the mouth. If this position is not possible, place the patient on his side to allow blood to drain from the mouth.

For injuries that penetrate the lip, place a rolled dressing between the lip and the gum. You can place another dressing on the outer surface of the lip. If the tongue is bleeding, apply a dressing and direct pressure. Applying cold to the lips or tongue can help reduce swelling and ease pain. If the bleeding cannot be controlled, obtain more advanced medical care.

If the injury knocked out one or more of the patient's teeth, control the bleeding and save any teeth so that they can be reinserted. To control the bleeding, roll a sterile dressing and insert it into the space left by the missing tooth. Have the patient bite down to maintain pressure (Figure 14–28). Put the tooth in milk, if available, and keep it with the patient. If there is no milk, wrap the tooth in a clean cloth or gauze along with some of the patient's own saliva. Seal the container with tape and label it with the name of the patient, date, and time. A dentist may be able to reinsert the tooth.

If the injury is severe enough for you to need to obtain more advanced medical care, give the tooth to the appropriate personnel. If the injury is not severe, the patient should immediately seek a dentist who can re-implant the tooth. Time is a critical factor if the tooth is to be successfully re-implanted. Ideally, it should be done within an hour after the injury.

Figure 14–28 If a patient has a knocked out tooth, he can bite down on a sterile dressing to maintain pressure.

Injuries serious enough to fracture or dislocate the jaw can also cause other head and/or spine injuries. Be sure to maintain an open airway. Check inside the mouth for bleeding. Control bleeding as you would for other head injuries.

SUMMARY

In this chapter, you have learned how to recognize and care for serious head and spine injuries and specific injuries to the head and face. To decide whether an injury is serious, you must consider its cause. If you think that an injury of this type might be serious, obtain more advanced medical care.

Like injuries elsewhere on the body, injuries to the head and spine often involve both soft tissues and bone. Control bleeding as necessary, usually with direct pressure on the wound. With scalp injuries, be careful not to apply pressure to a possible skull fracture. With eye injuries, remember not to apply pressure on the eyeball.

If you suspect that the patient may have a serious injury to the head and/or spine, minimize movement of the injured area when providing care. This is best accomplished by using in-line stabilization. Administer oxygen if it is available. Secure the patient to a backboard if you must move him.

As you read the next chapter about how to care for injuries to the chest, abdomen, and pelvis, remember the principles of care for head and spine injuries—serious injuries of the chest and abdomen can also affect the spine.

The man vomits while you are giving care. What do you do?

Chapter 15

Chest, Abdominal, and Pelvic Injuries

A man who has been shot is lying on a sidewalk in a busy urban setting. He is displaying an altered level of consciousness and is in considerable pain. There is blood on his shirt, and he makes an abnormal sucking sound when he tries to breathe. The scene has been deemed safe for you to approach. What do you do?

INTRODUCTION

Injuries to the chest and abdomen may include minor soft tissue injuries, internal organ damage, or fractures. Fractures and lacerations often occur in motor vehicle collisions to occupants not wearing safety belts. Falls, penetration by objects such as bullets, and other forms of trauma may also cause such injuries.

Injuries to the pelvis may be minor soft tissue injuries or serious bone and internal structure injuries. The pelvis includes a group of large bones that form a protective girdle around the organs inside. A great force is required to cause serious injury to the pelvis.

Because the chest, abdomen, and pelvis contain many organs important to life, injury to these areas can be fatal. A force that causes severe injury in these areas may also cause injury to the spine. Care for these injuries includes:

- Controlling external bleeding
- Limiting movement
- Minimizing shock
- Administering oxygen if available
- Obtaining more advanced medical care
- Providing ongoing survey and care

This chapter describes the signs and symptoms of and care for injuries to the chest, abdomen, and pelvis. In all cases, perform your scene and primary survey and then care for all life-threatening injuries first. *All injuries described in this chapter are serious enough that you should always obtain more advanced medical care immediately.*

CHEST INJURIES

Chest injuries are one of the leading causes of trauma deaths each year. Many traffic fatalities involve chest injuries. Injuries to the chest may also result from a wide variety of other causes, such as falls, sports mishaps, and crushing or penetrating forces (Figure 15–1).

Figure 15–1 Injuries to the chest may result from crushing forces, falls, or sports mishaps.

Chest wounds are either open or closed. Open chest wounds occur when an object, such as a knife or bullet, penetrates the chest wall. Fractured ribs may break through the skin to cause an open chest injury. A chest wound is closed if the skin is not broken. Closed chest wounds are generally caused by a blunt force, such as that from a fall or a motor vehicle collision.

Signs and Symptoms of Chest Injury

You should know the signs and symptoms of a serious chest injury. These may occur with both open and closed wounds. You will recognize some of these signs and symptoms from Chapter 6. They include:

- Difficulty breathing (dyspnea)
- Pain at the site of the injury that increases with deep breathing or movement
- Obvious deformity, such as that caused by a fracture
- Flushed, pale, or bluish discoloration of the skin
- Coughing up blood

NOTE:

If a patient has sustained a chest injury or is complaining of chest pain, the chest must be exposed for proper assessment, examination, and intervention.

Specific Types of Chest Injuries

Rib Fractures

Rib fractures are usually caused by a forceful blow to the chest (Figure 15–2). Although painful, a simple rib fracture is rarely life-threatening. Someone with a fractured rib often breathes shallowly because normal or deep breathing is painful. The person will usually attempt to ease the pain by leaning toward the side of the fracture and pressing a hand or arm over the injured area. Therefore, pain in the rib area, shallow breathing, and holding the area are signs and symptoms of a possible rib fracture.

However, serious rib fractures can be life-threatening. In severe blows or crushing injuries, multiple ribs can fracture in many places. This can produce a loose section of ribs that does not move normally with the rest of the chest during breathing. Usually, the loose section will move in the opposite direction from the rest of the chest; this is called paradoxical movement. The portion of chest wall lying between the fractures is called flail chest. When a flail chest involves the sternum, the breastbone is separated from the rest of the ribs.

Care for Rib Fractures

If you suspect a fractured rib or ribs, have the patient rest in a position that will make breathing easier. You can use an object, such as a pillow or rolled blanket, to

Figure 15–2 Forceful blows to the chest can cause rib fractures.

help support and immobilize the injured area. Serious fractures often cause severe bleeding and difficulty breathing (dyspnea); shock is likely to develop. Administer oxygen if it is available and provide ongoing survey and care.

Care for Flail Chest

Have the patient rest in a position that makes breathing easier, usually a semi-reclining position. Feel the chest area gently to locate the area of the flail segment and apply bulky dressings several centimetres thick.

Bandage the dressings in place with long strips of tape. If bulky dressings are not available, use a small pillow or other lightweight material. Do not try to bind, strap, or tape the flail section itself.

Puncture Injuries

Puncture wounds to the chest range in severity from minor to life-threatening. Stab and gunshot wounds are examples of puncture injuries. A forceful puncture may penetrate the rib cage and allow air to enter the chest through the wound (Figure 15–3). This prevents the

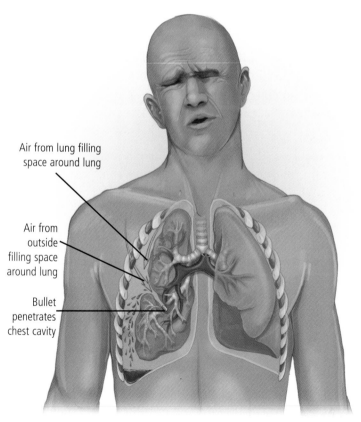

Air from lung filling space around lung

Air from outside filling space around lung

Bullet penetrates chest cavity

Figure 15–3 A puncture wound that penetrates the lung or the chest cavity surrounding the lung allows air to go in and out of the cavity.

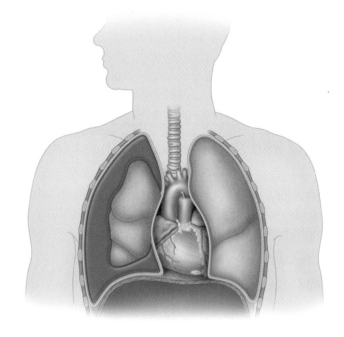

Figure 15–4 A hemothorax is bleeding into the pleural space.

lungs from functioning normally. The penetrating object can injure any structure within the chest, including the lungs, heart, or major arteries or veins.

Hemothorax

Hemothorax is bleeding into the pleural space (Figure 15–4). This can be caused by blunt or penetrating trauma resulting in a lacerated lung or laceration of a blood vessel to the chest. As the affected side of the chest begins to fill with blood, the person will have trouble breathing and will suffer from shock secondary to the blood loss. If bleeding continues, it will also create pressure on the heart and lungs.

Hemothorax can occur with closed or open chest wounds. The severity of the hemothorax depends on the amount of bleeding into the pleural space. Hemothorax is cared for by correcting the ventilatory and circulatory problems. High concentration oxygen should be administered, and if breathing is shallow or inadequate, ventilations should be assisted using a BVM. Control any external bleeding if necessary.

Pneumothorax

Pneumothorax is a condition caused by air entering the pleural space (Figure 15–5). It may occur as a

Figure 15–5 Pneumothorax is a condition caused by air entering the pleural space.

Figure 15–6 A tension pneumothorax is the continual flow of air into the pleural space, which cannot escape.

result of blunt or penetrating trauma or spontaneously in certain individuals. The lung may be partially or totally collapsed, depending on how much air has entered the pleural space. A person's signs and symptoms will also depend on how much air has entered the space. Signs and symptoms of pneumothorax may include the following:

- Pleuritic chest pain, pain that is made worse by coughing or deep breaths
- Difficult breathing (dyspnea) and rapid breathing (tachypnea)
- Decreased or absent breath sounds on the affected side

There is always the possibility that a pneumothorax can progress to a tension pneumothorax.

Tension Pneumothorax

Tension pneumothorax is the continual flow of air into the pleural space, which cannot escape (Figure 15–6). This usually occurs when lung tissue is torn and air leaks into the pleural space, causing pressure on the lung, heart, and major blood vessels. The lung will eventually collapse, thereby diminishing the amount of

air that can be inhaled or exhaled. As the condition worsens, the signs of hypoxia follow, and a breathing emergency is evident. Provide ongoing survey and care, administer oxygen, and ensure prompt transport to a medical facility.

Care for Puncture Injuries

Puncture wounds cause varying degrees of internal or external bleeding. If the injury penetrates the rib cage, air can pass freely in and out of the chest cavity and the patient cannot breathe normally. With each breath the patient takes, you may hear a sucking sound coming from the wound. This is the primary sign of a penetrating chest injury called a sucking chest wound.

Without proper care, the patient's condition will worsen quickly. The affected lung or lungs will fail to function, and breathing will become more difficult. Your main concern is the breathing problem. To care for a sucking chest wound, cover the wound with an occlusive dressing—one that does not allow air to pass through it. A plastic bag, a vinyl or nitrile glove, or a piece of plastic wrap or aluminum foil folded several times and placed over the wound can be substituted if a sterile occlusive dressing is not available. Tape the dressing in

a

b   Inhalation

c   Exhalation

Figure 15–7, a-c With a sucking chest wound, use an occlusive dressing: **a**, tape it on three sides; **b**, so air does not enter the chest cavity when the patient inhales; but **c**, air can escape when the patient exhales.

> ### NOTE:
> *Subcutaneous emphysema:*
> *If air or gas gets into the subcutaneous tissue of the body, the affected area may appear swollen and may make a "crackling" sound as air moves around.*

place, except for the side that is closest to the ground. This keeps air from entering the wound when the patient inhales but allows it to escape when he exhales and promotes drainage of any fluids from the chest wound (Figure 15–7, a-c). There are some commercially made occlusive dressings for chest wounds, such as an Asherman Chest Seal (Figure 15–8). Administer oxygen if available and take steps to minimize shock. Provide ongoing survey and care.

ABDOMINAL INJURIES

The abdomen is the area immediately under the chest and above the pelvis. It is easily injured because it is not surrounded by bones. It is protected at the back by the spine. The upper abdomen is only partially protected in front by the lower ribs. The muscles of the back and abdomen also help protect the internal organs, many of which are vital. Most important are the organs that are easily injured or tend to bleed profusely when injured, such as the liver, spleen, and stomach.

The liver is rich in blood. Located in the upper right quadrant of the abdomen, this organ is protected somewhat by the lower ribs. However, it is delicate and can be torn by blows from blunt objects or penetrated by a fractured rib. The resulting bleeding can be severe and can

Figure 15–8 A commercially available occlusive dressing.

quickly be fatal. The liver, when injured, can also leak bile into the abdomen, which can cause severe infection.

The spleen is located in the upper left quadrant of the abdomen, behind the stomach, and is protected somewhat by the lower left ribs. Like the liver, this organ is easily damaged. The spleen may rupture when the abdomen is struck forcefully by a blunt object. Since the spleen stores blood, an injury can cause a severe loss of blood in a short time and be life-threatening.

The stomach is one of the main digestive organs. The upper part of the stomach changes shape depending on its contents, the stage of digestion, and the size and strength of the stomach muscles. It is lined with many blood vessels and nerves. The stomach can bleed severely when injured, and food contents may empty into the abdomen and possibly cause infection.

Signs and Symptoms of Abdominal Injury

The signs and symptoms of serious abdominal injury include:

- Severe pain

- Bruising

- External bleeding

- Nausea and vomiting (sometimes vomit containing blood)

- Pale, moist skin

- Weakness

- Thirst

- Pain, tenderness, or a tight feeling in the abdomen

- Distension in the abdomen

- Organs possibly protruding from the abdomen

- Signs and symptoms of shock

Care for Abdominal Injuries

Like a chest injury, an injury to the abdomen is either open or closed. Even with a closed wound, the rupture of an organ can cause serious internal bleeding that can quickly result in shock. Injuries to the abdomen can be extremely painful. Serious reactions can occur if organs leak blood or other contents into the abdomen.

With a severe open injury, abdominal organs sometimes protrude through the wound (Figure 15–9, a). To care for an open wound in the abdomen, follow these steps:

1. Carefully position the patient on his back.

2. Bend the patient's knees slightly. This allows the muscles of the abdomen to relax. Place rolled-up blankets or pillows under the patient's knees. If the movement of the patient's legs causes pain, leave the legs straight.

3. Do not apply direct pressure.

4. Do not push organs back in.

5. Remove clothing from around the wound (Figure 15–9, b).

6. Apply moist, sterile dressings loosely over the wound. (Figure 15–9, c). (Warm tap water can be used to moisten the dressings).

7. Cover dressings loosely with plastic wrap if available.

8. Cover dressings lightly with a folded towel to maintain warmth (Figure 15–9, d).

9. Maintain normal body temperature.

10. Administer oxygen if available.

11. Obtain more advanced medical care.

12. Provide ongoing survey and care.

To care for a closed abdominal injury:

1. Carefully position the patient on her back.

2. Bend the patient's knees slightly. This allows the muscles of the abdomen to relax. Place rolled-up blankets or pillows under the patient's knees. If the movement of the patient's legs causes pain, leave the legs straight.

3. Do not apply direct pressure.

4. Administer oxygen if available.

5. Take steps to minimize shock.

6. Obtain more advanced medical care.

7. Provide ongoing survey and care.

Abdominal Aortic Aneurysm

In an abdominal aortic aneurysm, the wall of the aorta weakens and bulges (like a bulge in a garden hose) until the vessel thins and ruptures. The risk factors are the same as those for heart disease or stroke.

Signs and symptoms:

- Abdominal pain
- Abdominal rigidity
- Back pain
- Nausea and vomiting
- Pulsating mass in the abdomen
- Diminished or absent pulses in lower extremities
- Tingling or numbness in the lower extremities

PELVIC INJURIES

The pelvis is the lower part of the trunk and contains the bladder, the reproductive organs in females, and the lower portion of the large intestine, including the rectum. Arteries and nerves pass through the pelvis. The organs within the pelvis are well protected on the sides and back but not in front (Figure 15–10). Injuries to the pelvis may include fractures to the pelvic bone and damage to structures within. Fractured bones may puncture or lacerate internal organs. These organs can also be injured when struck by forceful blows from blunt or penetrating objects.

Signs and Symptoms of Pelvic Injury

Signs and symptoms of injury to the pelvis are very similar to those of abdominal injury. There may also be pain on palpation, as well as a grating, crackling, or popping sound (crepitus). Certain pelvic injuries may also cause loss of sensation in the legs or inability to move them. This may indicate an injury to the lower spine.

a

b

c

d

Figure 15–9, a-d **a**, Severe injuries to the abdominal cavity can result in protruding organs; **b**, remove clothing from around the wound; **c**, apply moist, sterile dressings loosely over the wound; and **d**, cover dressings lightly with a folded towel to maintain warmth.

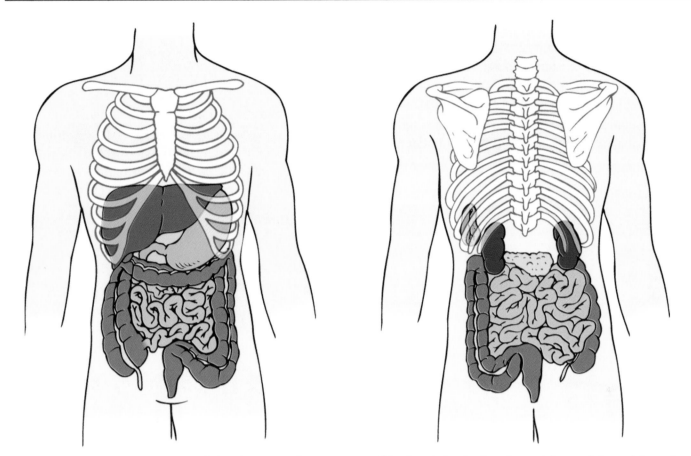

Figure 15–10 Unlike the organs of the chest or pelvis, organs within the abdominal cavity and front of the pelvic cavity are not well protected.

Care for Pelvic Injuries

Care for pelvic injuries in the same way as for abdominal injuries. Do not move the patient unless necessary and avoid putting any pressure on the pelvis. If possible, keep the patient lying flat. If not, help her become comfortable. Control any external bleeding and cover any protruding organs. Someone with a pelvic injury should be immobilized on a backboard. Always obtain more advanced medical care, administer oxygen if available, take steps to minimize shock, and provide ongoing survey and care.

An injury to the pelvis sometimes involves the genitals, the external reproductive organs. Genital injuries are either closed wounds, such as a bruise, or open wounds, such as an avulsion or laceration. Any injury to the genitals is extremely painful. It is also important to maintain the patient's privacy the best you can. Care for a closed wound as you would for any closed wound. If the injury is an open wound, apply a sterile dressing and

direct pressure with your hand or the patient's hand. If any parts are amputated, wrap them appropriately and make sure they are transported with the patient. Injuries to the genital area can be embarrassing for both the patient and the responder. Explain briefly what you are going to do and do it. Act in a confident manner; this will make the situation easier for you and the patient for whom you are providing care.

SUMMARY

Injuries to the chest, abdomen, or pelvis can be serious. They can damage soft tissues, bones, and internal organs. Although many injuries are immediately obvious, some may be detected only as the patient's condition worsens over time. Watch for signs and symptoms of serious injuries that require medical attention.

Care for any life-threatening condition, such as a breathing emergency, then give any additional care needed for specific injuries. For open wounds to the chest, abdomen, or pelvis, control bleeding. If you suspect a fracture, immobilize the injured part. Use special dressings for sucking chest wounds and open abdominal wounds when these materials are available. Always obtain more advanced medical care as soon as possible, administer oxygen if it is available, and take steps to minimize shock. This gives the patient with a serious injury the best chance for survival and full recovery.

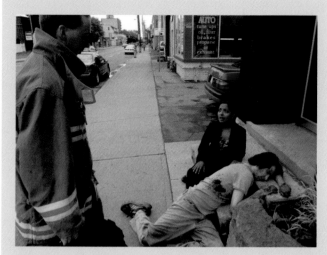

The man begins to find breathing more difficult. What do you do?

Medical Emergencies

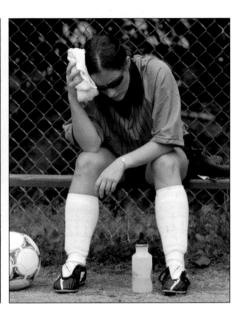

INTRODUCTION

You are summoned to assist with an emergency in an office building. When you arrive at the office, you find a middle-aged woman lying motionless on her side on the floor. A man is kneeling helplessly next to her; he identifies himself as her co-worker. Other co-workers are gathering, but no one is helping her. There is an empty pill bottle without a label on the floor beside her. You notice that her body is limp. Saliva is dribbling from her mouth. Her face seems distorted; her mouth droops to one side. The man tells you her name and then you speak to her, calling her name a few times and tapping her on the shoulder, but she doesn't respond. You observe that she is breathing rapidly. Her skin is cool, and she is sweating heavily.

You ask the man what happened and how long she has been lying like this, unresponsive. He says he's not sure. He came out of his office and found her lying face down on the floor. He then rolled her over. You obtain more advanced medical care. You ask the man and the bystanders if anyone knows whether she has any medical conditions, is taking any medications, or is allergic to anything. No one seems to know. You look for a MedicAlert® medical identification product but don't find one.

You scramble to think of all the possibilities to explain this woman's condition. Could she have had a heart attack? Could she have been poisoned? Did she have an allergic reaction? A stroke? A diabetic emergency? A head injury from a fall? Did she have a seizure?

You know that advanced medical care will arrive in about eight minutes. You try to remain calm. You ask bystanders for a blanket to help warm the woman's cool body and you cover her. You check to make sure her airway is clear. You administer oxygen. You don't move her but examine her carefully for any clues as to what the problem could be. You want to help the woman more, but because you do not know what the problem is, you are unsure about how to proceed. You feel as if you should do something. But what more should you do?

The Dilemma of Medical Emergencies

The dilemma in the preceding scenario is not rare. You could someday face a similar situation involving an unclear medical emergency. Unlike easily identifiable problems, such as external bleeding, medical emergencies are rarely as clear. Therefore, you may feel more uncertain about providing care.

When you face an emergency you do not understand, it is normal to feel helpless or indecisive. Yet, like everyone, you still want to help to the best of your ability. Take comfort from the fact that giving initial care, even for medical emergencies you do not understand, does not require extensive knowledge. You do not have to "diagnose" or choose among possible problems to be able to provide appropriate care. By conducting a proper assessment and using the guidelines for care in previous chapters, you can provide appropriate care until you are able to obtain more advanced medical care. Knowing this, you can approach an unclear medical emergency with confidence.

The woman could have been experiencing a stroke, a diabetic emergency, or some other medical emergency, but you could not have known this. None of the bystanders knew the nature of her problem, and she was not wearing a MedicAlert® medical identification product. Did it matter that you could not diagnose exactly what her condition was? Not at all. You correctly focused on the following basics of care:

- Monitor the ABCs. Keeping her positioned on one side kept her airway clear by letting fluid drain from her mouth so that it would not obstruct her airway. You could easily determine that she was breathing by watching and listening to her inhale and exhale. Since she was breathing, you knew she had a pulse. She did not have any severe external bleeding.

- Obtain more advanced medical care. This ensured a rapid response for a patient who needed more advanced attention.

- Do a secondary survey to check for any additional injuries. When you surveyed the woman's body looking for any clues to her condition or additional problems, you did not find any. Therefore, you did not need to give further care.

- Minimize shock. Maintaining normal body temperature with a blanket, keeping her positioned on the floor, and administering oxygen helped minimize shock.

In this instance, everything that needed to be done was done. What if other information had been available, such as a MedicAlert® medical identification product indicating that the woman had diabetes? Would that have helped you care for this patient? No; even if you had known she had diabetes, it would not have affected the care you provided. Since she was not conscious, your care would have been the same. Almost all the care you will give someone having a medical emergency is as simple as following these basics of care, whether the patient is conscious or unconscious.

The Onset of Medical Emergencies

Medical emergencies can be caused by widely varying conditions and illnesses. Some acute conditions can develop very rapidly, whereas chronic conditions may develop gradually and persist for a long time. Medical emergencies can result from illness, disease, or chronic problems caused by diseases such as heart and lung disease. Or they can involve hormone imbalances, such as diabetes. Sometimes a medical emergency can involve sudden unexplained conditions, such as fainting. A person may become seriously ill because of poisoning. Someone with epilepsy can become ill due to occasional seizures. In other instances, medical emergencies result from allergies, when someone is exposed to a certain substance that causes a severe reaction. Still other medical emergencies can be caused by serious illness brought on by overexposure to heat or cold.

Chapter *16*

Sudden Illnesses

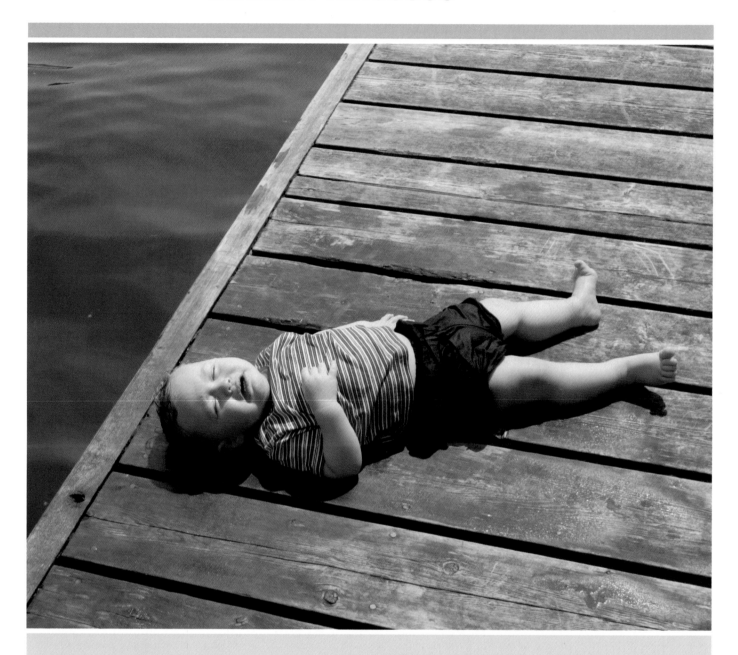

On a hot afternoon at the lake, a little boy staggers and falls into the water. The mother pulls him out onto the dock, where he begins to have a seizure. His arms and legs flail wildly about. What do you do?

INTRODUCTION

As a responder, you could someday face a situation involving an unidentifiable sudden illness, referred to as a medical emergency. In such a situation, you may feel uncertain about how to provide care.

When you face an emergency that is unclear, it is normal to feel indecisive. Yet, like any responder, you will still want to provide care to the best of your ability. You do not have to "diagnose" or choose among possible problems to provide appropriate care. By following a few basic guidelines for care, you can provide appropriate care until more advanced medical personnel arrive. Because you know these guidelines for care, you can approach any medical emergency with confidence.

Medical emergencies can develop rapidly (acute conditions) or gradually (chronic conditions) and may persist for a long time. Sometimes, there are no warning signs or symptoms to alert you or the patient that something is about to happen. At other times, the only symptoms the patient complains of are feeling "ill" or feeling that "something is wrong." Symptoms may also be atypical; older adults or those with diabetes, for example, may have a heart attack without experiencing chest pain.

Medical emergencies have a wide range of causes, including chronic problems from diseases such as heart disease and diabetes, allergies, or seizures from illnesses such as epilepsy or overexposure to heat or cold. Conditions such as diabetes, epilepsy, poisoning, shock, and high-altitude illness can cause a variety of signs and symptoms, including sudden, unexplained altered mental status. A patient may complain of feeling lightheaded, dizzy, or weak. The patient may also feel nauseated or may vomit. Breathing, pulse, and skin characteristics may change. Ultimately, if a patient looks and feels ill, there could be a medical emergency that requires immediate care (see Table 16–1).

GENERAL MEDICAL COMPLAINTS

Making the Assessment and Providing Care

The assessment and care of general medical complaints follow the same process as other conditions:

- Size-up the scene to ensure your own safety and the safety of others.

- Conduct your primary survey to identify and correct any immediately life-threatening conditions.

- Conduct a SAMPLE history and secondary survey to gather additional information whenever possible.

- Obtain more advanced medical care.

- Help the patient rest comfortably.

- Keep the patient from getting chilled or overheated; maintain normal body temperature.

- Provide reassurance.

- Prevent further harm.

- Administer emergency oxygen if it is available and indicated.

- Provide ongoing survey and care.

Altered Mental Status

Altered mental status can result from many causes. Some of these include the following:

- Fever

- Infection

- Poisoning or overdose, including substance abuse or misuse

- Blood sugar/endocrine emergencies

- Head injury

- Inadequate oxygenation or ventilation

- Any condition resulting in decreased blood flow or oxygen to the brain

- Cardiac emergencies

- Diabetic emergencies

- Shock

- Stroke

- Behavioural illness

- Seizures

Signs and Symptoms of Altered Mental Status

Altered mental status is one of the most common medical emergencies. It is often characterized by a sudden or gradual change in a person's level of consciousness (LOC), including drowsiness, confusion, and partial or complete loss of consciousness. Altered mental status is sometimes caused by a temporary reduction of blood flow to the brain, such as when blood collects or pools in the legs and lower body. When the brain is suddenly deprived of its normal blood flow, it momentarily shuts down. This condition is called fainting, or syncope.

Fainting can be triggered by an emotional shock, such as the sight of blood. It may be caused by pain, specific medical conditions like heart disease, standing for a long time, or overexertion. Some people, such as pregnant women or older adults, are more likely to faint when suddenly changing positions, for example, when moving from lying down to standing up. Whenever changes inside the body momentarily reduce the blood flow to the brain, fainting may occur.

A person may faint with or without warning. Often, the person may first feel light-headed or dizzy. There may be signs of shock, such as pale or ashen, cool, moist skin. The person may feel nauseated and complain of numbness or tingling in the fingers and toes. The person's breathing and pulse may become faster.

Providing Care for Altered Mental Status

To care for patients with altered mental status, complete primary and secondary surveys and history as needed. Perform ongoing assessments as you provide care. Make sure the airway is open, and place an unconscious patient in the supine (face-up) position. Have suction equipment available if needed. If the patient is conscious or becomes conscious, do not give anything to eat or drink. Eating or drinking can increase the chance of vomiting. If possible, attempt to get information from the patient, family members, or bystanders. This is important, as a patient's condition may deteriorate rapidly in these situations, making conversation impossible. Any information you can obtain may help with the patient's treatment upon arrival at the hospital.

Sometimes a patient may briefly faint and slowly begin to regain consciousness. Fainting often resolves itself when the patient moves from a standing or sitting position to a lying down position, as normal circulation to the brain often resumes. The patient usually regains consciousness within a minute.

Fainting itself does not usually harm the patient, but injury may occur from falling. Take spinal precautions if you suspect trauma. If you can reach a patient who is starting to collapse, lower the patient to the ground or another flat surface and position the patient on her back, lying flat. Monitor the patient's breathing and pulse. Loosen any restrictive clothing, such as a tie or collar. Do not splash water on the patient's face. Doing so does little to stimulate the patient, and the patient could aspirate the water. Administer emergency oxygen if it is available.

Although a fainting patient usually recovers quickly, you may not be able to determine if the fainting is associated with a more serious medical condition. For this reason, more advanced medical care is indicated and the EMS system should be activated.

Altered Mental Status in Pediatrics

Children who are experiencing altered mental status may exhibit a change in behaviour, personality, or responsiveness beyond what is expected at their age. These children may exhibit anxiety, agitation, aggression, and/or combativeness. Alternatively, they may be difficult to rouse, sleepy, or even unresponsive. It is not unusual for altered mental status to result in decreased muscle tone.

Common causes of altered mental status requiring immediate medical attention include respiratory failure, deficiency in oxygen concentration in arterial blood (hypoxemia), shock, hypoglycemia, brain injury (including shaken baby syndrome), seizures, poisoning, intentional overdose, sepsis, meningitis, hyperthermia, and hypothermia.

Left untreated, altered mental status can lead to life-threatening problems, including inefficient respiration, hypoxemia, airway obstruction, and respiratory failure. For care of children with altered mental status, take spinal precautions if the cause is not clear or trauma is suspected. Treat any breathing emergency and care for any other injuries or conditions found. Obtain more advanced medical care and provide ongoing assessment and care.

Diabetic Emergencies

To function normally, body cells need sugar as a source of energy. Through the digestive process, the body breaks down food into sugars, which are absorbed into

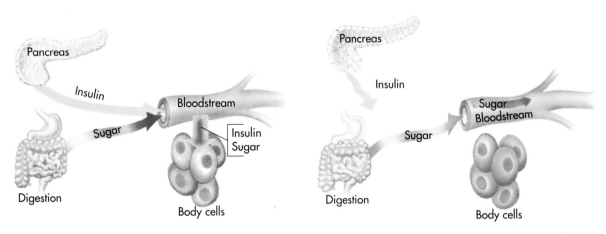

Figure 16–1 The hormone insulin is needed to take sugar from the blood into the body cells.

the bloodstream. However, sugar cannot pass freely from the blood into the body cells; it needs an escort. Insulin, a hormone produced in the pancreas, takes sugar into the cells. Without a proper balance of sugar and insulin, the cells will starve and the body will not function properly (Figure 16–1).

The condition in which the body does not produce enough insulin is called diabetes mellitus or sugar diabetes.

There are two major types of diabetes. Type 1, insulin-dependent diabetes, occurs when the body produces little or no insulin. Since this type of diabetes tends to begin in childhood, it is often called juvenile diabetes. Most people with insulin-dependent diabetes have to inject insulin into their bodies daily.

Type 2, non-insulin-dependent diabetes, occurs when the body produces insulin but not in a quantity sufficient for the body's needs, or the body does not properly use the insulin that it produces. This condition is called maturity-onset diabetes.

Anyone with diabetes must carefully monitor his diet and exercise. People with insulin-dependent diabetes must also regulate their use of insulin (Figure 16–2). When someone with diabetes fails to control these factors, either of two problems can occur: too much or too little sugar in the body. This imbalance causes illness, which can become a diabetic emergency.

When the insulin level in the body is too low, the sugar level in the blood is high. This condition is called hyperglycemia (Figure 16–3, a). Sugar is present in the blood but cannot be transported from the blood into the cells without insulin. When this occurs, body cells become starved for sugar. The body attempts to meet its need for energy by using other stored food and energy sources, such as fats. However, converting fat to energy produces waste products and increases the

Figure 16–2 People with insulin-dependent diabetes must regulate their use of insulin. They may need to check their blood glucose level frequently.

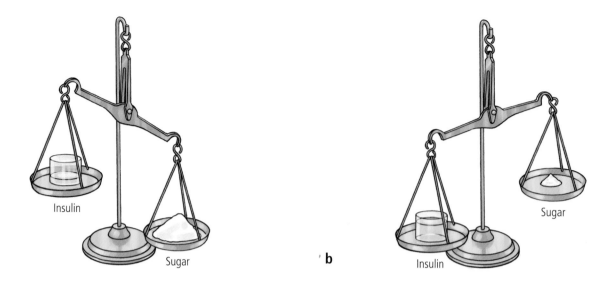

Figure 16–3, a-b a, Hyperglycemia occurs when there is insufficient insulin in the body, causing a higher level of sugar in the blood; **b,** hypoglycemia occurs when the insulin level in the body is high, causing a low level of sugar in the blood.

acidity level in the blood, causing a condition called acidosis. As this occurs, the person becomes ill. If it continues, the hyperglycemic condition deteriorates into its most serious form, diabetic coma.

On the other hand, when the insulin level in the body is too high, the person has a low sugar level. This condition is known as hypoglycemia (Figure 16–3, b). The sugar level can become too low if the person with diabetes:

• Takes too much insulin

• Fails to eat adequately

• Overexercises and burns off sugar faster than normal

• Experiences great emotional stress

In this situation, the small amount of sugar is used up rapidly and there is not enough for the brain to function properly. This results in an acute condition called insulin reaction, which can be life-threatening.

> **NOTE:**
>
> *Many people with diabetes carry a glucometer, a device with which they can test their blood sugar level.*

Diabetes and Special Populations

Children and Teens

People with Type 1 diabetes are usually diagnosed before the age of 30 years, most often during childhood or adolescence. Type 2 diabetes was once a disease that occurred primarily, if not exclusively, in adults. Today, however, the disease is increasingly appearing in adolescents and even in children. In 15 years, it is anticipated that the global incidence of Type 2 diabetes in children will have increased by up to 50%.[18]

Women

The burden of diabetes on women is unique because the disease can affect both mothers and their unborn children. Diabetes can cause difficulties during pregnancy, even miscarriage. For women who do not currently have diabetes, pregnancy brings the risk of gestational diabetes. Gestational diabetes develops in approximately 3.7% of all pregnancies (among non-Aboriginal women), but it usually disappears when the pregnancy is over. All pregnant women should be screened for gestational diabetes between 24 and 28 weeks of pregnancy. Women who have had gestational diabetes or who have given birth to a baby weighing more than four kilograms (nine pounds) are at an increased risk for developing Type 2 diabetes later in life.[19]

High-Risk Groups

People of Aboriginal, Hispanic, Asian, South Asian, or African descent are at particularly high risk for developing Type 2 diabetes. Diabetes can "run in families," meaning that heredity often makes someone more likely to develop diabetes. Researchers believe that certain genes affecting insulin function can contribute to the development of Type 2 diabetes and are present in high-risk populations.[20]

Signs and Symptoms of Diabetic Emergencies

The signs and symptoms of hyperglycemia and hypoglycemia differ somewhat, but the major signs and symptoms are similar. These include:

* Changes in the level of consciousness, including dizziness, drowsiness, and confusion

* Rapid breathing (tachypnea)

* Rapid pulse (tachycardia)

* Feeling and looking ill

It is not important for you to differentiate between insulin reaction and diabetic coma. The basic care for both conditions is the same.

Care for Diabetic Emergencies

First, do a primary survey and care for any life-threatening conditions. If the patient is conscious, do a secondary survey, asking and looking for anything visibly wrong. Ask if he has diabetes and look for a MedicAlert® medical identification product. If the patient is known to have diabetes and exhibits the signs and symptoms previously stated, then suspect a diabetic emergency.

If the patient is conscious and can take food or fluids, give him sugar (Figure 16–4). Most candy, fruit juices, and non-diet soft drinks have enough sugar to be effective. Common table sugar, either dry or dissolved

NOTE:

Glucose gel is a concentrated, rapidly absorbing glucose designed to treat low blood sugar. If the patient is unconscious, follow these steps to administer oral glucose gel:[21]

1. *Ensure that the patient is in the semi-prone position.*
2. *Remove the OPA if it will interfere with the administration of the oral glucose.*
3. *Place approximately 12 grams (half a tube) on the lower cheek.*
4. *You may use a tongue depressor to assist you in the administration of the oral glucose.*
5. *The longer you spread the glucose on the lower cheek, the quicker the absorption will be.*
6. *Repeat dosage in approximately 3–5 minutes.*

in a glass of water, can restore the blood sugar level to normal. Commercially available sugar sources also work well. Sometimes a patient who has diabetes will be able to tell you what is wrong and will ask for something with sugar in it. If the patient's problem is low sugar (hypoglycemia), the sugar you give will help

Figure 16–4 Examples of types of sugar that can be given to someone having a diabetic emergency.

quickly. If the patient already has too much sugar (hyperglycemia), the excess sugar will do no further harm.

Do not try to assist the patient by administering insulin. Maintain normal body temperature, obtain more advanced medical care, and administer oxygen if available. If the patient is conscious but does not feel better within approximately five minutes after taking sugar, obtain more advanced medical care. Oxygen should be administered if available. In both situations, provide ongoing survey and care.

Seizures

When the normal functions of the brain are disrupted by injury, disease, fever, infection, metabolic disturbances, or conditions causing a decreased oxygen level, a seizure may occur. A seizure is the result of abnormal electrical activity in the brain and causes temporary involuntary changes in body movement, function, sensation, awareness, or behaviour.

Types of Seizures

Generalized Seizures

Generalized tonic-clonic seizures, also called grand mal seizures, are the most well-known type of seizure. They involve both hemispheres (halves) of the brain and usually result in loss of consciousness. The seizure activity is known as tonic-clonic, which refers to the initial rigidity (tonic phase) followed by rhythmic muscle contractions (clonic phase), or convulsions. This type of seizure rarely lasts for more than a few minutes.

Before a generalized seizure occurs, the person may experience an unusual sensation or feeling called an aura. An aura can include a strange sound, taste, smell, or an urgent need to get to safety. If the person recognizes the aura, there may be time to warn bystanders and to sit or lie down before the seizure occurs.

Generalized seizures usually last one to three minutes and can produce a wide range of signs and symptoms. When a seizure occurs, the person loses consciousness and can fall, causing injury. The person may become rigid and then experience sudden, uncontrollable muscular contractions (convulsions) lasting several minutes. Breathing may become irregular and even stop temporarily. The person may drool and the eyes may roll upward. As the seizure subsides and the muscles relax, the person may lose bladder or bowel control.

The four stages of most generalized seizures are as follows:

1. **Aura phase**—person may sense something unusual (not all people will experience an aura)

2. **Tonic phase**—unconsciousness then muscle rigidity

3. **Clonic phase**—uncontrollable muscular contractions (convulsions)

4. **Post-ictal phase**—diminished responsiveness with gradual recovery and confusion (person may feel confused and want to sleep)

Partial Seizures

Partial seizures may be simple or complex. They usually involve only a very small area of one hemisphere of the brain. Partial seizures are the most common type of seizure experienced by people with epilepsy. Partial seizures can spread and become a generalized seizure. In simple partial seizures, the person usually remains aware. Complex partial seizures usually last for one to two minutes, though they may last longer and awareness is either impaired or lost while the person remains conscious.

In simple partial seizures, there may be involuntary muscular contractions in one area of the body, for example the arm, leg, or face. Some people cannot speak or move during a simple partial seizure, although they may remember everything that occurred. Simple partial seizures may produce a feeling of fear or a sense that something bad is about to happen. Simple partial seizures can also produce odd sensations such as strange smells or hearing voices. Rarely, feelings of anger and rage or joy and happiness can be brought on by the seizure. Auras are a form of simple partial seizure.

Complex partial seizures often begin with a blank stare followed by random movements such as smacking the lips or chewing. The person appears dazed, the movements are clumsy, and the person's activities lack direction. They may be unable to follow directions or answer questions. This type of seizure usually lasts for only a few minutes but may last longer. The person cannot remember what happened after the seizure is over and may be confused. This is called the post-ictal phase.

Absence (Petit Mal) Seizures

Individuals may also experience an absence seizure, also known as a petit mal seizure. These are most common in children. During an absence seizure, there is brief, sudden loss of awareness or conscious activity. This loss of awareness may be mistaken for daydreaming. There may be minimal or no movement, and the person may appear to have a blank stare. This type of seizure may also be referred to as a non-convulsive seizure, since the body remains relatively still during the episode, though eye fluttering and chewing movements may be seen. Most often these seizures last only a few seconds.

Febrile Seizures

Young children and babies may be at risk of febrile seizures, which are seizures brought on by a rapid increase in body temperature. They are most common in children under the age of five.

Febrile seizures are often caused by ear, throat, or digestive-system infections and are most likely to occur when a child or baby runs a rectal temperature of over 39°C (102°F). An individual experiencing a febrile seizure may experience some or all of the following symptoms:

- Sudden rise in body temperature
- Change in LOC
- Rhythmic jerking of the head and limbs
- Loss of bladder or bowel control
- Confusion
- Drowsiness
- Crying out
- Becoming rigid

- Holding the breath
- Rolling the eyes upward

Epilepsy

Epilepsy is a neurological disorder, estimated to affect approximately 0.6% of the Canadian population[22]. Epilepsy is not a specific disease but a term used to describe a group of disorders in which the individual experiences recurrent seizures as the main symptom. In about one third of all cases, seizures occur as a result of a brain abnormality or neurological disorder, but in two thirds of cases there is no known cause.

People of any age can be affected by epilepsy. The prevalence of epilepsy in young people (up to the age of 11) is approximately 0.3%. People aged 12 to 24 have a slightly higher rate of 0.6%, and the prevalence rises to 0.7% for those aged 25 and over.[23]

Most epileptic seizures last only a few seconds. People who have epilepsy can often control the seizures with medication. People whose seizures are difficult to control may also be treated with surgical resection, which can be curative, or with implanted devices, such as the vagus nerve stimulator, which help reduce their seizure frequency. While some people require life-long medical therapy, sometimes medication may be reduced or even eliminated over time. Some childhood epilepsies may resolve with age.

Care for Seizures

Seeing someone have a seizure may be intimidating, but you can easily care for the patient. The patient cannot control any muscular contractions that may occur, and it is important to allow the seizure to run its course because attempting to stop it or restrain the patient can cause musculoskeletal injuries.

Protecting the patient from injury and managing the airway are your priorities when caring for a patient having a seizure. To help avoid injury, you should move nearby objects, such as furniture, away from the patient.

People having seizures rarely bite the tongue or cheeks with enough force to cause any significant bleeding. Do not place anything in the mouth to prevent this type of injury. Foreign bodies in the mouth may cause airway obstruction. Do not put your fingers into the mouth of an actively seizing patient to clear the airway. After the seizure passes, position the patient on his side, if possible, so that fluids (saliva, blood, vomit) can drain from the mouth.

In many cases, the seizure will be over by the time you arrive. In this case, the patient may be drowsy and disoriented; this is the post-ictal phase. Check to see if the patient was injured during the seizure. Offer comfort and reassurance, especially if the seizure occurred in public, as the patient may feel embarrassed and self-conscious. If this is the case, keep bystanders well back to provide maximum privacy and stay with the patient until he is fully conscious and aware of the surroundings.

Care for a child or baby who experiences a febrile seizure is similar to the care for any other patient experiencing a seizure. Immediately after a febrile seizure, cool the body by removing excess clothing and giving the patient a sponge bath in lukewarm water. Cold water could lead to a rapid drop in body temperature, which could cause shivering and/or stimulate the nervous system, which could bring on another seizure. Rapid cooling with cold water could bring on other complications as well. Contact a healthcare provider before administering any medication, such as acetaminophen, to control fever. Do not give acetylsalicylic acid (ASA or Aspirin®) to any feverish patient under 18 years of age, as this has been linked to Reye's syndrome, an illness that affects the brain and other internal organs.

When to Call for More Advanced Medical Care

The patient will usually recover from a seizure in a few minutes. If you discover the patient has a history of seizures that is medically controlled, there may be no further need for medical attention. However, in the following cases, more advanced medical care should be provided:

- The seizure lasts more than five minutes or the patient has repeated seizures with no sign of slowing down (status epilepticus).
- The patient appears to be injured.
- You are uncertain about the cause of the seizure.
- The patient is pregnant.
- The patient is known to have diabetes.
- The patient is a child or baby, including a young child or baby who experienced a febrile seizure brought on by a high fever.
- The seizure takes place in water.
- The patient fails to regain consciousness after the seizure.
- The patient is an older adult and could have suffered a stroke.
- This is the patient's first seizure.

Status epilepticus is an epileptic seizure (or repeated seizures) that lasts longer than five minutes without any sign of slowing down. A status epilepticus seizure is a true medical emergency that may be fatal. If you suspect the patient is experiencing this type of seizure, call for more advanced medical care immediately. If the seizure passes, place the patient on his side and suction the patient's airway, if possible. If the patient is having difficulty breathing (dyspnea), administer ventilations with a bag-valve-mask resuscitator (BVM) along with emergency oxygen.

Appendicitis

Appendicitis is an acute inflammation of the appendix. This is a common abdominal emergency that occurs as a result of a viral or bacterial infection in the digestive tract or when the channel or cavity in the appendix becomes blocked. If untreated, the appendix may become gangrenous and rupture, which causes inflammation of the membrane that covers the abdominal wall (peritoneum).

The signs and symptoms of appendicitis include:

- Abdominal pain or cramping

- Nausea
- Vomiting
- Constipation
- Diarrhea
- Low-grade fever
- Abdominal swelling

The pain usually begins near the umbilical area and diffuses, later becoming intense and localized to the right lower quadrant. The pain becomes worse when moving, taking deep breaths, coughing, sneezing, and being touched in the area.

The goal of definitive care for appendicitis is surgical removal before rupture. Have the patient rest in a comfortable position and ensure prompt transport to a medical facility. Provide comfort measures by placing the patient in a comfortable position, prevent life-threatening complications such as shock or aspiration (remember to give nothing by mouth), and obtain more advanced medical care. Provide ongoing survey and care.

Bowel Obstruction

Bowel obstruction is an occlusion of the intestinal cavity that results in blockage of normal flow of intestinal contents. This condition may be caused by a number of factors, including adhesions, hernias, fecal blockage, and tumours. Bowel obstruction in the small intestine is usually caused by adhesions and hernias, whereas obstruction in the large intestine is usually caused by tumours and fecal obstruction. The signs and symptoms of a bowel obstruction include:

- Abdominal pain
- Constipation
- Abdominal distension

The time of onset depends on whether the obstruction is in the small or large bowel. A danger of an obstructed bowel is perforation with generalized inflammation of the peritoneum and infection (sepsis).

Definitive treatment includes fluid replacement and antibiotics. Frequently, surgery is necessary to correct the obstruction. Provide supportive treatment, care for

any life-threatening conditions, and ensure prompt transport to an appropriate medical facility. The patient should not eat or drink anything.

Gastroenteritis

Gastroenteritis often results from infection of the gastrointestinal tract. It is often caused by poor hygiene or improper water disinfection or food preparation.

To prevent gastroenteritis, keep hydrated, eat balanced meals, do not restrain bowel movements, and ensure that all water is disinfected, food is prepared and stored properly, and you wash your hands frequently.

Signs and symptoms of gastroenteritis may include:

- Nausea and vomiting
- Diarrhea
- Headache (due to dehydration)
- Abdominal cramps
- Possible fever
- Rapid onset/short duration
- Pain associated with diarrhea

Definitive treatment includes fluid replacement and possibly antibiotics (if not viral) or other medications prescribed at a medical facility.

Other conditions may be confused with gastroenteritis. If a patient has the following signs and symptoms, he is not suffering from gastroenteritis, and you should obtain advanced medical care (see abdominal injuries in Chapter 15):

- Localized and constant pain
- Slow pain onset
- Rebound tenderness
- Abdominal rigidity
- Signs of internal bleeding or shock

NOTE:

Finding out what the patient last ingested and if there is anyone else experiencing similar symptoms may give you a clue as to what the cause might be.

Kidney Stones

Kidney stones (renal colic) are solid concentrations of dissolved minerals found in the kidneys or ureters. These usually pass in the urine, but if they cause a blockage and obstruct the flow of urine, the patient can present with:

- Pain in the flank, lower abdomen, and groin (usually radiating from the back to the front)
- Nausea and/or vomiting
- Restlessness
- Possible blood in the urine (if urine is present)

Kidney stones cause severe pain, and the patient should be transported to a medical facility for removal of the stones, or wait until the stones pass.

Peptic Ulcers

A peptic ulcer is a small erosion in the gastrointestinal tract caused by destruction of the gastric or intestinal mucosal lining by hydrochloric acid. Infection by *Helicobacter pylori* is also thought to play a role, and ulcers caused by *Helicobacter pylori* are treated with medications prescribed by a doctor. Other major causes of ulcers include the chronic use of medications, such as ASA, and cigarette smoking.

The major symptom of an ulcer is a burning or gnawing feeling in the stomach area that lasts between 30 minutes and three hours. This pain is often misinterpreted as heartburn, indigestion, or hunger and usually occurs in the upper abdomen, although it may occur below the breastbone. In some individuals, the pain occurs immediately after eating; in others, it may not occur until hours after eating. The pain frequently awakens the person at night. Weeks of pain may be followed by weeks with no pain. Pain can be relieved by drinking milk, eating, resting, or taking antacids. Other symptoms include loss of appetite and weight loss.

Ulcers can also occur in the duodenum. People with duodenal ulcers may experience weight gain because they tend to eat more to help ease the discomfort. Other symptoms include recurrent vomiting, blood in the stool, and anemia.

More advanced medical care is required as prescription medication is often used to treat or relieve symptoms of ulcers.

Gastrointestinal Bleeding

There are multiple causes of gastrointestinal bleeding, and these tend to be classified as either upper or lower, depending on the location of the problem within the gastrointestinal tract. Bleeding in the upper gastrointestinal tract originates in the esophagus, stomach, or duodenum (the first part of the intestine) and may include such problems as peptic ulcers, gastritis, stomach cancer, or the ingestion of caustic poisons. Bleeding in the lower gastrointestinal tract originates in the small intestine, large intestine, rectum, or anus, and it includes diverticular disease, polyps, hemorrhoids, and anal fissures, as well as cancer and inflammatory bowel disease.

A patient with gastrointestinal bleeding may experience vomiting of blood, bloody bowel movements, or black, tarry stools. Symptoms that may accompany the bleeding include fatigue, weakness, abdominal pain, pale appearance, and shortness of breath.

Serious gastrointestinal bleeding can have a significant impact on vital signs—for example, causing blood pressure to drop sharply and heart rate to increase. Summon more advanced medical care, as the patient may require a blood transfusion or surgery.

Peritonitis

Peritonitis, an inflammation of the peritoneum, presents with acute abdominal pain and tenderness. Coughing, flexing the hips, and releasing manual pressure from the abdomen all tend to elicit more pain.

Peritonitis can be caused by infectious sources or non-infectious sources, such as sterile body fluids leaking into the peritoneum. Treatment includes rehydration, as well as possible antibiotics or surgery.

Urinary Tract Infection (UTI)

A urinary tract infection (UTI) is an infection at any site within the urinary tract, usually bacterial. It can affect the urethra, bladder, or kidney, as well as the prostate gland in men. These infections are very common. The signs and symptoms of a UTI include:

- An urgent need to urinate often
- Burning during urination
- Cloudy or foul-smelling urine
- Pain in the lower abdomen[24]

Those at greater risk of UTIs include females, because of their shorter urethra, paraplegics, and those with nerve disruption to the bladder, for example, people with diabetes. As well, those with urinary stasis (incomplete emptying of the bladder, which may serve as nutrition for pathogens) are also predisposed to the infection. This latter group includes pregnant women and people with neurological impairment. More advanced medical care is needed as medication will most likely be prescribed.

High-Altitude Illness

When travelling in mountainous areas, people can become sick due to the change in altitude. At higher altitudes, it is harder for the oxygen to enter the bloodstream due to the lower atmospheric pressure. When ascending quickly above 2,133 metres (7,000 feet), people can experience high-altitude illness.

It takes the body time to adapt physiologically to altitudes. Some of these changes take place within 10 days. Within the first 10 days, the body adapts to altitudes by increased respiratory rate, increased heart rate, and fluid shifts.

Other adaptations take longer for the body to make. Later changes occur after anywhere from 10 days to up to six weeks and include increased red blood cell production, increased active capillaries, and gradually decreasing heart rate.

High-altitude illness can take one of three forms: acute mountain sickness (AMS), high-altitude pulmonary edema (HAPE), and high-altitude cerebral edema (HACE).

Preventing High-Altitude Illness

If you are planning to climb to high altitudes, take the following steps to reduce the likelihood or severity of symptoms of high-altitude illness:

- Assess your ability to perform at high altitudes in advance.

- Plan your trip in stages, thereby allowing yourself time to acclimatize at specific sleeping elevations.

- Remember to descend to a lower altitude to sleep.

- Observe others in the party regularly, watching for signs and symptoms of altitude sickness.

- Drink up to four litres (four quarts) of fluid per day. (Keep urine colour light.)

- Avoid sleeping pills, alcohol, or any other respiratory depressants.

Signs and Symptoms of High-Altitude Illness
Acute Mountain Sickness

AMS is not a specific disease but a group of varied symptoms caused by altitude.

Signs and symptoms of AMS include:

- Headache and/or insomnia

- Vomiting and loss of appetite

- Coughing and/or tightness in the chest

- Irregular breathing or shortness of breath

- Swelling around the eyes and face

- Reduced urine output

- Weakness, fatigue, and lethargy

- Peripheral edema

- Cyanosis at nail beds and around the mouth

- Difficulty maintaining balance (ataxia)

High-Altitude Pulmonary Edema

HAPE is a progressive stage of AMS and usually occurs one to four days after arrival at altitude. It is a serious, life-threatening condition in which fluid begins pooling in the lungs. The result is a breathing emergency.

Signs and symptoms of HAPE include:

- Fatigue with difficulty breathing (dyspnea) at rest; wheezing

- General ache in the chest

- Continuous fast pulse

- Bluish colouring of the skin

- Gurgling cough accompanied by frothy sputum

- Mental confusion, delirium, and irrational behaviour (caused by reduced oxygen to the brain)

In more severe cases, the person may have a productive (fluid-generating) cough, extreme weakness, shortness of breath while at rest, heart rate greater than 110 at rest, breathing rate greater than 30 at rest, and frothy, blood-tinged sputum.

High-Altitude Cerebral Edema

HACE is another progressive stage of AMS and is an accumulation of fluid between the brain and skull. It occurs two to three days after arrival at altitude. It is a serious condition that is difficult to diagnose but will usually accompany HAPE.

Signs and symptoms of HACE include:

- Increasingly severe headache, convulsions, stupor
- Nausea and/or vomiting
- Dizziness and/or lack of coordination, mental confusion
- Unconsciousness
- Ataxia
- Vision disturbances
- Paralysis
- Seizures
- Hallucinations
- Cyanosis
- Increased blood pressure
- Decreasing heart rate

Care for High-Altitude Illness

Care for AMS includes the following:

- Check and record vital signs on a regular basis.
- Stop and rest, with light activity, allowing up to two days for acclimatization.
- If signs and symptoms persist, rapid descent is necessary.

Care for HAPE and HACE includes the following:

- Check and record vital signs on a regular basis.
- Descend, prepare for evacuation if necessary, and obtain more advanced medical care.

There are also steps you can take to help anyone with high-altitude illness of any type. First, descend to a significantly lower altitude. If available, and the patient's condition remains poor, place him in a portable altitude chamber (hyperbaric bag). It is also important to hydrate the patient regularly with four to six litres (four to six quarts) of fluids per day.

TABLE 16–1: SUMMARY OF SUDDEN ILLNESSES

Illness	Signs and Symptoms	Care
Appendicitis	• Abdominal pain or cramping, usually begins near umbilical area and diffuses, later becoming intense in the right lower quadrant • Pain is worse when moving, taking deep breaths, coughing, sneezing, or being touched in that area • Nausea, vomiting, constipation/diarrhea • Low-grade fever • Abdominal swelling	• Goal is surgical removal of appendix before rupture • Help ensure prompt transport to a medical facility • Provide comfort measures: place patient in a comfortable position, prevent shock or aspiration (give nothing by mouth) • Obtain more advanced medical care • Provide ongoing survey and care
Bowel Obstruction	• Abdominal pain • Constipation • Abdominal distension	• Treatment includes fluid replacement and antibiotics • Surgery is often necessary

		• Provide supportive treatment; care for any life-threatening conditions
		• Ensure prompt transport to a medical facility
		• Do not give the patient anything to eat or drink
Diabetic Emergencies	• Changes in LOC, including dizziness, drowsiness, and confusion • Rapid breathing (tachypnea) and rapid pulse (tachycardia) • Feeling and looking ill	• Do a primary survey and care for any life-threatening conditions • If patient is conscious, do a secondary survey • If patient is conscious and can take food or fluids, give sugar • No need to differentiate between insulin reaction and diabetic coma • Do not assist with giving insulin • Maintain normal body temperature • Obtain more advanced medical care, particularly if patient does not feel better five minutes after taking sugar
Altered Mental Status	• A sudden or gradual change in LOC, including drowsiness, confusion, and partial or complete loss of consciousness	• Administer oxygen if available • Complete primary and secondary surveys and history • Perform ongoing assessments • Make sure the airway is open • Place an unconscious patient in the supine (face-up) position • Have suction equipment available • Do not give anything to eat or drink • Attempt to get information from the patient, family members, or bystanders

	• Fainting:
	
	  ■ May occur without warning
	
	  ■ Light-headedness or dizziness
		• Fainting:
		
		  ■ If patient is collapsing, lower to the ground or other flat surface and position on the back

- Signs of shock (pale or ashen, cool, moist skin)

- Nausea

- Numbness or tingling in the fingers and toes

- Breathing and pulse may become faster

- If a head and/or spine injury is suspected, take spinal precautions

- Loosen restrictive clothing

- Monitor breathing and pulse

- Do not give anything to eat or drink

- Do not splash water on the patient's face

- Administer oxygen if available

- Obtain more advanced medical care

Gastroenteritis

- Nausea and vomiting

- Diarrhea

- Headache (due to dehydration)

- Abdominal cramps

- Possible fever

- Rapid onset/short duration

- Pain associated with diarrhea

- Treatment includes fluid replacement and possibly antibiotics or other medications prescribed at a medical facility

---

High-Altitude Illness

Acute Mountain Sickness:

- Headache and/or insomnia

- Vomiting and loss of appetite

- Coughing and/or tightness in the chest

- Irregular breathing or shortness of breath

- Swelling around the eyes and face

- Reduced urine output

- Weakness, fatigue, and lethargy

- Peripheral edema

- Cyanosis at nail beds and around the mouth

- Difficulty maintaining balance (ataxia)

High-Altitude Pulmonary Edema:

- Fatigue with difficulty breathing (dyspnea) at rest; wheezing

- Descend to a significantly lower altitude

- If condition remains poor, place patient in portable altitude chamber (hyperbaric bag), if available

- Hydrate regularly, with four to six litres (four to six quarts) of fluids per day

- Check and record vital signs regularly

- Stop and rest, with light activity, allowing up to two days for acclimatization

- If signs and symptoms persist, rapid descent is necessary

- Descend to a significantly lower altitude

- General ache in the chest

- Continuous fast pulse

- Bluish colouring of the skin

- Gurgling cough accompanied by frothy sputum

- Mental confusion, delirium, and irrational behaviour (caused by reduced oxygen to the brain)

- In more severe cases, productive cough; extreme weakness; shortness of breath at rest; heart rate greater than 110 at rest; breathing rate greater than 30 at rest; frothy, blood-tinged sputum

- If condition remains poor, place patient in portable altitude chamber (hyperbaric bag), if available

- Hydrate regularly, with four to six litres (four to six quarts) of fluids per day

- Check and record vital signs regularly

- Descend, prepare for evacuation if necessary, and obtain more advanced medical care

High-Altitude Cerebral Edema:

- Increasingly severe headache, convulsions, stupor

- Nausea and/or vomiting

- Dizziness and/or lack of coordination, mental confusion

- Unconsciousness

- Ataxia

- Vision disturbances

- Paralysis

- Seizures

- Hallucinations

- Cyanosis

- Increased blood pressure

- Decreasing heart rate

- Descend to a significantly lower altitude

- If condition remains poor, place patient in portable altitude chamber (hyperbaric bag), if available

- Hydrate regularly, with four to six litres (four to six quarts) of fluids per day

- Check and record vital signs regularly

- Descend, prepare for evacuation if necessary, and obtain more advanced medical care

Kidney Stones

- Pain (can be severe) in the flank, lower abdomen, and groin (usually radiating from back to front)

- Nausea, vomiting

- Transport to a medical facility for removal of stones or wait until stones pass

	• Restlessness	
	• Possible blood in urine	
Peptic Ulcers	• Burning or gnawing feeling in the stomach area lasting between 30 minutes and three hours; usually in upper abdomen but may occur below the breastbone	• Obtain more advanced medical care, as prescription medication is often used to treat or relive symptoms
	• Pain may occur immediately after eating or not until hours after	• Pain may be relieved by drinking milk, eating, resting, or taking antacids
	• May have weeks of pain followed by weeks of no pain	
	• Loss of appetite	
	• Weight loss	
	• For ulcers in duodenum: weight gain, recurrent vomiting, blood in the stool, anemia	
Peritonitis	• Acute abdominal pain and tenderness	• Rehydration
	• Increased pain with coughing, flexing of the hips, and releasing manual pressure from the abdomen	• Possible antibiotics or surgery
Generalized Seizures	**Before the seizure:** • May experience an unusual sensation or feeling (an aura) **During the seizure:** • Unconsciousness then muscle rigidity • Uncontrollable muscular contractions (convulsions) • Breathing may become irregular and even stop temporarily • Possible drooling and eyes may roll upward • Possible loss of bladder or bowel control **After the seizure:** • Diminished responsiveness and confusion	• Allow seizures to happen; do not attempt to stop or restrain the patient • Move nearby objects, such as furniture, away to protect patient from injury • After the seizure, position the patient on his side so fluids can drain from the mouth • Do not place anything in the patient's mouth • After the seizure, check if the patient has any injuries • Offer comfort and reassurance; stay with the patient until he is fully conscious and aware of surroundings • If the patient is known to have periodic seizures, you do not necessarily need to

		obtain more advanced medical care immediately
	• Drowsiness, disorientation, and desire to sleep • Embarrassment and self-consciousness	• Obtain more advance medical care if seizure lasts more than five minutes, the patient has repeated seizures, the patient appears injured, you are uncertain of the cause, the patient is pregnant, the patient has diabetes, the patient is a baby or child, the seizure takes place in water, the patient fails to regain consciousness afterward, or the patient has a febrile seizure and high fever or the patient is an older adult and could have had a stroke
Urinary Tract Infection	• Urgent need to urinate often • Burning during urination • Cloudy or foul-smelling urine • Pain in the lower abdomen	• Obtain more advanced medical care to get prescription medication

SUMMARY

Sudden illness can strike anyone at any time. The signs and symptoms for many of the sudden illnesses described in this chapter are very similar. Recognizing their general signs and symptoms, such as changes in the level of consciousness, sweating, confusion, weakness, and appearing ill, will indicate to you the necessary initial care you should provide. Usually, you will not know the cause of the illness. Diabetic emergencies, seizures, and fainting are all sudden illnesses, each with an individual, specific cause. Fortunately, you can provide proper care without knowing the cause. High-altitude illness may present with some of the same signs and symptoms but with a known cause. Performing a proper assessment and following the general guidelines of care for any emergency will help prevent the condition from becoming worse. When providing care for sudden illnesses, you should:

• Obtain more advanced medical care.

• Maintain normal body temperature.

• Administer oxygen if available.

• Provide ongoing survey and care.

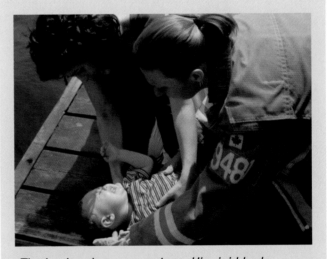

The boy's seizure soon stops. His rigid body goes limp. At this time, another responder asks if there is anything you would like her to do. What do you do?

Chapter *17*

Poisoning

You've been called to attend to a man feeling unwell, sitting on a bench in a shopping centre. You examine his leg where he says he's developed a rash. The centre of the rash is lighter in colour, and the outer edges are red and raised, giving the rash a bull's-eye appearance. He says he feels as if he's coming down with something, possibly the flu, but he's worried about the rash. What do you do?

INTRODUCTION

Poisoning is another type of sudden illness, but unlike sudden illnesses such as fainting and diabetic emergencies, poisoning results when an external substance enters the body. The substance may be a chemical, or it may be a germ or virus that enters the body through a bite or sting. In this chapter, you will learn how to recognize and care for poisoning.

PREVENTING POISONING

Thousands of Canadians are admitted to hospitals each year due to poisoning. The best approach to poisoning emergencies is to prevent them from occurring in the first place.

By following these general guidelines, people will be able to prevent most poisoning emergencies:

- Keep all medications and dangerous products well out of the reach of children.

- Use childproof safety caps on medication containers and other potentially dangerous products.

- Keep products in their original containers with the labels in place.

- Use poison symbols to identify dangerous substances.

- Dispose of outdated products.

- Use potentially dangerous chemicals only in well-ventilated areas.

- When working with a poisonous substance, wear clothing that can prevent contact with the substance.

- Wear appropriate clothing and footwear when in an area where bites from insects, spiders, ticks, and snakes are possible.

HOW POISONS ENTER THE BODY

A poison is any substance that causes injury or illness when introduced into the body. Some poisons can cause death. Poisons include solids, liquids, and fumes (gases and vapours). A poison can enter the body in four ways: ingestion, inhalation, absorption, and injection (Figure 17–1).

To ingest means to swallow. Ingested poisons include foods, such as certain mushrooms and shellfish;

substances, such as alcohol; medications, such as ASA; and household and garden items, such as cleaning products, pesticides, and plants. Many substances not poisonous in small amounts are poisonous in larger amounts.

Poisoning by inhalation occurs when a person breathes in toxic fumes. Inhaled poisons include:

- Gases such as carbon monoxide, from an engine or other combustion

- Gases such as carbon dioxide, which can occur naturally from decomposition

- Gases such as nitrous oxide, used for medical procedures

- Gases such as chlorine, found in commercial swimming facilities

- Fumes from household products, such as glues and paints

- Fumes from drugs, such as marijuana

An absorbed poison enters the body after coming into contact with the skin or other membranes (thin sheets of tissue that cover a structure or line a cavity, such as the mouth or nose). Absorbed poisons come from plants, such as poison ivy, poison oak, and poison sumac, and from fertilizers and pesticides used in lawn

Figure 17–1 A poison can enter the body by ingestion, inhalation, absorption, and injection.

and plant care. They can also come from drugs, such as cocaine, that can be absorbed through the mucous membranes in the mouth and nose.

Injected poisons enter the body through bites or stings of insects, spiders, ticks, snakes, and other animals or as drugs or medications injected with a hypodermic syringe.

SIGNS AND SYMPTOMS OF POISONING

The most important thing with a poisoning is to recognize that it may have occurred. As with other serious emergencies, such as severe chest pain or head and spine injury, evaluate the scene, the condition of the patient, and any information given by the patient or bystanders. If you then have even a slight suspicion that the patient has been poisoned, obtain more advanced medical care immediately.

As you approach the patient, survey the scene. Be aware of any unusual odours, flames, smoke, open or spilled containers, an open medicine cabinet, an over-turned or damaged plant, or other signs of possible poisoning.

When you reach the patient, do a primary survey. If the patient has no life-threatening conditions, do a secondary survey. Someone who has been poisoned generally displays signs and symptoms common to other sudden illnesses. These include nausea, vomiting, diarrhea, chest or abdominal pain, breathing difficulty, sweating, altered level of consciousness, and seizures.

Other signs of poisoning are burn injuries around the mouth or on the skin. You may also suspect a poisoning based on any information you have from or about the patient. Look also for any drug paraphernalia, such as pipes, paper for rolling, syringes, or containers.

If you suspect a poisoning, try to get answers to the following questions:

• What type of poison was taken?

• How much was taken?

• When was it taken?

This information will help you provide the most appropriate initial care and provide more advanced medical personnel with valuable information that may affect additional care.

POISON CONTROL CENTRES

A poisoning emergency can sometimes pose a unique problem for those trying to provide appropriate care. The severity of the poisoning depends on the type and amount of the substance, how it entered the body, and the patient's size, weight, and age. Some poisons act quickly and have characteristic signs and symptoms. Others act slowly and cannot easily be identified. Sometimes you will be able to identify the specific poison, sometimes not.

To help responders on all levels deal with poisonings, Poison Control Centres exist throughout Canada. Medical professionals in these centres have access to information about virtually all poisonous substances. They can tell you how to counteract the poison. You should know your closest Poison Control Centre number.

If the patient is unconscious, obtain more advanced medical care immediately. The dispatcher may be able to link you with the Poison Control Centre. The dispatcher may also monitor your discussion with the Poison Control Centre and provide additional information to the responding medical care personnel. In some instances, this eliminates the need for a second call and saves time.

CARE FOR POISONING

Follow these general principles for any poisoning emergency:

• Survey the scene to make sure it is safe to approach and gather clues about what happened.

• Remove the patient from the source of the poison.

• Do a primary survey to assess the patient's airway, breathing, and circulation.

• Care for any life-threatening conditions.

• If the patient is conscious, do a secondary survey to gather additional information. Look for containers, pills, etc.

• Contact the Poison Control Centre and/or obtain more advanced medical care.

• Follow the directions of the Poison Control Centre.

• Avoid giving the patient anything by mouth unless advised to do so by medical professionals. If the poison is unknown and the patient vomits, save some of the vomitus, which may be analyzed later to identify the poison.

- Provide ongoing survey and care.

Ingested Poisons

Besides following these general principles for any poisoning, you may also need to provide additional care for specific types of poisons. The Poison Control Centre may instruct you to induce vomiting. Unless local protol dictates otherwise, induce vomiting only upon the instruction of the Poison Control Centre.

The Poison Control Centre may ask you to neutralize the amount that remains with activated charcoal. Activated charcoal is available in both liquid and powder forms and may be part of your response equipment. Always follow local protocol and the directions from the Poison Control Centre.

If directed to do so by the Poison Control Centre, you can dilute some ingested poisons by giving the patient water to drink. Examples of such poisons are corrosive chemicals, such as acids or alkalis, which damage or destroy tissues. Vomiting these corrosives could burn the esophagus, throat, and mouth. Diluting the corrosive substance decreases the potential for damaging tissues.

Diluting poisons taken in tablet or capsule form is usually not a good idea. The increased fluid could dissolve them more rapidly in the stomach, speeding the body's absorption of the poison. As always, follow the advice of the Poison Control Centre or other medical professionals.

Inhaled Poisons

Toxic fumes come from a variety of sources. Hydrogen sulfide (H_2S), for example, is an inhaled poison given off by decomposing organic matter, some wells, and sewers. It is also found in the fumes from certain industrial and home spray chemicals.

A more common inhaled poison is carbon monoxide (CO). It is present in car exhaust and can be produced by defective cooking equipment, fires, and charcoal grills. A pale or bluish skin colour that indicates a lack of oxygen may signal carbon monoxide poisoning. For years, people were taught that carbon monoxide poisoning was indicated by a cherry-red colour of the skin and lips. This, however, is a poor initial indicator of carbon monoxide poisoning. The red colour occurs later, usually after death.

When someone has inhaled poison, the patient needs to be removed from the poison as soon as possible. First and foremost, ensure your own safety. Survey the scene to determine if it is safe for you to help. If you can remove the patient from the source of the poison without endangering your life, then do so. You can help a conscious patient by just getting her to fresh air and then obtaining more advanced medical care. Remove an unconscious patient from the environment and maintain an open airway. If the patient is not breathing, begin rescue breathing. Administer oxygen, if available, to anyone who has inhaled a poison.

Absorbed Poisons

People often come into contact with poisonous substances that can be absorbed into the body. Thousands of people each year suffer from contact with poison ivy (Figure 17–2, a), poison oak (Figure 17–2, b), and poison sumac (Figure 17–2, c). Other common poisons absorbed through the skin include dry and wet chemicals, such as those found in insecticides and toxic industrial chemicals, which may also burn the surface of the skin.

To care for poison contact, immediately wash the affected area with water. Rinse the area with cool water and pat dry. Keep the area clean and dry. Instruct the patient to see a doctor if the condition gets worse. If poisons such as dry or wet chemicals contact the skin, flush the affected area continuously with large amounts of water. Obtain more advanced medical care immediately. Continue to flush the area until care is obtained.

If running water is not available, brush off dry chemicals, such as lime. Take care not to get any in your eyes or the eyes of the patient or any bystanders. Dry chemicals are activated by contact with water, but if continuous running water is available, it will flush the chemical from the skin before activating it. Running water reduces the threat to you and quickly and easily removes the substance from the patient.

Injected Poisons

Insect and animal stings and bites are among the most common sources of injected poisons. This text cannot consider all possible types of stings and bites that could result in poisoning. The following sections describe the care for common stings and bites of insects, spiders, marine life, snakes, warm-blooded animals, and ticks.

Insects

Although insect stings are painful, they are rarely fatal. Some people, however, have a severe allergic reaction to

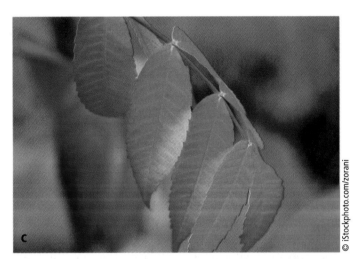

Figure 17–2, a-c a, Poison ivy; **b**, poison oak; and **c**, poison sumac.

Hantavirus

Hantavirus is found throughout North America, although it is most common in the southern United States. It is carried by various types of rodents. Hantavirus may be caused by inhaling microscopic particles of dried rodent saliva, urine, or feces. It can also be caused when someone touches her mouth or nose after handling contaminated materials. And it may occur after being bitten by a rodent.

There are steps to prevent acquiring hantavirus. Check sites for rodent droppings and burrows, avoid sleeping near areas where there may be rodents, and store food where rodents can't get at it. Thoroughly clean and disinfect areas (home, work, cabin, etc.) where there have been rodents, and use gloves if you have to pick up a rodent for any reason.

Signs and Symptoms of Hantavirus

A person with hantavirus will present with flu-like symptoms: fever, headache, muscle aches, nausea, and vomiting. This can progress to breathing difficulties.

Care for Hantavirus

The care for hantavirus is the same as care for other poisons.

an insect sting, resulting in the life-threatening condition anaphylaxis, discussed in Chapter 6.

To care for an insect sting, first examine the sting site to see if the stinger is in the skin. If it is, remove it to prevent any further poisoning. Scrape the stinger away from the skin with your fingernail or a plastic card, such as a driver's licence or credit card. Often the venom sac will still be attached to the stinger. Do not remove the stinger with tweezers since putting pressure on the venom sac can cause further poisoning.

Next, wash the site with soap and water. Cover it to keep it clean. Apply a cold compress to the area to reduce the pain and swelling. Observe the patient periodically for signs and symptoms of an allergic reaction.

Spiders

Few spiders in North America have venom that causes death. But the bites of the black widow and brown recluse spiders can be fatal. You can identify them by the unique designs on their bodies. The black widow spider is black with a reddish hourglass shape on its underbody (Figure 17–3). The brown recluse spider is light brown with a darker brown, violin-shaped marking on the top of its body.

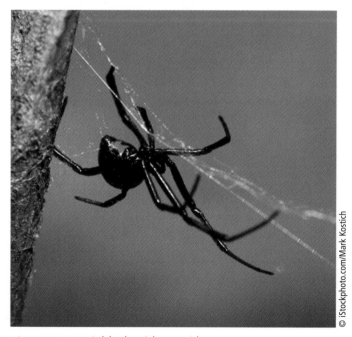

Figure 17–3 A black widow spider.

© iStockphoto.com/Mark Kostich

Both spiders prefer dark, out-of-the-way places where they are seldom disturbed. Bites usually occur on the hands and arms of people reaching into places such as wood, rock, and brush piles or rummaging in dark storage areas. Often the person will not know that she has been bitten until signs or symptoms develop.

If the spider is identified as either a black widow or brown recluse, the person should get immediate care at a medical facility. The wound will be cleansed and medication provided to reduce the pain and inflammation. An antivenin, a substance used to counteract or reduce the poisonous effects of snake or other venom, is available for particular spider bites.

Signs and symptoms of spider bites include:

- Nausea and vomiting
- Difficulty breathing (dyspnea) or swallowing
- Sweating and salivating profusely
- Irregular heart rhythms that can lead to cardiac arrest
- Severe pain in the sting or bite area
- Swelling on or around the site
- A mark indicating a possible bite or sting

To care for a spider bite, wash the wound and apply a cold compress to the site. A person who has these signs and symptoms needs to go to a medical facility.

Marine Life

Sting rays, sea anemones, certain fish, jellyfish, and some other marine animals can give painful stings that may cause serious problems, such as allergic reaction, paralysis, and cardiac and respiratory difficulties (Figure 17–4). Always remove the patient who has been stung from the water as soon as possible. Obtain more advanced medical care if the patient:

- Has a history of allergic reactions to marine life stings
- Is stung on the face or neck
- Develops severe problems, such as difficulty breathing (dyspnea)

If the sting is from a jellyfish, sea anemone, or man-of-war, soak the injured part in vinegar. Vinegar often works best to deactivate the toxin. Rubbing alcohol or baking soda may also be used. Do not rub the wound or apply fresh water or ammonia since this will increase pain.

If the sting is from a stingray, sea urchin, or spiny fish, flush the wound with sterile saline or water. Tap or ocean water may also be used. Immobilize the injured part, usually the foot, and soak the affected area in non-scalding hot water (as hot as the patient can stand) for about 30 minutes or until the pain subsides. Then carefully clean the wound and apply a bandage. Remind the patient to watch for signs of infection and check with a healthcare provider to determine if a tetanus shot is needed.

Snakes

Few people die of snakebites. Furthermore, a snakebite does not mean that venom is injected. Rattlesnakes account for most snakebites and nearly all deaths from snakebites. Most deaths occur because the person has an allergic reaction or a weakened body system or because significant time passes before the person receives medical care. Elaborate care is usually unnecessary because, in most cases, the person can reach advanced medical care within 30 minutes.

Follow these guidelines to provide initial care for someone bitten by a snake:

• Wash the wound.

• Immobilize the affected part.

• Keep the affected area lower than the heart if possible.

• Obtain more advanced medical care.

• Provide ongoing survey and care.

You should follow your local protocols regarding care for someone bitten by a snake.

When caring for a snakebite, avoid:

• Applying ice. Studies show that cooling the bite can cause as much harm as good.

• Cutting the wound. Cutting the wound can further injure the patient and has not been shown to remove any significant amount of venom.

• Applying a tourniquet. A tourniquet severely restricts blood flow to the extremity, which could result in the loss of the extremity.

NOTE:
If the patient's arm or leg is bitten by an elapid snake (coral family), the responder should wrap the entire extremity with an elastic bandage. The bandage should immobilize the extremity. It should be wrapped snugly enough to allow one finger to slip between the bandage and the skin.

Animals

The bite of a domestic or wild animal carries the risk of infection, as well as soft tissue injury. The most serious possible result is rabies, a disease transmitted through the saliva of diseased animals such as skunks, bats, raccoons, cats, dogs, cattle, and foxes.

Animals with rabies may act in unusual ways. For example, nocturnal animals, such as raccoons, may be active in the daytime. A wild animal that usually tries to avoid humans may not run away when you approach.

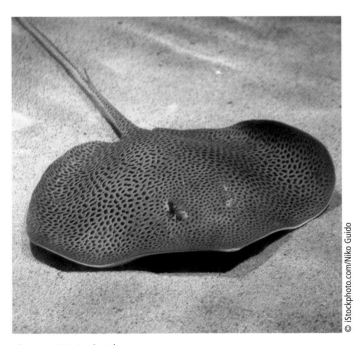

© iStockphoto.com/Niko Guido

Figure 17–4 A sting ray.

Figure 17–5 Ticks can be as small as a head of a pin.

Rabid animals may salivate, appear partially paralyzed, or act irritable, aggressive, or strangely quiet. Avoid petting or feeding wild animals and do not touch the body of a dead wild animal.

If not treated, rabies is fatal. Anyone bitten by an animal suspected of having rabies must get medical attention. To prevent rabies from developing, the patient receives a series of injections to build up immunity. In the past, caring for rabies meant a lengthy series of painful injections that had many unpleasant side effects. The vaccines used now require fewer injections and have less severe side effects.

If someone is bitten by an animal, try to get her away from the animal without endangering yourself. If possible, try to get a good description of the animal and the area in which it was last seen. If the wound is minor, wash it with soap and water and then control any bleeding. If the wound is bleeding profusely, control the bleeding first. The wound will be properly cleaned at a medical facility. Obtain more advanced medical care for any wounds with serious bleeding. Other authorities, such as animal control, may need to be notified. Any person who has been bitten by an animal must see her physician. Local laws or protocols may require you to report the bite to the proper authorities.

Ticks

Ticks can carry and transmit disease to humans. In the past, Rocky Mountain spotted fever was widely publicized as a tick disease. It is still occurring today,

but attention has been focused on another disease transmitted by ticks, known as Lyme disease or Lyme borreliosis. Lyme disease is an illness people get from the bite of an infected tick.

Not all ticks carry Lyme disease. Lyme disease is spread primarily by a type of tick that commonly attaches itself to field mice and deer. It is sometimes called a deer tick. This tick is found around beaches and in wooded and grassy areas. Like all ticks, it attaches itself to any warm-blooded animal that brushes by it, including humans.

Deer ticks are very tiny and difficult to see. They are much smaller than the common dog tick or wood tick. They can be as small as a poppy seed or the head of a pin (Figure 17–5). Even in the adult stage, they are only as large as a grape seed. A deer tick can attach to you without your knowledge. Many people who develop Lyme disease cannot recall having been bitten.

A person can get Lyme disease from the bite of an infected tick at any time of the year, but this occurs most often in summer, when ticks are most active and people spend more time outdoors.

The first sign of infection may appear a few days or a few weeks after a tick bite. Typically, a rash starts as a small red area at the site of the bite. It may spread up to 13 to 18 cm (5 to 7 in.) across. In fair-skinned

Figure 17–6 A rash in a bull's-eye pattern is a common sign of Lyme disease infection.

people, the centre is lighter in colour and the outer edges are red and raised, sometimes giving the rash a bull's-eye appearance (Figure 17–6). In dark-skinned people, the area may look black and blue, like a bruise.

Signs and symptoms of Lyme disease include fever, headache, weakness, and joint and muscle pain similar to the pain of "flu." These signals may develop slowly and may not occur at the same time as a rash. In fact, a person can have Lyme disease without developing a rash.

Lyme disease can get worse if not treated. In its advanced stages, it may cause arthritis, numbness, memory loss, problems seeing or hearing, high fever, and a stiff neck. Some of these symptoms could indicate nervous system problems. An irregular or rapid heartbeat could indicate heart problems.

If you find a tick, remove it by pulling steadily and firmly. Grasp the tick with fine-tipped tweezers (or a hook designed for tick removal), as close to the skin as possible, and pull slowly (Figure 17–7). If you do not have tweezers, use a glove, plastic wrap, a piece of paper, or a leaf to protect your fingers. If you use your bare fingers, wash your hands immediately. If you are unable to remove the tick or if its mouthparts stay in the skin, the patient should obtain medical care, such as from a family physician.

Once the tick is removed, wash the area immediately with soap and water. Unless the patient is allergic, if an antiseptic or antibiotic ointment is available, apply it to

prevent wound infection. The patient should be told to observe the site periodically thereafter. If a rash or flu-like symptoms develop, she should seek medical help. A physician will usually use antibiotics to treat Lyme disease. Antibiotics work best and most quickly when taken early. Treatment is slower and less effective in advanced stages.

SUBSTANCE MISUSE AND ABUSE

Alcohol and over-the-counter medications such as ASA, sleeping pills, and certain stimulants are among the most often misused or abused substances. The misuse or abuse of a substance results in the poisoning of the body.

Substance misuse is the use of a substance for unintended purposes or for appropriate purposes but in improper amounts or doses. Substance abuse is the deliberate, persistent, and excessive use of a substance without regard to health concerns or accepted medical practices. Many substances that are abused or misused are legal. Other substances are legal when prescribed by a physician. Some are illegal only for those under age. Figure 17–8 shows some commonly misused and abused legal substances.

Figure 17–8 Commonly misused and abused legal substances.

Figure 17–7 Remove a tick by grabbing it with tweezers as close to the skin as possible.

A drug is any substance other than food taken to affect body functions. A drug used to prevent or treat a disease or condition or otherwise enhance mental or physical well-being is a medication.

An overdose occurs if someone takes enough of a substance that it has toxic (poisonous) or fatal effects. An overdose may occur if the person takes more of a drug than is needed for medical purposes. It may occur unintentionally when someone takes too much medication at one time, for example, if an older adult forgets that she has already taken the medication and takes another dose. Or a person with failing eyesight may mistake one medication for another.

An overdose may also be intentional, such as in a suicide attempt. Sometimes the person takes a sufficient quantity of a substance to cause certain death. Other times, to gain attention or help, the person takes enough of a substance to need medical attention but not enough to cause death.

The term "withdrawal" describes the condition produced when someone stops using or abusing a drug to which she is addicted. Withdrawal may occur because of someone's deliberate decision to stop or because she is unable to obtain the specific drug. Withdrawal from certain substances, such as alcohol, can cause severe mental and physical discomfort and can become a serious medical condition.

Commonly Misused and Abused Substances

Substances are categorized according to their effects on the body. The basic categories are stimulants, hallucinogens, and depressants. The category to which a substance belongs depends mostly on the effects it has on the central nervous system. Some substances depress the nervous system, whereas others speed up its activity. Some are not easily categorized because they have various effects. Designer drugs, those that don't fit into one of the other three drug categories, are also commonly used. Figure 17–9 shows a variety of misused and abused substances.

Figure 17–9 Misused and abused substances.

Stimulants

Stimulants affect the central nervous system by speeding up physical and mental activity. They have limited medical value. They produce temporary feelings of alertness, improve task performance, and prevent sleepiness. They are sometimes used for weight reduction because they suppress appetite.

Many stimulants are ingested as pills, but some can be absorbed or inhaled. Amphetamine, dextroamphetamine, and methamphetamine are stimulants. There are many street, or slang, names for stimulants, for example, "speed."

Cocaine is one of the most publicized and powerful stimulants. Cocaine can be taken into the body in different ways. The most common is sniffing it in powder form. In this method, the drug is absorbed into the blood through the capillaries in the nose. A purer and more potent form of cocaine is crack. Crack is smoked. The vapours that are inhaled into the lungs reach the brain within 10 seconds, causing immediate effects. Crack poses a serious threat because it is highly addictive.

The most common stimulants are legal. Leading the list is caffeine, present in coffee, tea, many kinds of sodas, chocolate, diet pills, and pills used to combat fatigue. Next is nicotine, found in tobacco products. Other stimulants used for medical purposes are inhaled to treat asthma.

Hallucinogens

Hallucinogens, at present, have no medical uses. They cause changes in mood, sensation, thought, emotion, and self-awareness. They alter perception of time and space and produce delusions.

Among the most widely abused are LSD (lysergic acid diethylamide), commonly called acid; psilocybin, called mushrooms; and PCP (phencyclidine), also known as angel dust. These substances are usually ingested, but PCP is also often inhaled.

Hallucinogens often have physical effects similar to those of stimulants but are classified differently because of the other effects they produce. Hallucinogens can sometimes cause intense fear, panic, paranoid delusions, vivid hallucinations, profound depression, tension, and anxiety. The person may be irrational and feel threatened by any attempt others make to help.

Depressants

Depressants affect the central nervous system to slow down physical and mental activity. Unlike stimulants and hallucinogens, which have limited or no medical value, depressants are commonly used for medical purposes. Common depressants are barbiturates, benzodiazepines, narcotics, alcohol, and inhalants. Most depressants are ingested or injected.

All depressants alter consciousness to some degree. They relieve anxiety, promote sleep, relieve pain, and relax muscles, but they also depress respiration and impair coordination and judgment. Like other substances, the larger the dose or the stronger the substance, the greater its effects.

Alcohol is the most widely used and abused depressant in Canada. In small amounts, its effects are fairly mild. In higher doses, its effects can be toxic. Alcohol is like other depressants in its effects and the risks for overdose. Frequent drinkers may become dependent on the effects of alcohol and increasingly tolerant of them.

Alcohol taken in large amounts or frequently has many unhealthy consequences. The digestive system may be irritated. Alcohol can cause the esophagus to rupture or can injure the stomach lining, causing the person to vomit blood. This type of consumption is life-threatening. Chronic drinking can affect the brain and cause a lack of coordination, memory loss, and apathy. Other problems include liver disease, such as cirrhosis. In addition, many psychological, family, social, and work problems are related to chronic drinking.

Narcotics have effects similar to those of other depressants. They are powerful and are used to relieve anxiety and pain. All narcotics are illegal without a prescription, and some are not prescribed at all. The most common natural narcotics are morphine and codeine. Most other narcotics, including heroin, are synthetic.

Substances inhaled to produce an intoxicating effect are called inhalants. Inhalants also have a depressing effect on the central nervous system. In addition, inhalant use can damage the heart, lungs, brain, and liver. Solvents, such as acetone, toluene, butane, gasoline, kerosene, lighter fluid, paints, nail polish and remover, and aerosol sprays, have been inhaled for their effects. The effects are similar to those of alcohol. The user, at first, appears to be drunk.

Designer Drugs

Designer drugs are substances that do not fit neatly into any of the three categories mentioned previously.

Designer drugs are variations of medically prescribed substances such as narcotics and amphetamines. Through simple and inexpensive methods, the molecular structure of substances produced for medicinal purposes can be modified by street chemists into extremely potent and dangerous street drugs—hence the name designer drug. One such designer drug, a form of the commonly used surgical anaesthetic fentanyl, can be made 2,000 to 6,000 times stronger than its original form.

When the chemical makeup of a drug is altered, as with designer drugs, the user may experience a variety of unpredictable and dangerous effects. In many cases, the chemist has no knowledge of what the effects of the new designer drug could be.

Signs and Symptoms of Substance Misuse or Abuse

Like other poisons, the general signs and symptoms of substance misuse and abuse are similar to those of other medical emergencies. The misuse or abuse of stimulants can have many unhealthy effects on the body. These can include moist or flushed skin, sweating, chills, nausea, vomiting, fever, headache, dizziness, rapid pulse (tachycardia), rapid breathing (tachypnea), high blood pressure, and chest pain. In some instances, it can cause a breathing emergency, disrupt normal heart rhythms, or cause death. The person may appear very excited, restless, talkative, irritable, or combative or may suddenly lose consciousness.

Specific signs and symptoms of hallucinogen abuse may include sudden mood changes and a flushed face. The person may claim to see or hear something not present. She may be anxious and frightened.

Specific signs and symptoms of depressant misuse or abuse may include drowsiness, confusion, slurred speech, slow heart and breathing rates, and poor co-ordination. An alcohol abuser may smell of alcohol. A person who has consumed a great deal of alcohol in a short time may be unconscious or hard to arouse. The person may vomit violently. Someone suffering alcohol withdrawal, a potentially dangerous condition, can be confused and restless. She may also tremble and experience hallucinations.

You may be able to find clues that suggest the nature of the problem. Often these clues will come from the patient, bystanders, or the scene itself. Look for containers, drug paraphernalia, and signs and symptoms of other medical problems. Try to get information from the patient or from any bystanders or family members. Since many of these physical signs and symptoms of substance abuse mimic other conditions, you may not be able to determine that a patient has overdosed on a substance.

To provide care for the patient, you need only recognize abnormalities in breathing, pulse, skin colour, temperature, moisture, and behaviour that may indicate a condition requiring professional help.

Care for Substance Misuse or Abuse

As with other medical emergencies, you do not have to diagnose substance abuse or misuse to provide care. Your initial care does not require that you know the specific substance taken. Since substance misuse or abuse is a form of poisoning, care follows the same general steps as for other types of poisoning:

- Survey the scene to be sure it is safe to help the person.

- Do a primary survey and care for any life-threatening conditions.

- Contact the Poison Control Centre and/or obtain more advanced medical care.

- Question the patient or bystanders during your secondary survey to try to find out what substance was taken, how much was taken, and when it was taken.

- Try to keep the patient calm by minimizing movement, loud noises, etc.

- If the patient is unconscious, maintain an open airway.

- Maintain normal body temperature.

- If the patient vomits or has vomited, place her on one side and clear any matter out of the mouth. Save a sample of the vomitus, if possible.

- Withdraw from the area if the patient becomes violent or threatening.

- If you suspect that someone has used a designer drug, tell the responding advanced medical care personnel. This is important because someone who has overdosed on a designer drug frequently does not respond to usual medical treatment.

- Provide ongoing survey and care.

SUMMARY

Poisonings can occur in four ways: ingestion, inhalation, absorption, and injection. Substance misuse and abuse are types of poisoning that can occur in any of these ways. Substance misuse and abuse can produce a variety of signs and symptoms, most of which are common to other types of poisoning. You do not need to be able to determine the cause of a poisoning to provide appropriate initial care. If you see any of the signs and symptoms of sudden illness, ensure your own safety and follow the basics of care for any sudden illness.

For suspected poisonings, contact your local or regional Poison Control Centre and/or obtain more advanced medical care. Beyond following the general guidelines for giving care for a suspected poisoning, medical professionals may advise you to provide some specific care, such as inducing vomiting. The best way to avoid poisoning is to take steps to prevent it.

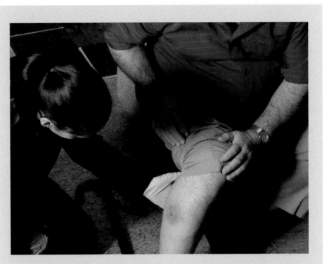

On questioning, the man tells you he was recently hiking in the woods and was not wearing long pants. Knowing this and his signs and symptoms, what do you do?

Heat- and Cold-Related Emergencies

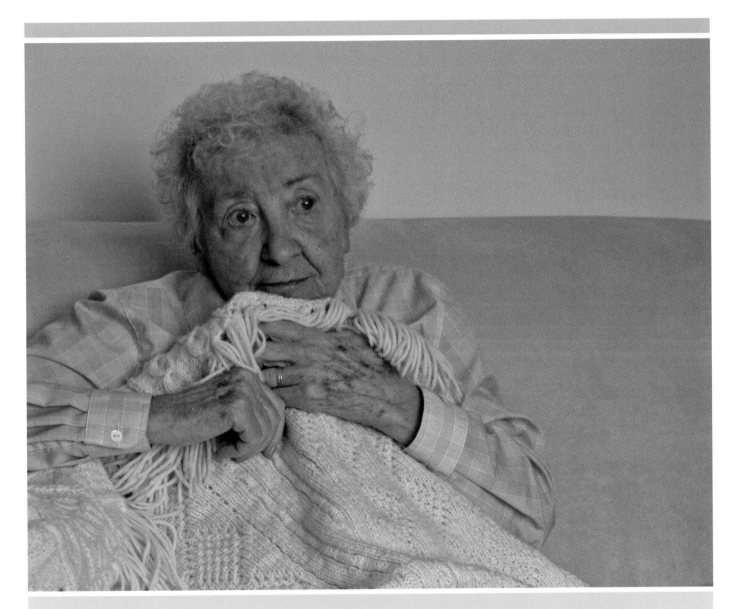

On a winter morning, you are summoned to the home of an older woman by her daughter, who tells you that her mother must have become confused the night before and had been wandering out in the cold overnight. When the daughter arrived in the morning to check on her, she found her mother sitting on the snowy steps, barely awake. She managed to wake her mother up and bring her into the house, where she covered her in blankets. You speak to her and ask how she is. She appears disoriented and responds weakly. She is shivering uncontrollably. What do you do?

INTRODUCTION

The lead runner enters his final lap and is approaching the finish line. You are part of the mobile aid team that has been following the front runners throughout the race. A few laps back, you remember seeing the person who is now in first place and noticing that he looked fresh and ready for the final few laps. You knew he had trained hard for this race. But now you observe that he looks exhausted. Urged forward by the cheering crowd, he appears to summon up his last reserves of energy to push ahead, but, instead, his legs begin to falter. He looks ill, and you suddenly see him shiver, even though the day is hot. Others begin to pass him. You hear him say he is dizzy and feeling nauseated.

Later, he says he can't remember falling. He barely remembers hearing voices shouting for help and people sponging him with cool water. He says things are now coming into focus. The sounds around him are becoming clearer. He says he hears a siren very near. Suddenly, he realizes he is the one in trouble. He is on his way to the hospital in an ambulance. His moment of glory ended just short of the finish line. He has fallen ill from the heat.

The human body is equipped to withstand extremes of temperature. Usually, its mechanisms for regulating body temperature work very well. However, when the body is overwhelmed by extremes of heat and cold, illness occurs.

Extreme temperatures can occur anywhere, both indoors and outdoors, but a person can develop a heat- or cold-related illness even if temperatures are not extreme. The effects of humidity, wind, clothing, living and working environments, physical activity, age, and an individual's health are all factors in heat- and cold-related illnesses.

Illnesses caused by exposure to temperature extremes are progressive and can become life-threatening. Once the signs and symptoms of a heat- or cold-related illness begin to appear, a person's condition can rapidly deteriorate and lead to death. If the person shows any of the signs and symptoms of sudden illness, notice the weather conditions and decide if they suggest the possibility of a heat- or cold-related emergency. If so, give the appropriate care. Immediate care can prevent the illness from becoming life-threatening. In this chapter, you will learn how extremes of heat and cold affect the body, how to recognize temperature-related emergencies, and how to provide care.

HOW BODY TEMPERATURE IS CONTROLLED

Body temperature must remain constant for the body to work efficiently. Normal body temperature is 37°C (98.6°F). Body heat is generated primarily through the conversion of food to energy. Heat is also produced by muscle contractions, as in exercise or shivering.

Heat always moves from warm areas to cooler ones. Since the body is usually warmer than the surrounding air, it tends to lose heat to the air. The body maintains its temperature by constantly balancing heat loss with heat production. The heat produced in routine activities is usually enough to balance normal heat loss.

When body heat increases, the body removes heat through the skin. Blood vessels near the skin dilate (widen) to bring more warm blood to the surface. Heat then escapes, and the body cools (Figure 18–1, a).

The body is also cooled by the evaporation of sweat. When the air temperature is very warm, dilation of blood vessels is a less effective means of removing heat. Therefore, sweating increases. But when humidity is high, sweat does not evaporate as quickly. It stays on the skin longer and has little or no cooling effect.

When the body reacts to cold, blood vessels near the skin constrict (narrow), which moves warm blood to the centre of the body. Thus, less heat escapes through the skin, and the body stays warm. When constriction of blood vessels fails to keep the body warm, shivering results (Figure 18–1, b). Shivering produces heat through muscle action.

Three external factors affect how well the body maintains its temperature: air temperature, humidity, and wind. Humidity and wind multiply the effects of heat or cold. Extreme heat or cold accompanied by high humidity hampers the body's ability to effectively maintain normal body temperature (Figure 18–2). A cold temperature combined with a strong wind rapidly cools exposed body parts. The combination of temperature and wind speed forms the "wind chill factor."

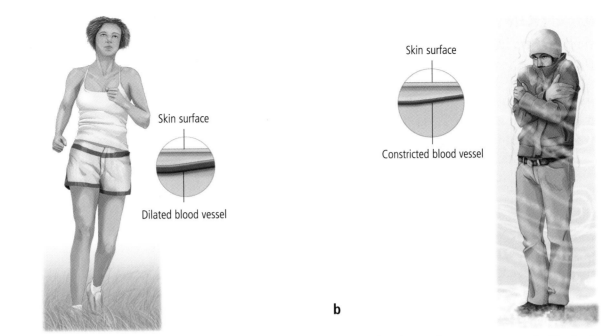

Figure 18–1, a-b a, The body stays cool by dilating blood vessels near the skin so heat can escape; **b,** The body stays warm by constricting blood vessels close to the skin. If this does not work, it begins to shiver.

Other factors, such as the clothing you wear, how often you take breaks from exposure to extreme temperature, how much and how often you drink water, and how intense your activity is, also affect how well your body manages temperature extremes. These are all factors you can control to prevent heat- or cold-related emergencies.

PREVENTING HEAT- OR COLD-RELATED EMERGENCIES

Generally, emergencies caused by overexposure to extreme temperatures are preventable. To prevent heat- or cold-related emergencies from happening to you or anyone else, follow these guidelines:

- Avoid being outdoors in the hottest or coldest part of the day.
- Change your activity level according to the temperature.
- Take frequent breaks.
- Dress appropriately for the environment.
- Drink large amounts of fluids.

The easiest way to prevent emergencies caused by temperature extremes is to avoid being outside during the time of day temperatures are most intense. For instance, if you plan to work outdoors in hot weather, plan your activity for the early morning and evening hours, when the sun is not as strong. Likewise, if you must be outdoors on cold days, plan your activities for the warmest part of the day.

However, not everyone can avoid temperature extremes. Often work or other situations require exposure to extreme conditions. But you can take additional precautions, such as changing your activity level and taking frequent breaks. For instance, in very hot conditions, exercise only for brief periods; then rest in a cool, shaded area. Frequent breaks allow your body to readjust to normal body temperature, enabling it to better withstand brief periods of exposure to temperature extremes. Avoid intense exercise during the hottest or coldest part of the day. Extremes of temperature promote fatigue, which hampers the body's ability to adjust to the temperature.

Always wear clothing appropriate to the environmental conditions and your activity level. When possible, wear light-coloured cotton clothing in the heat. Cotton absorbs perspiration and lets air circulate through the material. This lets heat escape and perspiration evaporate, cooling the body. Light-coloured clothing also reflects the sun's rays.

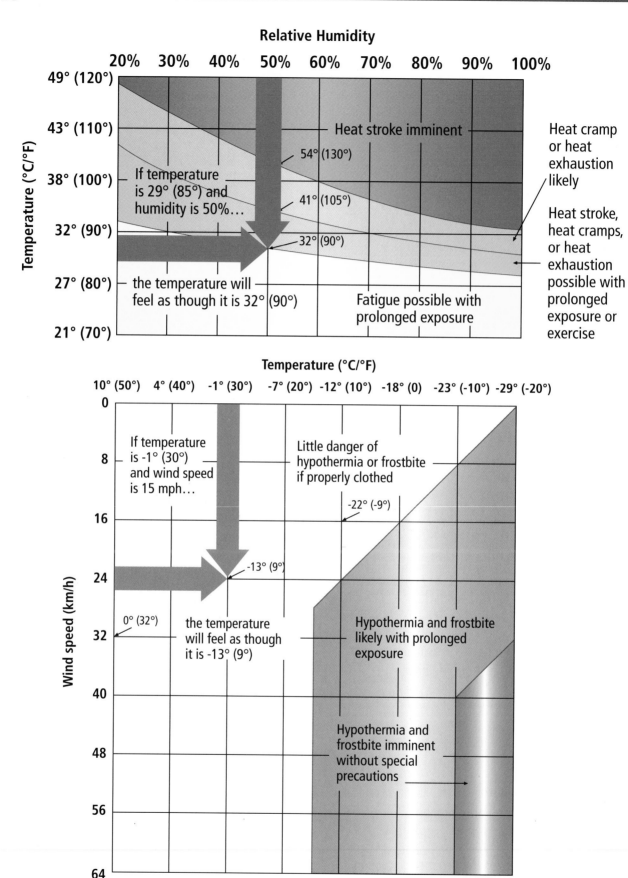

Figure 18–2 Extreme heat accompanied by humidity, or cold accompanied by wind, can hamper the body's ability to maintain normal body temperature.

When you are in the cold, wear layers of clothing made of tightly woven fibres, such as wool, that trap warm air against your body. Wear a head covering in both heat and cold. A hat protects the head from the sun's rays in the summer and prevents heat from escaping in the winter. Also protect other areas of the body, such as the fingers, toes, ears, and nose, from cold exposure by wearing protective coverings.

Whether you're in heat or cold, always drink enough fluids. Drinking plenty of fluids is the most important thing you can do to prevent heat- or cold-related illnesses. Plan to drink fluids when you take a break. Just as you would drink cool fluids in the summer, drink warm fluids in the winter. Cool and warm fluids help the body maintain a normal temperature. If cold or hot drinks are not available, drink plenty of plain water. Avoid drinking beverages containing caffeine or alcohol, as these beverages hinder the body's temperature-regulating mechanism.

PEOPLE AT RISK FOR HEAT- OR COLD-RELATED EMERGENCIES

People at a higher risk for heat- or cold-related emergencies include:

- Those who work or exercise strenuously outdoors or in unheated or poorly cooled indoor areas

- Older adults

- Young children

- Those with health problems

- Those who have had a heat- or cold-related illness in the past

- Those who have respiratory or cardiovascular disease or other conditions that cause poor circulation

- Those who take medications to eliminate water from the body (diuretics)

Usually, people seek relief from an extreme temperature before they begin to feel ill. However, some people do not or cannot easily escape these extremes. Athletes and those who work outdoors or in hot, humid indoor conditions often keep working even after they develop the first signs or symptoms of illness, which they may not even recognize (Figure 18–3).

Figure 18–3 Athletes and those who work in hot, humid conditions often keep going after they develop the first signs or symptoms of heat illness.

Heat- and cold-related emergenices occur more frequently in older adults, especially those living in poorly ventilated and insulated buildings or in buildings with poor heating or cooling systems. Young children and people with health problems are also at risk because their bodies do not respond as effectively to temperature extremes.

HEAT-RELATED EMERGENCIES

Heat cramps, heat exhaustion, and heat stroke are conditions caused by overexposure to heat. Heat cramps are the least severe but are often the first indicator of a problem. Heat exhaustion and heat stroke are more serious conditions.

Heat Cramps

Heat cramps are painful spasms of skeletal muscles. The exact cause is not known, although it is believed to be a combination of fluid and salt loss caused by heavy sweating. Heat cramps develop fairly rapidly and usually occur after heavy exercise or work outdoors in warm or even moderate temperatures. Heat cramps are characterized by severe muscle contractions, usually in the legs and the abdomen, but can occur in

Figure 18–4 Resting and lightly stretching the affected muscle may help relieve heat cramps.

any voluntary muscle. Body temperature is usually normal, and the skin is moist. However, heat cramps may also indicate that a person is in the early stages of a more severe heat-related emergency.

To care for heat cramps, have the patient rest comfortably in a cool place. Provide cool water or a commercial sports drink. Usually, rest and fluids are all the body needs to recover. Lightly stretch the muscle and gently massage the area (Figure 18–4).

Once the cramps stop and there are no other signs or symptoms of illness, the patient can usually resume activity. Caution the patient to be aware of signs and symptoms of developing heat-related illness. Tell the patient to continue to drink plenty of fluids during and after activity.

Heat Exhaustion

Heat exhaustion is the early stage and the most common form of heat-related illness. It typically occurs after long periods of strenuous exercise or work in a hot environment. Although heat exhaustion is commonly associated with athletes, it also affects firefighters, construction workers, factory workers, and others who work and wear heavy clothing in a hot, humid environment. Heat exhaustion is an early indication that the body's temperature-regulating mechanism is becoming overwhelmed. It is not always preceded by heat cramps. Over time, the person loses fluid through sweating, which decreases blood volume. Blood flow to the skin increases, reducing blood flow to the vital organs. Because the circulatory system is affected, the person goes into mild shock.

The signs and symptoms of heat exhaustion include:

• Normal or slightly raised body temperature (higher than 37°C or 98.6°F)

• Cool, moist, pale skin (skin may be red in the early stage, immediately following exertion)

• Headache

• Nausea

• Dizziness and weakness

• Exhaustion

In its early stage, heat exhaustion can usually be reversed with prompt care. Often the patient feels better when he rests in a cool place and drinks cool water. If heat exhaustion is allowed to progress, the patient's condition will worsen. Body temperature will continue to climb. The patient may vomit and begin to show changes in his level of consciousness. Without prompt care, heat exhaustion can quickly advance to a more serious stage of heat-related illness—heat stroke.

Heat Stroke

Heat stroke is the least common and most severe heat-related illness. It most often occurs when people ignore the signs and symptoms of heat exhaustion. Heat stroke develops when body systems are overwhelmed by heat and begin to stop functioning. Sweating stops because body fluid levels are low. When sweating stops, the body cannot cool itself effectively, and body temperature rapidly rises. It soon reaches a level at which the brain and other vital organs, such as the heart and kidneys, begin to fail. If the body is not cooled, seizures, coma, and death will result. Heat stroke is a serious medical emergency. You must recognize the signs and symptoms of this later stage of heat-related illness and provide care immediately.

The signs of heat stroke include:

- High body temperature (often as high as 41°C or 106°F)
- Red, hot, dry skin
- Progressive loss of consciousness
- Rapid, weak pulse
- Rapid, shallow breathing

Someone with heat stroke may at first have a strong, rapid pulse as the heart works hard to rid the body of heat by dilating blood vessels and sending more blood to the skin. As consciousness deteriorates, the circulatory system begins to fail and the pulse becomes weak and irregular. Without prompt care, the person will die.

Care for Heat-Related Emergencies

When signs or symptoms of sudden illness develop and you suspect the illness is caused by overexposure to heat, follow these general care steps immediately:

1. Cool the body.
2. Give fluids.
3. Minimize shock.
4. Provide ongoing survey and care.

When you recognize heat-related illness in its early stages, you can usually reverse it. Remove the patient from the hot environment and give him cool water to drink. Moving the patient out of the sun or away from the heat allows the body's own temperature-regulating mechanism to recover, cooling the body more quickly.

Remove any tight or heavy clothing. Cool the body by any means available (Figure 18–5). This can be done by applying cool, wet cloths, such as towels or sheets, to the skin or immersing the body in cool water from the neck down. You can also fan the patient to help increase evaporation. If you only have ice or cold packs, place them on areas such as the patient's wrists and ankles, in each armpit, and on the neck to cool the large blood vessels. Do not apply rubbing (isopropyl) alcohol. Alcohol closes the skin's pores and prevents heat loss.

If the patient is conscious, have him drink cool water slowly. This will help replenish the vital fluids lost through sweating. The patient is likely to be nauseated,

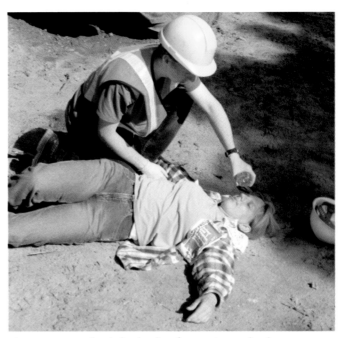

Figure 18–5 Cool the body of a patient who has a heat-related emergency.

and water is less likely than other fluids to cause vomiting. It also is more quickly absorbed into the body from the stomach. Do not let the patient drink too quickly. Give one half-glass (approximately 125 mL) about every 15 minutes. Let the patient rest in a comfortable position and watch carefully for changes in his condition. A patient with a heat-related emergency should not resume normal activities the same day.

Refusing water, vomiting, and changing level of consciousness are signs that the patient's condition is worsening. Obtain more advanced medical care immediately, if you have not already done so. If the patient vomits, stop giving fluids and position the patient on one side. Make sure the airway is clear. Keep the patient lying down and continue to cool the body as quickly as possible, which may involve safely immersing the body in cool water from the neck down. Someone with heat stroke may experience respiratory or cardiac arrest. Be prepared to do rescue breathing or CPR. Provide ongoing survey and care.

COLD-RELATED EMERGENCIES

Frostbite and hypothermia are two types of cold-related emergencies. Frostbite occurs in body parts exposed to the cold. Hypothermia is a general cooling of the body that develops when the body can no longer generate sufficient heat to maintain a normal temperature.

Frostbite

Frostbite is the freezing of body tissues. It usually occurs in exposed areas of the body, depending on the air temperature, length of exposure, and wind. Frostbite can affect superficial or deep tissues. In superficial frostbite, the skin is frozen, but the tissues below are not. In deep frostbite, also called freezing, both the skin and underlying tissues are frozen. Both types of frostbite are serious. The water in and between the body's cells freezes and swells. The ice crystals and swelling damage or destroy the cells. Frostbite can cause the loss of fingers, hands, arms, toes, feet, and legs.

The signs and symptoms of frostbite include:

- Lack of feeling in the affected area
- Skin that appears waxy
- Skin that is cold to the touch
- Skin that is discoloured (flushed, white, yellow, blue, or black)

Frost nip

Frost nip is a superficial injury caused by the freezing of the skin. The skin may appear pale, and there may be pain or stinging in the area. Treat it similarly to frostbite.

Care for Frostbite

When caring for frostbite, handle the area gently. Never rub an affected area. Rubbing causes further damage because of the sharp ice crystals in the skin.

Warm the area gently by soaking the affected part in water no warmer than 38° to 40°C (100° to 104°F). Use a thermometer to check the water, if possible. If not, test the water temperature yourself. If the temperature is uncomfortable to your touch, the water is too warm. Keep the affected body part away from the bottom or sides of the container (Figure 18–6, a). Keep the frostbitten part in the water until it appears red and feels warm. Bandage the area with a dry,

sterile dressing. If fingers or toes are frostbitten, place cotton or gauze between them (Figure 18–6, b). Avoid breaking any blisters. The patient should seek professional medical attention as soon as possible and will experience significant pain as the affected areas warm.

Do not thaw the area if transport may be delayed or if there is a possibility of the area refreezing. Provide ongoing survey and care.

Hypothermia

In hypothermia, the entire body cools when its warming mechanisms fail. The person will die if not given care. In hypothermia, body temperature drops below 35°C (95°F). Hypothermia progresses from mild to severe stages (Table 18–1). As the body temperature cools, the heart begins to beat erratically and eventually stops. Death then occurs.

Some signs and symptoms of hypothermia include:

- Shivering (may be absent in later stages)
- Slow, irregular pulse
- Numbness
- Glassy stare
- Apathy and decreasing level of consciousness
- Changes in skin colour
- Decreased blood pressure
- Slowly responding pupils
- Decreasing motor and/or sensory function

The air temperature does not have to be below freezing for people to develop hypothermia. Older adults in poorly heated homes, particularly people who have poor nutrition and get little exercise, can develop hypothermia at higher temperatures. People who are homeless or ill are at risk. Certain substances, such as alcohol and barbiturates, can also interfere with the body's normal response to cold, causing hypothermia to occur more easily. Medical conditions such as infection, insulin reaction, stroke, and brain tumours make a person more susceptible. Anyone remaining in cold water or wet clothing for a prolonged time may easily develop hypothermia.

38°–40°C
(100°–104°F)

a

b

Figure 18–6, a-b a, Warm the frostbitten area gently by soaking the area in water; **b**, after rewarming, bandage the area with dry, sterile dressings. Place gauze between frostbitten fingers or toes.

TABLE 18–1: PROGRESSION OF CLINICAL SIGNS AND SYMPTOMS OF HYPOTHERMIA

| Class | Core Temperature | | Signs and Symptoms |
	°C	°F	
Mild	36	96.8	Increased metabolic rate, maximum shivering, thermogenesis
Moderate	34	93.2	Impaired judgment, slurred speech
	30	86.0	Respiratory depression, irregular heart rhythms
Severe	<30	<86.0	Loss of deep tendon reflexes, fixed and dilated pupils, spontaneous ventricular fibrillation

Note: Normal body temperature is 37°C (98.6°F)

Care for Hypothermia

To care for hypothermia, do a primary survey and care for any life-threatening conditions. Obtain more advanced medical care. Remove any wet clothing and dry the patient.

Warm the body gradually by wrapping the patient in blankets or putting on dry clothing and moving him to a warm environment. Hot water bottles, heating pads (if the patient is dry), or other heat sources can aid in rewarming the body. Keep a barrier, such as a blanket, towel, or clothing, between the heat source and the patient to avoid burning him. If the patient is alert, give warm liquids to drink. Do not warm the patient too quickly by immersing in warm water, for instance. Rapid rewarming can cause dangerous heart rhythms. Be extremely gentle in handling the patient.

In cases of severe hypothermia, shivering will cease and the patient may be unconscious. Breathing may have slowed or stopped. The pulse may be slow and irregular. The body may feel stiff as the muscles become rigid. Rescue breathing should be started immediately if the patient is not breathing. Be prepared to start CPR. Before starting CPR, check the patient's signs of circulation, including pulse, for up to 45 seconds. If you cannot detect signs of circulation, begin CPR. Obtain more advanced medical care. Provide ongoing survey and care.

SUMMARY

Overexposure to extreme heat and cold may cause a person to become ill. The likelihood of illness also depends on factors such as physical activity, clothing, wind, humidity, working and living conditions, and a person's age and physical condition.

Heat cramps are an early indication that the body's normal temperature-regulating mechanism is not working efficiently. They may signal that the person is in the early stage of a heat-related illness. For heat-related emergencies, it is important to stop physical activity, cool the body, and obtain more advanced medical care.

Frostbite and hypothermia are serious cold-related emergencies, and the person experiencing either needs professional medical care. Hypothermia can be life-threatening. For both hypothermia and frostbite, it is important to warm the patient. For hypothermia, warm the entire body. For frostbite, warm the affected area.

As you assess the woman, you find that she has an irregular pulse. What do you do?

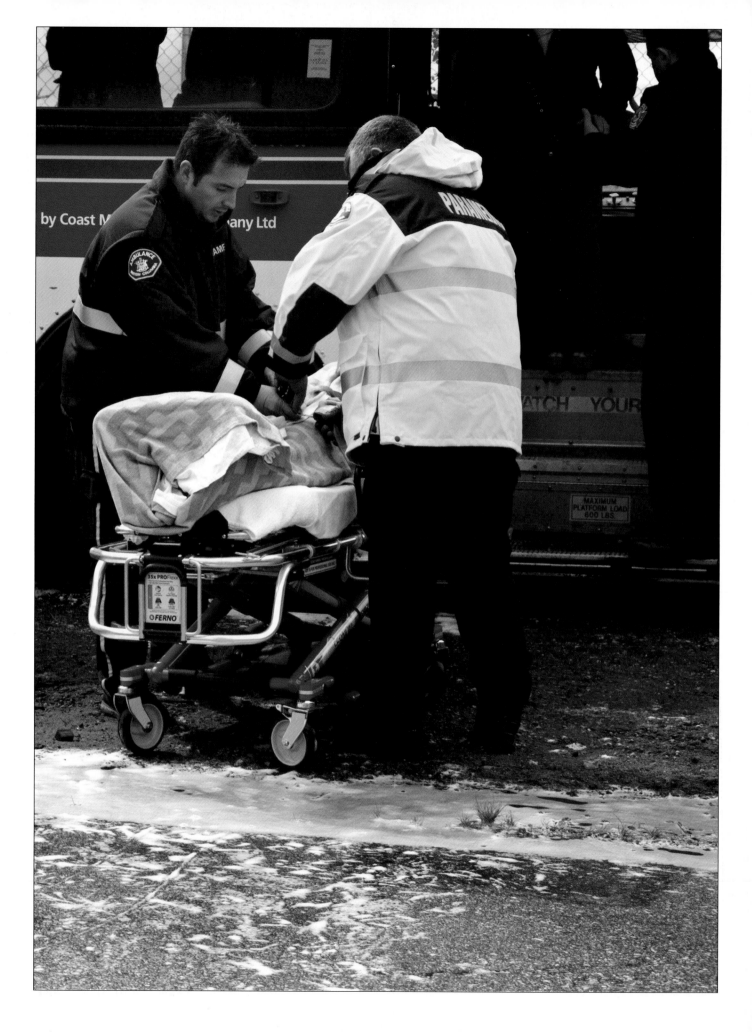

Part 5
Special Populations and Situations

Chapter 19

Special Populations and Crisis Intervention

You're called to the scene at a playground where a young girl has been struck in the face by a moving swing seat. The girl's sister brings the bleeding child toward you. The child is crying and is bleeding from a laceration on her cheek. What do you do?

INTRODUCTION

You are summoned to assist an older woman who says she hasn't been feeling well. As you question her, you notice she seems distracted and her answers don't exactly fit with your questions. Is some condition causing her to be disoriented? Is she fully conscious? Is this the way she normally behaves? Are you missing something?

A seven-year-old boy has crashed his bicycle into a parked car. He was thrown to the ground, landing on his head. As you approach, you notice him clinging to his mother and he appears lethargic. Does he have a head injury? Is this a reaction to a stranger or normal behaviour for him?

As a responder, you are likely to encounter individuals who fit the description of "special populations." What makes these people special are their needs and considerations. This chapter focuses on three special populations: children, older adults, and people with mental or physical impairments or disabilities. By being able to understand the special needs of a particular patient, you will be better able to communicate with him. As a result, you will be able to provide more effective care.

As a responder, you will also frequently encounter people in crisis. In one way or another, a serious injury, sudden illness, or death has an emotional impact on everyone involved: the patients, family, friends, bystanders, responders, and others. The degree of impact varies from person to person. For some, the impact is minimal, and they can accept an injury or illness that results in hospitalization, disability, or even death and handle it well. For others, however, even a minor injury can create an extreme emotional crisis, a highly emotional state resulting from stress. The way a person responds to an emergency largely depends on his emotional makeup and patterns of response. Therefore, the way one person responds to a stressful situation can differ substantially from the response of another person in a similar situation.

Sometimes it is not the fact that injury or illness has occurred that triggers emotional distress but how it occurred. The nature of an event, such as a sexual assault, can cause great emotional turmoil. A person's realization that he has been sexually violated can cause extreme stress. Events such as a suicide, self-inflicted death, or attempted suicide can cause great stress to the family and friends of the person. They often feel as if they could have done more or should have been able to help.

Besides providing care for any specific injury or illness, you may also need to provide emotional support to patients experiencing an emotional crisis. In some instances, the patient will be so distraught that he will be entirely dependent on you and your directions. Being able to understand some of what the patient is feeling can help you cope with the situation.

THE ILL OR INJURED CHILD

At some time, you will probably be summoned to assist an ill or injured child. If you are, you must keep several considerations in mind. The most important is that children are not simply small adults. They have unique needs and require special care. They do not readily accept strangers. This can make it difficult to accurately assess a child's condition. Young children can be especially difficult to assess since they often will not be able to tell you what is wrong.

It is often difficult for adults to imagine how a young child with a serious illness or injury feels. One of a child's primary emotions is fear. A child is afraid of the unknown. He is afraid of being ill or hurt, of being touched by strangers, and of being separated from his parents. Being aware of the fears of a child and knowing how to cope with them will enable you to provide more effective care.

Assessing the Child

When assessing a child, follow the same steps as for an adult. However, remember to get consent from the child's parent or guardian. Do the primary survey first. Any problems that threaten the child's airway, breathing, and circulation must be taken care of as soon as he is found. Once you have completed the primary survey, you can begin the secondary survey.

Keep in mind that there are differences in babies and children compared with adults (Table 19–1).

During the secondary survey, you will interview the child and any bystanders, such as the child's parent or guardian. How you interact with the child and the

TABLE 19–1: ANATOMICAL AND PHYSIOLOGICAL DIFFERENCES IN BABIES AND CHILDREN COMPARED WITH ADULTS[25]

Body System	Differences	Clinical Significance
Respiratory	Tongue is larger	Can cause airway to become blocked
	Airway is smaller	Can become easily blocked
	Secretions are abundant	Can block airway
	Nose and face are flatter	Makes it more difficult to obtain good airway seal with mask
	Trachea is shorter and narrower and cartilage development is incomplete	Can close off trachea if overextended
	Respiratory rate is faster	Muscles become easily fatigued
	Breathing is done primarily through the nose (newborns)	Airway is more easily blocked
	Abdominal muscles are used for breathing	Evaluating breathing is more difficult
	Ribs are more flexible	Less protection for lungs; may have significant injuries without external signs
Circulatory	A faster heart rate can be sustained for a longer time	Can compensate longer before signs of shock are evident; usually decompensates faster and more suddenly
Nervous	Brain tissue is thinner and softer	Head injury is considered more serious
Thermoregulatory	Body surface is larger	More prone to hypothermia
Integumentary	Skin is thinner	Burns are considered more serious
Musculoskeletal	Head is larger (proportionally)	Causes neck flexion or head to be displaced anteriorly when supine; increases potential for head injuries in trauma cases
	Neck is shorter	Stabilization is difficult
	Bones are softer	Bend and fracture easily

parent or guardian is very important. You must establish a good rapport. This means reducing anxiety and panic in both the child and the parent or guardian. There are a few basic guidelines that will help you assess an injured or ill child:

- Observe the child before touching him. Information can be obtained before actually touching the child. Look for signs that indicate changes in the level of consciousness, any breathing difficulty, and any apparent injuries or conditions. All may change as soon as you touch the child because he may become anxious or upset.

- Communicate clearly with the parent or guardian and the child. If the family is excited or agitated, the child is likely to be so, too. When you can calm the family, the child will often calm down as well. Explain what you wish to do. Get at eye level with the child (Figure 19–1). Talk slowly and use simple words when speaking with the child. Ask questions that can be easily answered.

- Remain calm. Caring for children, especially those who are seriously ill or injured, can be very stressful. Calmness on your part will show confidence and help keep the child and parent or guardian calm.

- Keep the child with loved ones, unless it's necessary to separate them. This is especially true for younger children (under age seven or eight). Often a parent or guardian will be holding a crying child. In this case, you can assess the child's condition while the parent or guardian continues to hold the child.

- Gain trust through your actions. Explain to the child and parent or guardian what you are going to do before you do it. Be sure to use terms and language appropriate for the child's age.

In performing the secondary survey, it is often easier to do the head-to-toe examination before you check vital signs. Furthermore, the head-to-toe examination is often better performed in reverse order, as a toe-to-head examination, on a conscious child. The child is more likely to accept you first touching the feet and progressing to the head. You should still look and feel for the same things.

Children up to one year of age are commonly referred to as babies. Young babies, those less than six months old, are relatively easy to examine. Your presence will not generally bother this age group. Older babies, however, will often exhibit "stranger anxiety." They are uncomfortable around strangers and may cry and cling to a parent or guardian.

Children one to three years of age are called toddlers. These children are frequently uncooperative. As a result, they are often best examined in the parent's or guardian's lap. A toddler will be concerned that he will be separated from his parent or guardian. Reassurance that this will not happen will often comfort a concerned child of this age.

Children aged three to five are generally referred to as preschoolers. Children in this age group are usually easy to examine if approached properly. Use their natural curiosity. Allow them to inspect equipment or supplies, such as oxygen tubing or bandages. This can allay many fears and distract them during your assessment.

School-aged children are those between 5 and 12 years of age. They are usually cooperative and can be a good source of information regarding what happened. You should be readily able to converse with them. Children in this age group are becoming conscious of their bodies and do not like exposure. Respect the child's modesty.

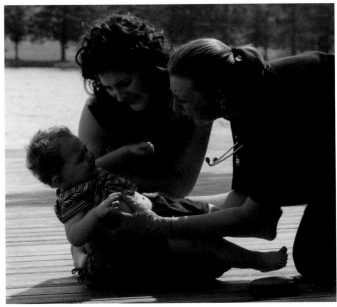

Figure 19–1 When communicating with a child, get down to his eye level.

Adolescents are between 13 and 18 years of age. They are typically more of an adult than a child. Direct questions to them instead of toward parents or guardians. However, allow input from a parent or guardian. Occasionally, in the presence of a parent or guardian, it may not be possible to get an accurate history. Adolescents do not like having their bodies exposed and often respond better to a caregiver of the same gender. Respect the adolescent's modesty.

When checking a child's vital signs, such as breathing and pulse, during the secondary survey do not be alarmed at finding faster rates. A child's resting pulse and breathing are normally faster than those of an adult. A normal resting heart rate for an adult ranges from 60 to 100 beats per minute. Babies and toddlers, on the other hand, have normal resting heart rates from approximately 100 to 160 beats per minute. As the child ages, his resting heart rate will become slower. By the time the child reaches adolescence, his resting heart rate will be approximately the same as an adult's.

This is also true for a child's breathing rate. In response to a heart that is beating faster, the child also breathes faster. Average resting breathing rates for preadolescent children are 20 to 40 breaths per minute.

Special Problems

Common Childhood Conditions

Chickenpox (contagious viral infection)—A child with chickenpox is most contagious for one to two days before and for approximately five days after the onset of the rash, or until the chickenpox lesions are crusted. The contagious period may be prolonged in an immune-compromised person.[26] The child may have a fever, rash, possibly with fluid-filled blisters, and itchiness.

Dehydration (not contagious)—Suspect dehydration if the child's diaper stays dry longer than usual; the child wets fewer than the usual number of diapers in 8 to 10 hours; or the child has a dry mouth and tongue, no tears when crying, or sunken eyes. In babies, the soft spot on the top of the head may be sunken.

Diarrhea (underlying condition may be contagious)—Diarrhea is characterized by unusually frequent, liquid bowel movements, blood in the stool, pain in the abdomen, other signs of illness, and dehydration, which can be suspected if the child is passing less urine than usual.

Earaches (not contagious)—A child with an earache may be worried; may pull at his ear or cover it with his hand; may have sore ears or fluid discharging from the ear; and may develop fever, chills, deafness, dizziness, and/or nausea.

Eczema (not contagious)—A child with eczema may have inflamed skin and one or a combination of rashes, pimples, scaly skin, and scabs. The skin may also be dry or have a watery discharge, and the skin may burn or itch.

Impetigo (contagious bacterial infection)—Impetigo is contagious and can spread to anyone who comes into contact with the infected skin or other items, such as clothing, towels, and bed linens, that have been touched by the infected skin.[27] The child will have inflamed skin and crusted, broken clusters of pimples around the mouth and nose that may be flat and pitted (filled with straw-coloured fluid).

Ringworm (contagious fungal infection)—Ringworm is characterized by red, scaling rings on the skin. A child with ringworm is contagious until 48 hours after treatment begins.[28]

Scabies (contagious skin parasite)—A child with scabies will have many tiny blisters, scratch marks, and scaly crusts (found mainly in skin folds), as well as extreme itchiness. Scabies is highly contagious.[29]

Persistent vomiting (underlying condition may be contagious)—Child will have nausea and stomach pain.

Prickly heat rash (not contagious)—Presents as a rash of tiny, pinpoint blisters surrounded by blotches of pink skin, and it may appear on the face or on the parts of the body most heavily clothed. It occurs in hot weather or whenever a baby or child is overdressed.

Pink eye (contagious)—The white of the eye looks pink, the eyelids are usually swollen, pus may form, and eyes are itchy or sensitive. Pink eye is contagious until 24 hours after treatment is started.[30]

Pinworms (contagious)—The child will be constantly scratching around the anus and is unusually irritable.

Injury

Injury remains the number one cause of death for children in Canada. Many of these deaths result from incidents involving motor vehicles. The greatest dangers to a child involved in a vehicle incident that results in serious injury are airway obstruction and bleeding. Because a child's head is usually large in proportion to the rest of the body, the head is often injured.

To prevent some of the needless deaths children suffer as a result of motor vehicle incidents, laws requiring safety seats and seat belts have been imposed. As a result, more lives will be saved, but also more injured children will need to be cared for while in car seats (Figure 19–2). A car seat does not normally pose any problem when you are trying to assess a child. A child involved in a motor vehicle crash and found in a car seat should be left in the car seat if the device has not been damaged. If the child is to be transported to a medical facility for evaluation, he can be easily secured in the car seat by putting rolled towels on each side of the head and wrapping two strips of tape around the car seat and the head—one over the forehead and one over the upper lip. Pad any spaces with blankets or towels.

High Fever

A high fever in a child indicates some type of infection. Because a young child's temperature-regulating mechanism has not fully developed, even a minor infection can result in a rather high fever. This is often defined as a temperature above 39°C (102°F). In this case, prolonged or excessively high fever can result in seizures known as febrile seizures. Obtain more advanced medical care. Your initial care for a child with high fever is to gently cool the child. This includes removing excessive clothing or blankets and sponging lukewarm water on the child. Provide ongoing survey and care.

Breathing Emergencies

Infections of the respiratory system are more common in children than in adults. These can range from minor infections, such as the common cold, to life-threatening infections that block the airway. Signs and symptoms of a breathing emergency in children include:

Figure 19–2 Children may need to be cared for while they are in a car seat.

- Unusually fast or slow breathing
- Noisy breathing
- Skin discoloration
- Retraction of the spaces between the ribs during breathing
- Diminished level of consciousness

Croup is a common childhood illness that causes a breathing emergency. It is a viral infection that causes swelling of the tissues below the vocal cords. Besides the basic signs and symptoms of a breathing emergency and a cough that sounds like the bark of a seal, croup is often preceded by one or two days of illness, sometimes with a fever. Croup occurs more often in the winter months, and the signs and symptoms of croup are often more evident in the evening. It is generally not life-threatening. The child will often improve when exposed to cool air, such as the air outdoors or cool steam from a vaporizer.

Another childhood problem is epiglottitis, a bacterial infection that causes severe inflammation of the epiglottis. The epiglottis is a flap of tissue above the vocal cords that protects the airway during swallowing. When it becomes infected, it can swell to a point at which the airway is completely obstructed. The child with epiglottitis will appear quite ill and have a high fever. He will often be sitting up and straining to breathe. The child will be very frightened. Saliva will often be drooling from his mouth. This is because swelling of the epiglottis prevents the child from swallowing.

You will not need to distinguish between croup and epiglottitis since the care you provide will be the same for either illness. To care for a child in a breathing emergency, allow him to remain in the most comfortable position for breathing and administer oxygen. Do not attempt to place any object in the child's mouth or examine the mouth. Obtain more advanced medical care immediately. This is extremely important because the child needs immediate transport to a medical facility. Provide ongoing survey and care.

Child Abuse

Child abuse is unfortunately an all-too-common occurrence in our society. Child abuse commonly refers to the physical, psychological, or sexual assault of a child, resulting in injuries and/or emotional trauma. Children of all ages and backgrounds are victimized. You should suspect child abuse if a child's injuries are not consistent with the explanation you are given by the child or parent or guardian as to what happened.

The child abuser can come from any geographic, ethnic, religious, occupational, or socio-economic background. The abuser is often a person that the child or family knows and trusts. The signs of child abuse include:

- Obvious fractures in a child less than two years of age

- Signs of shaken baby syndrome

- Injuries in various stages of healing, especially bruises and burns

- More injuries than are usually seen in a child of the same age

- Injuries located in suspect parts of the body, such as the back, buttocks, genitals, upper thighs, torso, head, upper arms, or neck

- An injury that does not fit the description of what caused the injury

When caring for a child who may have been abused, always care for the child's injuries first. An abused child may be frightened, hysterical, or withdrawn. He may be unwilling to talk about the incident in an attempt to protect the abuser. As you provide care for any injuries, attempt to reassure the child and listen calmly and openly to what he tells you. Do not ask questions or make any accusations. Instead, explain your concerns to responding law enforcement or EMS personnel and follow organizational policies regarding making a report of child abuse. In all provinces and most territories in Canada, suspected child abuse must be reported to the appropriate child protection agency or police. When in doubt, ask your local police department or child protection agency for advice. As a follow-up, accurately complete an incident report, noting in detail anything you were told and any injuries you noted when you first examined the child. Also ensure that you record any instructions provided by police or the child protection agency.

Sudden Infant Death Syndrome (SIDS)

Sudden infant death syndrome (SIDS) is defined as the sudden death of a seemingly healthy baby that occurs during the baby's sleep and without evidence of disease. Usually, a thorough medical examination fails to reveal a cause of death. SIDS is sometimes mistaken for child abuse because of the unexplained death of an otherwise normal child and the bruise-like blotches on the baby's body. However, SIDS is not related to child abuse. It is not caused by vomiting or aspiration of stomach contents. It is also not believed to be hereditary but does tend to recur in families. What causes SIDS is not yet clear. You will not be able to "diagnose" SIDS. When the baby is found, he will be in cardiac arrest. You should care for the baby as you would anyone in cardiac arrest.

Shaken Baby Syndrome

When a baby won't stop crying, some people get so angry and frustrated that they shake the baby. This can cause fractures, heavy bleeding, bruising, and brain swelling, which stops oxygen from getting to the brain. Treat the baby for the injuries found and obtain more advanced medical care. Treat the situation as a case of suspected child abuse.

TABLE 19–2: SUMMARY OF CHILDHOOD INJURIES AND ILLNESSES

Injury or Illness	Description
Injury	• Number one cause of death for children in Canada • Many result from motor vehicles incidents, which can cause airway obstruction and bleeding; the head is often injured
High Fever	• Defined as a temperature above 39°C (102°F) • Indicates infection • Can be caused by even a minor infection • When prolonged or excessively high, can result in febrile seizures

Breathing Emergencies	• Often caused by infections of the respiratory system (more common in children than in adults)
	• Croup:
	  ■ Viral infection that causes swelling of tissues below the vocal cords
	  ■ Often preceded by one or two days of illness, sometimes a fever
	  ■ Child has a cough that sounds like the bark of a seal
	  ■ Occurs more often in winter months
	  ■ Generally not life-threatening
	• Epiglottitis:
	  ■ Bacterial infection
	  ■ Causes severe inflammation of the epiglottis; can obstruct the airway
	  ■ Child appears quite ill and has a high fever; child will often be straining to breathe, frightened, and drooling because swelling of the epiglottis prevents swallowing

Child Abuse	• Refers to physical, psychological, or sexual assault of a child, resulting in injuries and/or emotional trauma • Children of all ages and backgrounds are victimized • Suspect child abuse if child's injuries are inconsistent with explanation of what happened • Child abuser can come from any background and is often someone the child or family knows and trusts
Sudden Infant Death Syndrome	• The sudden death of a seemingly healthy baby that occurs during the baby's sleep and without evidence of disease • Usually, a thorough medical exam fails to reveal cause of death; cause is unknown • Sometimes mistaken for child abuse but is not related • Not caused by vomiting or aspiration of stomach contents • Not believed to be hereditary but tends to recur in families • Baby will be found in cardiac arrest
Shaken Baby Syndrome	• Result of someone shaking the baby through anger and frustration, often because the baby won't stop crying • Causes fractures, heavy bleeding, bruising, and brain swelling, which stops oxygen from getting to the brain

OLDER ADULTS

Older adults are generally considered those 65 years of age and over. These individuals are quickly becoming the fastest growing population group in Canada. A major reason for this is an increase in life expectancy because of advances in health care. Since 1900, there has been a 53% increase in life expectancy. For example, in 1900, the average life expectancy was 49 years. Today, the average life expectancy exceeds 75 years.

Many changes occur with age (Table 19–3). Overall, there is a general decline in body function, with some changes beginning as early as age 30. One of the first body systems affected by age is the respiratory system. The capacity of the respiratory system begins to decrease around age 30. By the time we reach age 65, our respiratory system may be only half as effective as it was in our youth. The heart also suffers the effects of aging. The amount of blood pumped by the heart with each beat decreases, and the heart rate slows. The blood vessels harden, causing increased work for the heart. The number of functioning brain cells also decreases with age. Hearing and vision usually decline, often causing some degree of sight and hearing loss. Reflexes become slower, and arthritis may affect joints, causing movement to become painful.

As a result of slower reflexes, failing eyesight and hearing, arthritis, and problems such as numbness related to blood vessels, older adults are at increased risk of injury from falls. Falls frequently result in fractures because bone density decreases. Bones become weaker and more brittle with age.

An older adult is also at increased risk of serious head injuries due to trauma. This is primarily because of the difference in proportion between the brain and the skull. As we age, the size of the brain decreases, which results in increased space between the surface of the brain and the inside of the skull (Figure 19–3). This allows more movement of the brain within the skull, which can increase the likelihood of serious head injury. Occasionally, an older adult may not develop the symptoms of a head injury until days after a fall. Therefore, you should always suspect a head injury as a possible cause of unusual behaviour in an older adult, especially if there is a history of a fall or blow to the head. Burns are a special concern to older adults as their skin is thinner and more fragile. Their immune system is less effective in fighting infection, so infections become more frequent and the potential for localized infection becomes widespread. Bowel obstructions are common due to the weak muscles of the bowel. Older people are susceptible to problems involving the system that regulates body temperature, called the thermoregulatory system.

Alzheimer's Disease

Older adults are also prone to nervous system disorders. One of the most common of these disorders in older adults is stroke, discussed in Chapter 8. In addition, older adults are at increased risk of altered thinking patterns and confusion. Some deterioration in mental function caused by aging is normal.

Another common nervous system disorder is Alzheimer's disease, a progressive, degenerative disease that affects the brain. It results in impaired memory, thinking, and behaviour.

If you are providing care for a confused older adult, try to determine whether the confusion is the result of injury or a pre-existing condition. Get at the patient's eye level so he can see and hear you more clearly. Sometimes confusion is actually the result of decreased vision or hearing.

Figure 19–3 The size of the brain decreases as we age.

TABLE 19–3: AGE-RELATED SYSTEMIC CHANGES

Body System	Changes with Age	Clinical Significance
Respiratory	Respiratory muscles are weaker and less coordinated Lung function decreases Cough and gag reflex are reduced	More likely to have respiratory failure
Circulatory	Arteries harden and lose their elasticity Changes in heart rate, rhythm, efficiency Decrease in blood volume and/or red blood cells	Hypertension is common Higher potential for strokes/heart attacks More likely to have bleeding from minor trauma Recuperates more slowly from illness/injury Greater risk of complications from trauma
Nervous	Brain tissue shrinks Memory declines Clinical depression is common Altered mental status is common Balance is impaired Pain perception decreases Reaction time decreases	Symptoms from head injury may be delayed May be more difficult to assess More prone to falls
Endocrine	Lowered estrogen production (women) Decline in insulin sensitivity Increase in insulin resistance Decrease in glucose metabolism Less effective pituitary gland	Increased risk of fractures (bone loss) and heart disease Diabetes mellitus common and more likely to have hyperglycemia Decrease in energy
Gastrointestinal	Digestive functions are less effective	Constipation is common More likely to suffer from malnutrition Vitamin and mineral deficiencies
Thermoregulatory	Reduced sweating Decreased shivering	Decreased heat/cold tolerance
Integumentary	Skin becomes thinner and more fragile	Skin is more subject to tears and sores Bruising more common Heals more slowly
Musculoskeletal	Bones become weaker (osteoporosis) Joints become weaker and less flexible (osteoarthritis)	More prone to fractures Slower healing More prone to falls
Renal	Kidneys get smaller and function less effectively	Increased problems with drug toxicity
Genitourinary	Loss of bladder function Prostate enlarges	Increased urination/incontinence Increased urinary tract infection Urinary retention
Immune	Poorer immune response	More susceptible to infections Doesn't respond effectively to vaccines

Care for older adults requires you to keep in mind the special problems and concerns of older adults and to communicate appropriately. Often an older adult's problem will seem insignificant to him—he may not recognize the signs or symptoms of a serious condition. For example, an older adult may complain of weakness. On further questioning, you may learn that he has been having fainting episodes with periods of numbness and tingling in one side of the body. Some older adults may purposely minimize their symptoms for fear of losing their independence or of being placed in a nursing home or similar institution. If the patient takes medications, you should gather them and see that they are with the patient if he is being taken to a medical facility.

Elder Abuse

Elder abuse is a growing problem in our society. Elder abuse involves any of four types of abuse: the infliction of pain or injury (physical abuse), mental anguish or suffering (psychological abuse), financial or material abuse, or unnecessary confinement or willful deprivation (neglect) by an older adult's caretaker. Typically, the abuser is a relative and lives with the abused elder.

The signs and symptoms of elder abuse generally include any unexplained injury or any physical situation in which older adults seem to be neglected. Provincial/territorial laws may require the reporting of such abuse if suspected, so follow your local protocol.

THE TERMINALLY ILL PATIENT

As a responder, you will respond to calls involving terminally ill patients. Terminal illness can happen to anyone, at any age. Often these situations are emotionally charged and require empathy and compassion toward the patient and his family and friends at the scene.

Cancer

Cancer is the general term used for a group of diseases in which there is an increased growth of cells in one or more organs or tissues. These cells most commonly develop in major organs such as the breasts, intestine, skin, lungs, stomach, brain, and pancreas but can also develop in cell-forming tissues of the bone marrow, muscle, or bone.

Not all people diagnosed with cancer become terminally ill; however, those who have cancer will often become very ill. The signs and symptoms will usually depend on the type, extent, and location of the disease. When responding to a patient with cancer, try to obtain a thorough history from the patient, including a list of all his medications. Caring for a terminally ill patient also requires that you offer comfort and support for the patient as well as his family and friends at the scene.

PATIENTS WITH PHYSICAL OR MENTAL DISABILITIES

Other special populations include those with physical or mental disabilities. The terms "physical disability" and "mental disability" mean different things to different people. What comes to mind when you hear these words? A person who uses a wheelchair? An amputee? Someone with a mental health impairment?

A person who suffers a serious injury that results in the loss of a limb or who is born lacking a limb is often referred to as having a physical impairment. So is someone who suffers the paralyzing effects of a stroke.

A person with a mental disability has an impairment of mental function that may interfere with normal activity and participation in life. Anyone at any age can find himself challenged by a physical or mental impairment that may interfere to some degree with normal activities, causing an activity limitation or participation restriction.

Visual Impairment

People who are unable to see adequately, or at all, are often called blind or partially blind. These people are also said to have a visual impairment. Blindness can occur from many causes. Some people are born blind. Others are born with the ability to see and then subsequently lose that ability through injury or illness. Visual impairment is not necessarily a problem in the eyes. It can occur because of problems in the visual centres of the brain.

People with a visual impairment usually adapt well to their condition. It should be no more difficult to communicate with a patient who has a visual impairment than with a patient who has full sight. It is not necessary to speak loudly or in overly simple terms. In fact, your

Figure 19–4 You can help a patient with a visual impairment by having her hold onto your arm.

assessment of the patient with a visual impairment should be little different from that of other patients. The patient may not be able to tell you certain things about how an injury occurred but can generally give you a good description based on her interpretation of sounds and touch.

If you are called to assist someone who has a visual impairment, explain to her what is going on and what you are doing. This will help alleviate anxiety. It will also allow the patient to orient herself to the environment and then provide you with information regarding her care. If you must move a patient with a visual impairment who can walk, stand beside the patient and have her hold on to your arm (Figure 19–4). Walk at a normal pace and alert her to any hazards, such as stairs, as you move. If the patient has a guide dog, try to keep the dog with her. These dogs are usually not aggressive.

Hearing Impairment

People with partial or complete deafness are referred to as having a hearing impairment. Deafness can occur as a result of injury or illness affecting the ear, the nerves leading from the ear to the brain, or the brain itself. As with blindness, deafness can be present at birth or can develop later because of injury or illness. Some responders become anxious when called to treat a patient with a hearing impairment. This anxiety is unfounded. Patients with a hearing impairment should be cared for in basically the same manner as other patients. You may only have to modify your assessment somewhat so that you can obtain necessary information.

You may not even be aware initially that a patient has a hearing impairment. Often the patient will tell you. Others may point at their ear and shake their head, "No." A child may carry a card stating that he has a hearing impairment. You may see a hearing aid in a patient's ear.

The biggest obstacle you must overcome in caring for the patient who has a hearing impairment is how to best communicate. Most people have adapted to their hearing loss by learning to speak, lip read, sign, or any combination of these.

Don't assume that people with a hearing impairment can't speak; many can, although their speech may be unclear. If you do not understand what the patient is saying, ask him to repeat it. Do not pretend that you understand.

Often the patient will be able to read lips. If the patient's illness or injury does not detract from the ability to read your lips, then communicate in this manner. Position yourself where the patient can see you, look at the patient when you speak, and speak slowly and enunciate carefully (Figure 19–5, a).

Some people who have a hearing impairment communicate using sign language. Communicate in this way if you are able to (Figure 19–5, b).

If the patient cannot speak, read lips, or communicate through sign language, you can write messages on paper and have the patient respond (Figure 19–5, c). This system is slow but effective. Some people have a machine called a Telecommunications Device for the Deaf (TDD), which is generally used for telephone communication. You can use this device to type messages and questions to the patient, and the patient can type replies to you.

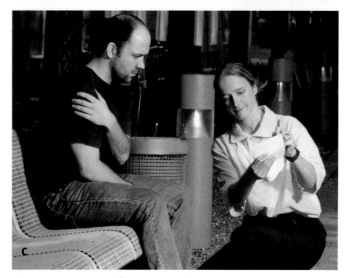

Figure 19–5, a-c There are many ways you can communicate with someone who has a hearing impairment: **a**, allow him to read your lips; **b**, use sign language; and **c**, write down what you want to say.

Physical Disability

A person who is restricted with a physical condition is referred to as having a physical disability. The impairments causing a disability can be diverse. Physical impairments are generally the result of problems with the muscles or bones or the nerves controlling them. Causes include stroke, cerebral palsy, multiple sclerosis, muscular dystrophy, and brain and spinal cord injuries. Depending on the nature and severity of the problem, you may care for the patient who has a physical disability in much the same way you would care for anyone else. In some situations, you will need to adapt to complex problems that may call for extra patience and compassion on your part. Many people have adapted to life without assistance, so be careful not to make assumptions about a patient's ability.

The patient with a physical disability who is injured poses unique problems because it may be difficult to determine which problems are new and which are pre-existing conditions. If this situation occurs, care for any detected problems as if they are new.

Developmental Disability

Impairment of mental function occurs with greater frequency than you might expect. A person with a mental health impairment may be referred to as having a developmental disability. As with physical impairments, mental impairments also can be diverse. Some types of mental impairment, such as Down's syndrome, are genetic. Others result from injuries or infections that occur during pregnancy, after birth, or later in life. Some occur from undetermined causes.

Often you will be able to determine easily whether a patient has a developmental disability. However, in some situations, you will not be able to tell. Always approach the patient as you would any other patient in his age group. When you speak, try to determine the patient's level of understanding. If the patient is confused, rephrase your statement or question in simpler terms. Listen carefully to what the patient is saying. A sudden illness or injury can interrupt the order in the patient's life and cause a great deal of anxiety and fear. You should expect this and offer reassurance. Take time to explain to the patient who you are and what you are going to do. Try to gain the patient's trust.

If a parent or guardian is present, ask him to assist you in providing care.

Behavioural or Psychiatric Disorders

Responding to an emergency involving someone with a behavioural or psychiatric disorder provides challenges that you should try to be equipped to handle. These people may be out of touch with reality, withdrawn, or even suicidal. As a responder, it is not your responsibility to diagnose a psychiatric disorder. In any behavioural emergency, first ensure the safety of responders and the scene. After determining that the scene is safe, your most important responsibility is to identify and care for any potentially life-threatening medical conditions the person may have.

The Person with a Behavioural or Psychiatric Disorder

Behavioural or psychiatric emergencies are those in which the person's chief complaint is some disorder of mood, thought, or behaviour that is dangerous or disturbing to the person or those around him. The cause of the disorder, either behavioural or psychiatric, can be classified into three categories:

1. Situational

2. Organic

3. Psychiatric

Situational disturbances can affect anyone if subjected to enough stress, but some people are more vulnerable than others. When a person's basic needs are threatened, that person faces a crisis. The severity of the crisis will depend on his ability to deal with his own feelings.

Organic disturbances can result in significant changes in behaviour. Examples include:

• Substance abuse

• Trauma

• Illness (e.g., diabetes, electrolyte imbalance, infection, tumour, dementia)

It is important for you to consider the possibility of organic causes in all behavioural emergencies.

Psychiatric problems may result in behavioural disturbances, that is, problems that arise within the mind of the person, by mechanisms we do not yet understand fully. Conditions that fall into this category are psychosis, anxiety, and depression.

Psychiatric disorders can also present with the appearance of a medical problem. For example, a person with an anxiety disorder may experience a panic attack, with signs and symptoms of hyperventilation and rapid heart rate and even chest pain, which suggests a medical emergency. Also, a person with a history of mental illness may experience a situational or physical problem unrelated to his psychiatric history.

In any behavioural emergency, first ensure the safety of responders and the scene. You may need to take special precautions for concerns that pose a threat to you or other responders. Then identify and care for the patient's potentially life-threatening medical conditions. If the patient has no obvious life-threatening conditions, take extra time to calm the patient and develop a rapport before proceeding with your assessment. Avoid making judgments or subjective interpretations of the patient's behaviour. You may need to look beyond the obvious to determine the true nature of the problem.

A good secondary survey will help you determine whether an underlying medical emergency exists and how to proceed. Transport decisions should be made in accordance with local protocols and based on medical control orders. Throughout management and transport, reassess the patient's ABCs and mental status at frequent intervals.

Psychosis

Psychosis is a severe mental condition characterized by a loss of touch with reality. An individual who is suffering from psychosis is tuned into his internal reality of ideas and feelings, which he may mistake for the reality of the real world. The internal reality may make him belligerent and angry toward others. Or the individual may become mute and withdrawn as he gives all his attention to the voices and feelings within. Signs and symptoms of psychosis may include:

• Loss of touch with reality

• Hallucinations

• Mania

- Confusion
- Depression
- False beliefs

As you assess the patient, his responses to your questions may reveal bizarre or disorganized thought processes, memory disturbance, and an inability to concentrate. Dealing with a patient who is suffering from psychosis is often difficult. An attempt to reason with the patient may be ineffective. Aggressive behaviour can also occur during psychotic episodes. Before approaching the patient, assess the potential for violence. Consider the possibility of requesting police back-up or other support when necessary.

Schizophrenia

This is a group of mental disorders that may present with distortions in language and thought. The person may also have delusions, hallucinations, and social withdrawal.

Anxiety

Anxiety is a term for mental disorders in which the dominant mood is fear and apprehension. All of us experience anxiety from time to time, and a certain amount of anxiety is useful and even necessary in helping us adjust to stress. But a person with an anxiety disorder may experience persistent, incapacitating anxiety in the absence of external threat. There are several types of anxiety disorders, but the two you are most likely to encounter are panic disorder and phobia.

Panic disorders, often called panic attacks, are unpredictable feelings of terror that strike suddenly and repeatedly. They can occur at any time, even during sleep. Signs and symptoms of panic attacks may include:

- Hyperventilation
- Feelings of weakness or faintness
- Chest discomfort
- Dizziness
- Rapid heart rate
- Sweating
- Nausea

- Smothering sensations
- Fear of loss of control

A phobia is a constant, irrational fear of something that compels a person to avoid it, causes stress, and impairs a person's ability to function normally. Phobias produce anxiety that is out of proportion to the actual threat. Signs and symptoms of phobias may include:

- Anxiety produced by exposure to an object or situation of phobia that may be overwhelming
- Sweating
- Rapid heart rate
- Feelings of weakness, cowardice

Calming and reassuring the patient may be the only treatment necessary for a panic attack or phobia. However, a complete medical history may be necessary to rule out the possibility of an underlying disease. For example, the rapid heart rate often associated with panic attacks or phobias may indicate a pulmonary embolism.

Depression

Depression or depressive behaviour in a person is often identified by a sad expression, bouts of crying, and listless or apathetic behaviour. Major depression, or clinical depression, is a mood disorder. The person may express feelings of worthlessness, hopelessness, guilt, and pessimism. Individuals with depression may also experience fatigue, a change in appetite with weight gain or loss, disruption of sleep patterns, and recurring thoughts of death or suicide. He may have difficulty concentrating or making decisions and may be restless or irritable. The person may want to be left alone, asserting that no one understands or cares. A depressive reaction can also arise in the wake of a stressful event, such as the loss of a close friend or relative.

Care for a patient with depression includes calmly talking to the patient about his interests and trying to direct responsiveness. Individuals experiencing depression are at risk for suicide. Any statements about suicide attempts or suicidal ideation should be taken seriously, documented, and reported to the receiving facility.

PEOPLE IN CRISIS

Specific Emotional Crises

Many different situations can result in an emotional crisis for people or bystanders. Examples commonly encountered by emergency personnel include attempted suicide, sexual or physical assault, the sudden death of a loved one, or a dying person.

Suicide

Suicide is more common in Canada than people may realize. It is one of the leading causes of death among people aged 15 to 19, although it is common among adults and older adults as well. Many people who attempt suicide suffer from some form of mental or emotional problem or illness. Substance misuse or abuse, primarily of alcohol and barbiturates, plays a major role in attempted suicides.

What motivates a person to try to commit suicide? It is often a combination of unbearable underlying tensions caused by a major event in a person's life, such as:

- A failing or failed relationship with a spouse, other family member, or friend
- Serious illness or death of a close family member or friend
- Serious, prolonged, or chronic personal illness
- A long period of failure at work or school
- A long period of unemployment
- Failure to achieve sufficient occupational, educational, or financial success
- Dramatic change in the economy

Assault

Assault is an all-too-common occurrence in our society. It can be physical, sexual, or both. It results in injury and, often, emotional distress to the person.

Sexual Assault

Sexual assault occurs when one person takes advantage of another by rape or forces a person to take part in any unwanted sexual act. Sexual assault is a crime of violence, or one committed under threat of violence, that involves a sexual attack. A sexual assault is a devastating experience for the person. People who have been raped often feel degraded, extremely frightened, and at further risk of attack. They require significant emotional support.

Besides providing emotional support, you must care for any injuries the patient may have received. When caring for a patient who has been sexually assaulted, do the following:

- Cover the patient and protect her from unnecessary exposure.
- Clear the area of any bystanders, except those friends or family able to help provide emotional support.
- Remove articles of clothing only if absolutely necessary to provide care for injuries.
- Care for any physical injuries.
- Discourage the patient from bathing, showering, or douching before a medical examination can be performed.
- Treat the area as a crime scene; mentally note all elements at the scene and, at the appropriate time, document all information.
- Do not question the patient about the specifics of the assault.
- Obtain more advanced medical care and summon law enforcement personnel.

Physical Assault

Physical assault on a child, spouse or partner, or older adult occurs more frequently than reported. Unfortunately, when you are summoned, the assault has often resulted in more serious injuries. The emergency scene where a physical assault has occurred is not always safe. The attacker may still be present or nearby. If the scene involves domestic violence, it may not be clear what has happened. Substances such as alcohol may be involved. Remember that your first concern is always your own safety. If you are not trained in law enforcement, do not approach the scene until it is determined to be safe. Wait for additional personnel. As with sexual assault, the scene is a crime scene. Therefore, do not handle items unrelated to the patient's care. Reassure and comfort the patient while providing care.

Death and Dying

You may be summoned to an emergency in which one or more people have died or are dying. Although your responses will vary according to the situation, you must recognize that death will have an emotional impact on you, as well as on others involved. Be prepared to handle your feelings and the feelings of others. Remember that reactions to death and dying range from anxiety to acceptance. How well you and others handle the situation will depend on both personal feelings about death and the nature of the incident. One of the most disturbing situations is when there is sudden death. This could involve someone who suffers a sudden illness, becomes unconscious, and later dies. It could also be someone involved in what appeared to be a minor motor vehicle collision; the person may be alert and talkative when you arrive but then suddenly suffers a cardiac arrest. Especially disturbing to new parents is the sudden unexplained death of a baby in the first few weeks of life. In situations such as these, there is no time to prepare for what has happened. Suddenly, a man, woman, or child who was alive only minutes earlier is now dead.

Sometimes you may be in a situation in which you think someone has been dead for a while and you are unsure whether you should attempt to resuscitate the person. The general rule is to always attempt to resuscitate and continue efforts to resuscitate until advanced medical personnel advise you to stop.

There are protocols to follow to determine whether a patient is dead. When it is determined that the patient has no heart rhythm, no pulse, no respiration, and no blood pressure, the patient is declared dead by the appropriate authority. In some instances, this will be after prolonged resuscitation attempts. At other times, additional signs—such as decapitation, transection, gross evisceration, rigor mortis, lividity, and decomposition—may cause resuscitation attempts to be withheld (it is important to be familiar with legislative protocols).

Some patients may have living wills, which are written legal documents saying that they do not wish to be resuscitated or kept alive by mechanical means. In most instances, the wishes of the patient expressed in writing

STAGES OF GRIEF

Everyone involved in a sudden, unexpected, and undesired event, such as a life-threatening illness or injury or the death of a loved one, experiences grief. The grieving process involves an outpouring of emotions that often follows a common pattern with various stages. These stages are not separate entities and do not necessarily follow one after the other. Instead, they often blend together. These stages include:

- Anxiety—a stage characterized by a feeling of worry, uncertainty, and fear. Signs and symptoms include rapid breathing (tachypnea) and pulse, increased activity, rapid speech, loud talking or screaming, and agitation.

- Denial/disbelief—a stage in which a person refuses to accept the fact that the event, such as the death of a loved one or suffering a debilitating injury, has occurred.

- Anger—a stage that involves the expression of aggressive verbal or physical behaviour. It is sometimes the result of the frustration of not being able to accept the event or a feeling that not enough was done or is being done to help.

- Bargaining—a stage that involves an unspoken promise of something in exchange for an extension of life or return to the pre-event condition.

- Guilt/depression—a stage that involves placing the blame for what happened on oneself, resulting in feelings of guilt or depression. A parent will often feel guilty for the event involving his child. A family member may feel guilty for not being of help to another family member who committed suicide.

- Acceptance—the final stage in the grieving process is when the pain and discomfort are eased. The person accepts the event and the outcome. For some people, arriving at the stage of acceptance takes weeks, months, or even years. For others, such as friends or family members who are aware that a person's condition is terminal, this stage can occur much more rapidly.

should be honoured. However, since provincial/territorial and local laws about these situations vary, you should obtain more advanced medical care immediately.

If you must confront the individual, his family and friends, or bystanders during or after a situation in which death is probable, be cautious about what you say. Avoid making statements about the patient's condition. You can provide comfort with positive statements such as "We are doing everything we can."

CRISIS INTERVENTION

Regardless of the nature of the incident, caring for someone experiencing an emotional crisis involves offering emotional support, as well as caring for any specific injury. The most important initial step you can take is to communicate with the patient in an open manner. Communication can be both verbal and nonverbal.

Nonverbal communication refers to your actions, posture, facial expression, and tone of voice. Sometimes your actions (body language) say more than you intend. You should always be aware of the messages you are sending with your body. General body posture is an important aspect of nonverbal communication. Begin by assuming a non-threatening posture. This involves getting at eye level with the patient and looking at him as you talk (Figure 19–6). Also, avoid positions such as placing your arms across your chest, your hands on your hips, pointing at the patient, or leaning over and looking down at the patient.

As you begin to communicate verbally, remember that communication involves stimulating discussion and listening as much as talking. When you do talk, speak in a calm, reassuring manner. Ask the patient his name and use it frequently in conversation. One technique used to help you more fully communicate is "active listening." The process of active listening requires you to listen closely to what the patient is saying. It involves four behaviours:

1. Making every effort to understand fully what the patient is trying to say.

2. Repeating back to the patient, in your own words, what he said.

3. Avoiding criticism, anger, or rejection of the patient's statements.

4. Using open-ended statements/questions such as "You appear to be very sad" or "What problems are you having?" Generally, avoid questions that can be answered with "yes" or "no."

Patients in emotional crisis may be withdrawn or hysterical. Some may be entirely dependent on you to help. Avoid being judgmental. Do not place blame on the patient. The patient needs to be cared for gently and with respect. If care is needed for a minor injury, try to get the patient to help you (Figure 19–7). By encouraging the patient to participate, you may help her regain a sense of control.

Figure 19–6 Assuming a non-threatening posture and getting at eye level are examples of nonverbal communication.

Figure 19–7 Having a patient help care for her own injury may give her a sense of regained control.

Do not be fooled into thinking you can manage a situation involving emotional crisis yourself. A suicidal patient or someone who has been raped needs professional counselling. Obtain more advanced medical care. This could include law enforcement, EMS, or local mental health or rape crisis centre personnel. While waiting for others to arrive, continue to talk with the patient. Never leave the patient alone unless there is a threat to your safety.

SUMMARY

As a responder, you will likely be called to assist a wide variety of special populations. When dealing with children, remember that they are not small adults. They must be approached gently and in a manner appropriate for their age. You need to recognize and try to alleviate their fears. Your assessment will be modified slightly because of the special needs of children. Certain illnesses, such as croup and epiglottitis, can cause a breathing emergency that should be cared for promptly. When caring for the child, do not forget the parent or guardian. They can make your job easier, so allow them to remain with the ill or injured child and to assist in care when appropriate.

Besides the ill or injured child, you are likely to encounter an older adult or a patient of any age with a physical or mental disability. Remember to care for these individuals based on individual need. You should recognize their limitations and work around them. As with the ill or injured child, proper communication will be the most important thing for you to establish.

An emotional crisis is often the result of an unexpected, shocking, and undesired event, such as the sudden loss of a loved one. Although people react differently in different situations, each experiences some or all of the stages associated with grieving. By considering the nature of the incident, you can begin to prepare yourself to deal with its emotional aspects. Regardless of the nature of the event, however, the care you provide to patients in any emotional crisis is very similar. Your care involves appropriate verbal and nonverbal communication. It also requires you to understand that in some cases death is inevitable.

After a little while, the girl stops crying, and she seems to be getting tired. What do you do?

Chapter 20

Childbirth

A 24-year-old woman believes she is in labour. She says that this will be her third child and labour came on so fast she didn't have a chance to get to the hospital. She says she feels the need to move her bowels. Contractions are frequent, about two minutes apart. What do you do?

INTRODUCTION

A woman calls the local EMS number and asks for an ambulance. She says she is expecting a baby and is in labour now. She thinks the baby is coming fast. The woman lives in a rural area, and it will take the ambulance nearly 25 minutes to get there. A police officer nearby is dispatched to help until ambulance personnel arrive.

The officer knocks on the door, and there is no answer. She tries the door and finds it unlocked, so she enters the house and finds the woman lying on the floor, in obvious pain. She sees bloody fluid on the floor. When she examines the woman, she sees the baby's head at the opening of the birth canal and realizes that the birth is imminent. She knows that the baby will be born before the ambulance crew arrives. She prepares to help deliver the baby.

Someday you may be faced with a similar situation, requiring you to assist with childbirth. If you have never seen or experienced childbirth, your expectations probably consist of what others have told you.

Terms such as exhausting, stressful, exciting, fulfilling, painful, and scary are sometimes used to describe a planned childbirth, one that occurs in the hospital or at home under the supervision of a healthcare provider. If you find yourself assisting with the delivery of a baby, however, it is probably not happening in a planned situation. Therefore, your feelings, as well as those of the expectant mother, may be intensified by fear of the unexpected or the possibility that something might go wrong.

Take comfort in knowing that things rarely go wrong. Childbirth is a natural process. Thousands of children all over the world are born each day, without complications, in areas where no medical assistance is available during childbirth.

By following a few simple steps, you can effectively assist in the birth process. This chapter will help you better understand the birth process, how to assist with the delivery of a baby, how to provide care for both the mother and the newborn, how to recognize complications, and what complications could require more advanced medical care.

PREGNANCY

Pregnancy begins when an egg (ovum) is fertilized by a sperm, forming an embryo. The embryo implants itself within the mother's uterus, a pear-shaped organ that lies at the top centre of the pelvis. The embryo is surrounded by the amniotic sac. This is a fluid-filled sac also called the "bag of waters." The fluid is constantly renewed and helps protect the baby from injury and infection.

As the embryo grows, its organs and body parts develop. After about eight weeks, the embryo is called a fetus. To continue to develop properly, the fetus must receive nutrients. The fetus receives these nutrients from the mother through a specialized organ attached to the uterus called the placenta. The placenta is attached to the fetus by a flexible structure called the umbilical cord. The fetus will continue to develop for approximately 40 weeks (about nine months), at which time the birth process will begin (Figure 20–1).

THE BIRTH PROCESS

The birth process begins with the onset of labour. Labour is the final phase of pregnancy. It is a process in which many systems work together to bring about birth. Labour begins with a rhythmic contraction of the uterus. As these contractions continue, they dilate the

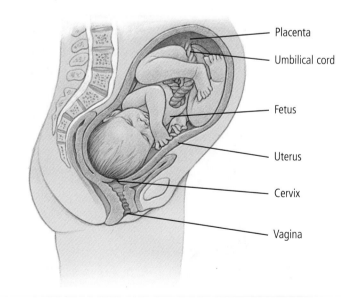

Figure 20–1 Mother and fetus at 40 weeks.

- Placenta
- Umbilical cord
- Fetus
- Uterus
- Cervix
- Vagina

cervix—a short tube of muscle at the upper end of the birth canal, the passageway from the uterus to the vaginal opening. When the cervix is sufficiently dilated, it allows the baby to travel from the uterus through the birth canal. The baby passes through the birth canal and emerges from the vagina, the lower end of the canal, to the outside world. For first-time mothers, this process normally takes between 12 and 24 hours. Subsequent babies are usually delivered more quickly.

The Labour Process

The labour process has four distinct stages. The length and intensity of each stage vary.

Stage One—Preparation

In the first stage, the mother's body prepares for the birth. This stage covers the period of time from the first contraction until the cervix is fully dilated. A contraction is a rhythmic tightening of the muscles in the uterus. It is like a wave. It begins gently, rises to a peak of intensity, and then drops off and subsides. The muscles then relax, and there is a break before the next contraction starts. As the time for delivery approaches, the contractions become closer together, last longer, and feel stronger. Normally, when contractions are less than three minutes apart, childbirth is near.

Stage Two—Delivery of the Baby

The second stage of labour involves the actual delivery of the baby. It begins once the cervix is completely dilated and ends with the birth of a baby. The baby's

Figure 20–2 When crowning begins, birth is imminent.

head will become visible as it emerges from the vagina. When the top of the head begins to emerge, it is called crowning (Figure 20–2). When crowning occurs, birth is imminent, and you must be prepared to receive the baby.

Stage Three—Delivery of the Placenta

Once the baby's body emerges, the third stage of labour begins. During this stage, the placenta usually separates from the wall of the uterus and exits from the birth canal. This process normally occurs within 20 minutes of the delivery of the baby.

Stage Four—Stabilization

The final stage of labour involves the initial recovery and stabilization of the mother after childbirth. Normally, this stage lasts for approximately one hour. During this time, the uterus contracts to control bleeding, and the mother begins to recover from the physical and emotional stress that occurred during childbirth.

Assessing Labour

If you are called to assist a pregnant woman, you will want to determine whether she is in labour. If she is in labour, you should determine how far along she is in the birth process and whether she expects any complications. You can determine these factors by asking a few key questions and making some quick observations. Ask the following:

- Is this your first pregnancy? The first stage of labour normally takes longer with first pregnancies than with subsequent ones.

- Has the amniotic sac ruptured? When this happens, fluid flows from the vagina in a sudden gush or a trickle. Some women think they have lost control of their bladder. The breaking of the sac usually signals the beginning of labour. People often describe the rupture of the sac as "the water breaking."

- What are the contractions like? Are they very close together? Are they strong? The length and intensity of the contractions will give you valuable information about the progress of labour. As labour progresses, contractions become stronger, last longer, and are closer together.

- Is there a bloody discharge? This pink or light red, thick discharge from the vagina is the mucous plug that falls from the cervix as it begins to dilate, also signalling the onset of labour.

- Does she have an urge to bear down? If the expectant mother expresses a strong urge to push, this signals that labour is far along.

- Is the baby crowning? If the baby's head is visible, the baby is about to be born.

PREPARING FOR DELIVERY

Preparing Yourself

There comes a time when you realize that you are about to assist with childbirth. Although this is often exciting, it is rarely comforting. Childbirth is messy. It involves a discharge of watery, sometimes bloody fluid at stages one and two of labour and what appears to be a rather large loss of blood after stage two. Try not to be alarmed at the loss of blood. It is a normal part of the birth process. Only bleeding that cannot be controlled after the baby is born is a problem. Take a deep breath and try to relax. Remember that you are only assisting in the process; the expectant mother is doing all the work.

Helping the Mother Cope With Labour and Delivery

Explain to the expectant mother that the baby is about to be born. Be calm and reassuring. A woman having her first child often feels fear and apprehension about the pain and the condition of the baby. Labour pain ranges from discomfort similar to menstrual cramps to intense pressure or pain. Many women experience something in between. Factors that can increase pain and discomfort during the first stage of labour include:

- Irregular breathing

- Tensing up because of fear

- Not knowing what to expect

- Feeling alone and unsupported

You can help the expectant mother cope with the discomfort and pain of labour. Begin by reassuring

her that you are there to help. Explain what to expect as labour progresses. Suggest specific physical activities that she can do to relax, such as regulating her breathing. Ask her to breathe in slowly and deeply through the nose and out through the mouth. Ask her to try to focus on one object in the room while regulating her breathing. By staying calm, firm, confident and offering encouragement, you can help reduce fear and apprehension. This will aid in reducing pain and discomfort.

The use of slow, deep breathing through the mouth during labour can help in several ways:

- Aids muscle relaxation

- Offers a distraction from the pain of strong contractions as labour progresses

- Ensures adequate oxygen to both the mother and the baby during labour

Taking childbirth classes, such as those offered at local hospitals, can help you become more competent in techniques used to help the expectant mother relax.

ASSISTING WITH DELIVERY

It is difficult to predict how much time you have before the baby is delivered. However, if the expectant mother says that she feels the need to push or feels as if she has to have a bowel movement, delivery is near.

You should time the expectant mother's contractions from the beginning of one contraction to the beginning of the next. If they are less than two minutes apart, prepare to assist with the delivery of the baby.

Assisting with the delivery of the baby is often a simple process. The expectant mother is doing all the work. Your job is to create a clean environment and to help guide the baby from the birth canal, minimizing the possibility of injury to the mother and baby. Begin by positioning the mother. She should be lying on her back, with her head and upper back raised, not lying flat. Her legs should be bent, with the knees drawn up and apart. Positioning the mother in this way will make her more comfortable.

Next, establish a clean environment for delivery. Use items such as clean sheets, blankets or towels. To make

Figure 20–3 Place clean sheets, blankets, towels, or even clothes under the mother.

the area around the mother as sanitary as possible, place these items over the mother's abdomen and under her buttocks and legs (Figure 20–3). Keep a clean, warm towel or blanket handy to wrap the newborn. Because you will be coming in contact with the mother's and baby's body fluids, be sure to wear appropriate PPE.

Other items that can be helpful include a bulb syringe to suction secretions from the baby's mouth and nose, gauze or sanitary pads to help absorb secretions and vaginal bleeding, a large plastic bag or towel to hold the placenta after delivery, and oxygen if available.

As crowning occurs, place a hand on the top of the baby's head and apply light pressure (Figure 20–4). In this way, you allow the head to emerge slowly, not forcefully. This will help prevent tearing of the vagina and injury to the baby. At this point, the expectant mother should stop pushing. Instruct the mother to concentrate on her breathing techniques. Have her "pant like a dog." This technique will help her stop pushing and help prevent a forceful birth.

As the head emerges, the baby will turn to one side (Figure 20–5). This will enable the shoulders and the rest of the body to pass through the birth canal. Support the baby's head and check to see if the umbilical cord is looped around the baby's neck. If it is, gently slip it over the baby's head. If this cannot be done, slip it over the baby's shoulders as they emerge. The baby can slide through the loop.

Guide one shoulder out at a time. Do not pull the baby. As the baby emerges, she will be wet and slippery. Use a clean towel to catch the baby. Place the baby on its side, between the mother and you. In this way, you can provide initial care without fear of dropping the newborn. If possible, note the time the baby was born.

Leave the cord in place and do not pull on it. Clamp or tie the cord while waiting for the placenta to be delivered. Use strips of sterile cloth tied tightly at two different locations 10 and 15 cm (4 and 6 in.) away from the baby. Do not cut the cord.

Figure 20–4 Place your hand on top of the baby's head and apply light pressure.

Figure 20–5 As the baby emerges, support the head.

COMPLICATIONS REQUIRING ADVANCED MEDICAL CARE

Complications During Pregnancy

Complications during pregnancy are rare. Since the nature and extent of most complications can only be determined by medical professionals during or after examination, you should not be concerned with trying to "diagnose" a particular problem. Instead, concern yourself with recognizing signs and symptoms that suggest a serious complication during pregnancy. You should be concerned with two important signs and symptoms: vaginal bleeding and abdominal pain.

Any persistent or profuse vaginal bleeding, or bleeding in which tissue passes through the vagina during pregnancy, is abnormal, as is any abdominal pain. For an expectant mother exhibiting these signs and symptoms, obtain advanced medical care quickly. While waiting or en route, take steps to minimize shock. These include:

- Helping the woman into the most comfortable position
- Controlling bleeding
- Maintaining normal body temperature
- Administering oxygen, if available

Miscarriage

Miscarriage is the spontaneous termination of pregnancy from any cause before 20 weeks of gestation. This is a common cause of vaginal bleeding in the first trimester of pregnancy. This condition occurs in about 1 in 10 pregnancies. Signs and symptoms of miscarriage to check for include the following:

- Often the woman is anxious and apprehensive
- Vaginal bleeding, which may be minor or profuse
- "Cramp-like" pain that is similar to the pain of labour or menstruation

When assessing the woman, you should be sensitive and obtain a detailed history, which should include:

- Time of onset of pain and bleeding
- Amount of blood loss
- Whether the woman passed any tissue during the bleeding episodes

Often the woman will tell you that she feels an urge to go to the bathroom. If this happens, make sure you check the contents for tissue or clot-like matter. You should collect and transport any tissue found to the hospital for analysis.

Pre-hospital management of all first-trimester emergencies includes close observation of vital signs for signs of shock from blood loss. If the woman is not in shock, have her rest in a comfortable position.

Administer supplemental oxygen as necessary.

Premature Labour

Labour that begins between the 20th and 37th week of gestation is called premature or preterm labour and frequently requires medical intervention. It can be due to problems with the mother, baby, or placenta.

Many factors increase the chance of having a preterm birth, including a history of preterm births or miscarriages, carrying multiple babies, and poor nutrition, as well as certain diseases and abnormalities.

Common signs and symptoms are:

- Contractions every 10 minutes (or less)
- Dull backache
- Feeling as if the baby is pushing down or has "dropped"
- "Cramp-like" pain that is similar to the pain of menstruation or abdominal pain
- Possible diarrhea
- Cramps in the bowel
- Vaginal bleeding or discharge (out of the normal)

Treat as a regular childbirth.

For the premature baby, provide the following care:

- Keep the baby warm with a blanket or swaddle.
- Keep the baby's mouth and nose clear of fluids by gently suctioning with a bulb syringe.
- Prevent bleeding from the umbilical cord.

- Administer passive oxygen, if local protocols permit, by blowing the oxygen gently across the baby's face.
- Do not let anyone breathe into the baby's face (to prevent infection).
- Obtain more advanced medical care.

Ectopic Pregnancy

An ectopic pregnancy is the leading cause of maternal death in the first trimester, which usually results from hemorrhage. It occurs when a fertilized ovum implants anywhere other than in the uterus. This occurs in about one in every 200 pregnancies. There are numerous causes of ectopic pregnancy; however, most involve factors that delay or prevent passage of the fertilized ovum to its normal place of implantation in the uterus. Predisposing factors include previous surgery, previous ectopic pregnancy, or blocked tubes as a sterilization method. When conducting a secondary survey, it is important to get a thorough history from the woman. Most ruptures occur by 2 to 12 weeks of gestation.

The signs and symptoms of ectopic pregnancy include:

- Abdominal pain
- Referred pain to the shoulder
- Vaginal bleeding (spotty, minimal, or severe)
- Nausea
- Vomiting
- Fainting spells
- Signs of shock

A ruptured ectopic pregnancy is a true emergency. When administering care for a woman with a ruptured ectopic pregnancy, maintain the ABCs (which may deteriorate rapidly), administer supplemental oxygen, and help ensure prompt transport to the medical facility. Remind the woman to take nothing by mouth in case she requires surgery. Provide ongoing survey and care.

Third Trimester Bleeding

Third trimester bleeding occurs in a very small percentage of pregnancies and is never normal. The causes of third trimester bleeding are usually abruptio placentae, placenta previa, or uterine rupture. Abruptio placentae

is a partial or complete detachment of a normally implanted placenta at more than 20 weeks' gestation. Placenta previa is a condition in which the placenta is attached in the lower uterus, encroaching on the opening to the cervix. Uterine rupture is a spontaneous or traumatic rupture of the uterine wall. This condition may be a result of a previous scar from a Caesarean birth, prolonged or obstructed labour, or direct trauma.

The signs and symptoms of third trimester bleeding may include:

- Vaginal bleeding (may be sudden and/or painless)
- Uterine cramping
- Back pain

Treat the woman for shock, administer supplemental oxygen, and maintain the ABCs. Place the woman in the recovery position and help ensure prompt transport to the medical facility. Remind the woman to take nothing by mouth as she may require surgery. Provide ongoing survey and care.

Complications During Childbirth

The vast majority of births occur without complication. However, this fact is reassuring only if the one you are assisting with is not complicated. For the few that do have complications, delivery can be stressful and even life-threatening for the expectant mother and the baby. In all of these cases, obtain advanced medical care.

The most common complication of childbirth is persistent vaginal bleeding. Besides obtaining more advanced medical care, you should take steps to minimize shock. Other childbirth complications include prolapsed cord, premature birth, breech birth, shoulder dystocia, and multiple births.

Prolapsed Cord

A prolapsed cord occurs when a loop of the umbilical cord protrudes from the vagina while the baby is still in the birth canal (Figure 20–6). If this occurs, it can threaten the baby's life. As the baby moves through the birth canal, the cord will be compressed against the unborn baby, and the birth canal and blood flow to the baby will stop. Without this blood flow, the baby will die

Figure 20-6 A prolapsed cord.

Figure 20-7 The knee-chest position will take pressure off the cord.

within a few minutes from lack of oxygen. If you notice a prolapsed cord, have the expectant mother assume a knee-chest position (Figure 20–7). This will help take the pressure off the cord. Administer oxygen to the mother if it is available. Obtain more advanced medical care if you have not done so already.

Breech Birth

Most babies are born headfirst. However, on rare occasions, the baby is delivered feet- or buttocks-first. This condition is commonly called breech birth. If you encounter a breech delivery, support the baby's body as she exits the birth canal while you are waiting for the head to deliver. Do not pull on the baby's body. This will not help to deliver the head.

If, after about three minutes, the head has not delivered, you will need to help create an airway so the baby can breathe. Because the weight of the baby's head lodged in the birth canal will reduce or stop blood flow by compressing the cord, the baby will be unable to get any oxygen. Should the baby try to take a spontaneous breath, she will also be unable to breathe because her face will be pressed against the wall of the birth canal.

To help with a breech delivery, place the index and middle fingers of your gloved hand into the vagina next to the baby's mouth and nose. Spread your fingers to form a "V" (Figure 20–8). Although this will not lessen the compression on the umbilical cord, it may allow air to enter the baby's mouth and nose. You must

maintain this position until the baby's head is delivered. Administer oxygen to the mother if it is available. Obtain more advanced medical care.

Multiple Births

Although most births involve only a single baby, a few will involve delivery of more than one. If the mother has had proper prenatal care, she will probably be aware that she is going to have more than one baby. Multiple births should be handled in the same manner as single

Figure 20-8 During a breech birth, position your index and middle fingers to allow air to enter the baby's mouth and nose.

births. The mother will have a separate set of contractions for each child being born. There may also be a separate placenta for each child, although this is not always the case.

Limb Presentation

In most births, the baby's head presents first and the rest of the body follows. Less frequently, the baby's arms or legs may present first, preventing the possibility of a normal delivery (Figure 20–9). This kind of delivery can be fatal. Never pull on the baby's arms or legs. This type of birth is an emergency, and you must transport the mother to the hospital without delay.

Postpartum Bleeding

Postpartum bleeding is excessive bleeding after the birth. It may be caused by the uterine muscles not contracting fully after birth, pieces of placenta or membranes left in the uterus, or vaginal or cervical tears during delivery.

The signs and symptoms of postpartum bleeding include excessive bleeding (more than 500 mL or 17 oz.) after giving birth. It frequently occurs within the first few hours after delivery but can be delayed for up to 24 hours after delivery.

If a woman experiences postpartum bleeding, care for any external bleeding from perineal tears. Do not attempt vaginal packing to control internal bleeding. Position the woman for shock and maintain her ABCs. Remind the woman to take nothing by mouth. Help ensure prompt transport to the medical facility. Provide ongoing survey and care.

CARING FOR THE NEWBORN AND MOTHER

Caring for the Newborn

The first few minutes of the baby's life are a difficult transition from life inside the mother's uterus to life outside. You have two priorities at this point. Your first is to see that the baby's airway is open and clear. Since a newborn baby breathes primarily through the nose, it is important to immediately clear the mouth and nasal passages. You can do this by using your finger, a gauze pad, or a bulb syringe (Figure 20–10).

Most babies begin crying and breathing spontaneously. If the baby has not made any sounds, stimulate her to elicit the crying response by flicking your fingers on the soles of the baby's feet. Crying helps clear the baby's airway of fluids and promotes breathing. If the baby

Figure 20–9 Limb presentation prevents the possibility of a normal birth and could be fatal. This type of birth is an emergency and the mother requires immediate transport.

Figure 20–10 A bulb syringe can be used to clear the baby's mouth and nose of any secretions.

TABLE 20–1: THE APGAR SCORE

Element	0	1	2	Score
Activity (muscle tone)	Limp	Some flexion of extremities	Active movement, flexed arms and legs	
Pulse	Absent	Below 100 bpm	100 bpm or above	
Grimace (irritability)	No response	Grimace	Cough, sneeze, cry	
Appearance (skin colour)	Body and extremities blue; pale	Body pink, extremities blue	Completely pink	
Respiration	Absent	Slow and irregular	Strong, crying	
			Total Score =	

Assessing the Newborn

If the newborn's respiratory rate does not increase to a normal range with tactile stimulation, assess the heart rate. Do so using a stethoscope, feeling a pulse at the base of the umbilical cord, or palpating the brachial or femoral artery. Optimally, the heart rate should be between 140 and 160 bpm (normal is 100 to 180 bpm). If the pulse is in the normal range, continue to assess. If it is less than the normal range, or there is cyanosis around the chest and abdomen (after 100% oxygen has been administered), artificial ventilation is called for.

Newborns should be assisted to achieve between 40 and 60 breaths per minute. It may be necessary to place a cloth or small towel under the newborn's shoulders to maintain proper positioning. Use an appropriate BVM for ventilations; never use mechanical ventilation.

If the newborn's pulse rate is less than 60 bpm and she is not responding to ventilations, begin CPR. Continue to reassess frequently.

does not begin breathing on her own within the first minute after birth, begin rescue breathing. If the baby's pulse rate is less than 60 bpm and she is not responding to ventilations, begin CPR. Continue to reassess frequently. You can review these techniques in Chapters 6 and 8.

If the baby is having difficulty breathing, additional oxygen would be beneficial. If you have oxygen available, you can attach a section of tubing to the flowmeter and deliver oxygen at 4 litres per minute to the newborn. Do this by holding the other end of the tubing near the baby's face.

Your second responsibility is to maintain normal body temperature. Newborns lose heat quickly; therefore, it is important to keep her warm. Dry the newborn and wrap her in a clean, warm towel or blanket. If possible, record an initial set of vital signs. Most important are breathing, heart rate, and skin colour. You can review vital signs in Chapter 5.

The APGAR score is a numerical system of rating the condition of the newborn (Table 20–1). It evaluates the newborn's heart rate, respiratory rate, muscle tone, reflex irritability, and colour. It is done at one minute after birth and five minutes after birth. A normal score is 7 to 10, 4 to 6 is fairly low, and 0 to 3 is critically low.

Caring for the Mother

You can continue to meet the needs of the newborn while caring for the mother. Allow the mother to begin nursing the newborn. This will stimulate the uterus to contract and help slow bleeding. The placenta will still be in the uterus, attached to the baby by the umbilical cord. Contractions of the uterus will usually expel the placenta within 20 minutes of delivery. Catch the placenta in a clean towel or container. Do not separate the placenta from the newborn or cut the clamped/tied umbilical cord. Leave the placenta attached to the newborn and place it in a plastic bag or wrap it in a towel for transport to the hospital.

Expect some additional vaginal bleeding when the placenta is delivered. Using gauze pads or clean towels, gently clean the mother. Place a sanitary pad or towel over the vagina. Do not insert anything inside the vagina. Have the mother place her legs together. Feel for a grapefruit-sized mass in the lower abdomen. This is the uterus. Gently massage the lower portion of the abdomen. Massage will help eliminate any large blood clots within the uterus, cause the uterus to contract, and slow bleeding.

Many new mothers experience shock-like signs or symptoms, such as cool, pale, moist skin; shivering; and slight dizziness, after childbirth. Keep the mother positioned on her back. Administer oxygen if available. Maintain normal body temperature and monitor vital signs.

SUMMARY

Ideally, childbirth should occur in a controlled environment under the guidance of healthcare professionals trained in delivery. In this way, the necessary medical care is immediately available for mother and baby should any problem arise. However, there will always be unexpected deliveries occurring outside the controlled environment that may require your assistance. By knowing how to prepare the expectant mother for delivery, assist in the delivery, and provide proper care for the mother and baby, you will be able to successfully assist in bringing a new child into the world.

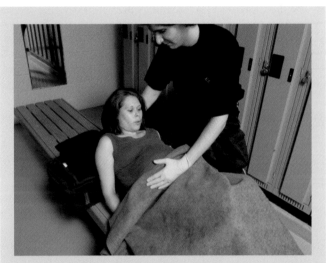

The woman's contractions are about two minutes apart. Now she tells you she feels a powerful urge to push. What do you do?

Chapter 21

Reaching and Moving Patients

You arrive on the scene of a two-vehicle collision. Both people inside the smaller car appear to be unconscious and are bleeding. What do you do?

INTRODUCTION

You have learned how to care for patients when it is safe to do so; sometimes, however, you will not have easy access to the patient. At other times, the patient may be in a dangerous situation and must be moved before you provide care. In this chapter, you will learn how to quickly and safely reach and move patients.

GAINING ACCESS

One of your primary responsibilities as a responder is to provide care for a patient. Sometimes, however, providing care is not possible because the patient is inaccessible. One example is a situation in which someone is able to call EMS/9-1-1 or another local emergency number for help but is unable to unlock the door of the home or office to let in the responders. This is also true in a large number of motor vehicle collisions. Vehicle doors are sometimes locked or crushed, windows may be tightly rolled up, or the vehicle may be unstable. In other instances, fire, water, or other elements may prevent you from reaching the patient.

In these cases, you must immediately begin to think of how to safely gain access to the patient before you can begin to provide care. If you cannot reach the patient,

you cannot help her. But remember, when attempting to reach a patient, your safety is the most important consideration. Protect yourself and the patient by doing only what you are trained to do and by using equipment and clothing appropriate for the situation (Table 21–1). Items such as helmets, face shields, safety goggles, gloves, blankets, and heavy clothing will help keep you safe. Items such as reflective markers or flares, and flashlights will help keep the scene, as well as the patient, safe as you attempt to gain access to someone who is trapped. Simple tools such as a screwdriver, hammer, pocket knife, vehicle jack, rope, hatchet, pry bar, and chains can also be helpful. It is also important to take precautions to not cause the patient further injury. Stay with the patient and try to keep her calm—explain what is going on and monitor the patient closely. It is also important to keep the spine immobilized during the extrication. If glass needs to be broken, ensure your safety and the safety of the patient by using a thick blanket, tarp, or other object to prevent glass from being thrown at you or the patient.

During any extrication, or when attempting to gain access to a patient, ensure that all team members communicate clearly and develop a plan so that each team member knows the role she will play.

TABLE 21–1: RECOMMENDED EQUIPMENT AND CLOTHING FOR RESPONDERS

Warning Devices	Protective Items	Breaking Windows
• Flares	• Helmet	• Pry bar
• Reflective markers	• Safety goggle	• Hammer or hatchet
• Flashlights	• Face shield	• Window punch
	• Gloves	
	• Heavy clothing	
	• Blanket	

Motor Vehicles

As with any emergency situation, begin by surveying the scene to see if it is safe. If it is not safe, determine whether you can make it safe so that you can attempt to gain access to the injured person. Well-intentioned responders and others are injured or killed every year while attempting to help injured people out of motor vehicle collisions. Often these responders are struck by oncoming vehicles. Such unfortunate instances can be prevented if you take adequate measures to make the scene safe before trying to gain access and provide care.

Upright Vehicles

Fortunately, most motor vehicle collisions you encounter will involve upright, stable vehicles. These vehicles are unlikely to move while you attempt to help their occupants. However, there are times when the vehicle will not be stable. Environmental factors can influence the stability of the vehicle. Vehicles on slippery surfaces, such as ice, water, or snow, or on inclined surfaces need to be stabilized. In addition, vehicles positioned where oil has been spilled should also be stabilized.

Stabilizing an upright vehicle is a simple task. Placing blocks or wedges against the wheels of the vehicle will greatly reduce the chance of the vehicle moving. This process is called chocking (Figure 21–1). You can use items such as rocks, logs, wooden blocks, and spare tires. If a strong rope or chain is available, these can be attached to the frame of the car and then secured to strong anchor points such as large trees, guard rails, or another vehicle. Letting the air out of the car's tires also reduces the possibility of movement.

Once you are certain the vehicle is stable, you should attempt to enter it. Begin by checking all the doors to see if they are unlocked. Although it may seem obvious to check the doors, sometimes in the excitement it is easy to forget this simple, time-saving step. If the doors are locked, the people inside may be able to unlock at least one door for you. If the windows are open, you may be able to unlock the door yourself.

Sometimes locked or jammed doors require you to enter the vehicle through a window. If the window is open or can be rolled down by someone inside the car, this is not a problem. If the window is rolled up, you can use specific equipment and techniques to get into the car (Figure 21–2). Once inside the vehicle, you can further stabilize it by placing the vehicle in "park," turning the key to the off position, and setting the parking brake.

Figure 21–1 Chocking is used to stabilize a vehicle.

Figure 21–2 There is specific equipment that can be used to get into a car.

Overturned Vehicles

It is unusual to find a vehicle overturned or on its side. Consider any vehicle found in either position to be unstable. Although a vehicle on its side or overturned can be stabilized by using spare tires, jacks, wooden blocks, or other items, it is unlikely that you can adequately stabilize the vehicle.

NOTE:

It is important to beware of airbags.
If they haven't gone off already, they may still be charged and ready to inflate. Ensure your own safety.

Vehicles and Electrical Hazards

When a vehicle is in contact with an electrical wire, you must consider the wire to be energized until you know otherwise. When you arrive on the scene, your first priority is to ensure your safety and that of others in the immediate area. A safety area should be established at a point twice the length of the span of the wire. Attempt to reach and move people only after the power company has been notified and has removed any electrical current from the downed wire. Do not touch any metal fence, metal structure, or body of water in contact with the downed wire. People inside the vehicle should be told to remain in the vehicle. You can tell them how to provide care for any injured people in the vehicle. Do not attempt to deal with electrical hazards unless you are specifically trained to do so.

Once the current has been removed from the wire, you can safely approach the vehicle. Since the vehicle and possibly the injured person/people were in contact with the current, electrical injury is possible.

NOTE:

When approaching any scene, you should be aware of dangers involving chemicals. Whether a motor vehicle collision or an industrial emergency is involved, you should be able to recognize clues that indicate the presence of hazardous materials. For more information on hazardous materials, see Chapter 25.

WATER EMERGENCIES

Drowning

Drowning is a form of suffocation caused by being immersed in water or other liquid. The process of drowning begins whenever small amounts of water are inhaled into the lungs. This happens when a person is gasping for air while struggling to stay afloat. Stimulation by the water causes spasms of the muscles of the larynx, which closes the airway (laryngospasm). This is a natural body response to prevent more water from entering the lungs. As a result, the lungs of most people who drown or survive a drowning incident are relatively dry unless the people are submerged for a long time. However, the spasms that block the airway to prevent water from entering also prevent air from entering. Without air, the person suffocates and soon becomes unconscious. At some point after unconsciousness, the muscles relax, and the person spontaneously breathes. If the person is submerged, more water can enter the lungs.

Assisting a Conscious, Drowning Patient

The responder should get to the person as soon as possible without risking personal safety. The safest methods are throwing, reaching, and wading assists. In most cases, at least one of these methods will succeed.

You must always remember not to endanger yourself. Rescues that involve swimming to a person require special training, such as Red Cross Lifeguard training. If you swim to a person without this training, you are not likely to save the person. In fact, you only put yourself in danger and thus risk two lives. Likewise, leaping into water, even shallow water, to help someone may seem courageous, but choosing a less dramatic method is safer and usually more effective. You can help a person only if you remain safe yourself and in control of the situation. The throwing, reaching, and wading methods presented here help you do both.

Throwing Assists

With a throwing assist, you throw a heaving line, ring buoy, throw bag, rescue tube, or any other device that the patient can grab to help stay afloat. If a line is attached, you can pull the patient to safety. When throwing a device, follow these general principles:

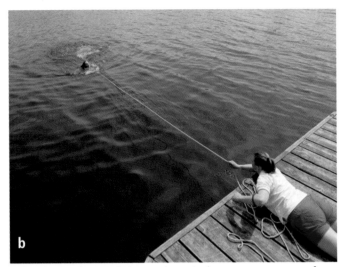

Figure 21–3, a-b When using a throwing assist: **a**, try to throw the device beyond the patient; **b**, keep your centre of gravity low when pulling the patient back in.

- Get into a safe position where you can keep your balance—keep low to the ground.
- Secure the non-throwing end of the line.
- Try to throw the device beyond the patient (Figure 21–3, a).
- Throw the device so that the wind or current will bring it back within the patient's reach.
- Once the patient has grasped the device, slowly pull her to safety. Lie down or lean your body away from the patient as you pull so that you are less likely to get pulled into the water (Figure 21–3, b).
- If there is no line on the device, tell the patient to hold on and kick to safety.

Reaching Assists

With a reaching assist, you reach out to the patient in the water while remaining in a safe position. First, firmly brace yourself. Extend your reach with any object that will reach the patient, such as a pole, oar or paddle, tree branch, shirt, belt, or towel (Figure 21–4).

If you have no objects to extend your reach, try to extend your arm and grasp the patient or to extend your foot to the patient. To avoid going into the water, lie flat on a pool deck or pier and reach with your arm or leg.

Wading Assists

If you can enter the water without danger from currents, objects on the bottom, or an unexpected drop-off, wade in and reach to the patient. If possible, extend your reach using a floatable item, such as a rescue tube, a ring buoy, a buoyant cushion, a raft, a kickboard, a personal flotation device (PFD), or a lifejacket. If you do not have a buoyant object, reach out with a tree branch, a pole, or another object.

Whatever object you have, use it for support in the water. Let the patient grasp the other side of it. You can then pull the patient to safety, or you can let go of an object that floats and tell the patient to kick with it toward safety. Keep the safety device between you and the patient so that a panicked patient cannot grab you and pull you under.

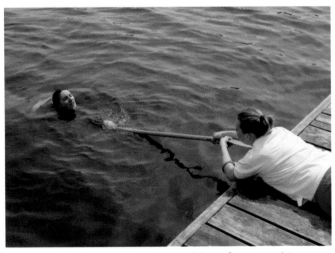

Figure 21–4 You can use many things for a reaching assist such as a paddle, tree branch, belt, or towel.

After Reaching the Patient

After reaching the patient, remove her from the water as quickly as possible. If you suspect that the patient may have a head and/or spine injury, you must support her head and neck and keep it aligned with the body. If it is necessary to turn the patient on her back, the head, neck, chest, and the rest of the body must be aligned, supported, and turned as a unit. The patient should be floated, on her back, onto a firm support, such as a backboard, before being moved from the water.

Once the patient is out of the water, open the airway and check for breathing. Begin ventilations if the patient is not breathing. If you are unable to get air into the patient, the airway is probably obstructed. In this case, follow the procedure for an obstructed airway. Once you are able to get your air in, check for signs of circulation. If you cannot detect a pulse, start CPR.

Basic life support should be continued until more advanced medical care is available. Every patient who survives a drowning incident, regardless of how rapid the recovery, should be transported to a medical facility immediately for follow-up care.

You should attempt to resuscitate the patient even if she has been submerged for a prolonged period. Patients have been successfully resuscitated even after being submerged in cold water for longer than 30 minutes. Continue CPR until advanced care can be started.

NOTE:

For more information and training on in-water rescues for suspected head and/or spine injuries, take a Red Cross Lifeguard Course.

Self-Rescue

Besides knowing the skills needed to rescue someone in trouble in the water, you should know what to do to help yourself if you suddenly get into trouble in the water. Whenever you attempt a water rescue in a dangerous water environment, you should wear a PFD/lifejacket.

However, if you unexpectedly fall into the water without a PFD/lifejacket, you may need to remove clothing to swim or float. But some clothing, such as a long-sleeved shirt that buttons, will actually help you float and protect you from cold. If your shoes are light enough for you to swim comfortably, leave them on. If they are too heavy, remove them.

Tread water to stay in an upright position while you signal for help or wait for rescue. You may need to tread water while you arrange your clothing to help you float. To tread water, stay vertical and submerge to your chin. Move your hands back and forth and use a kick that you can do effectively and comfortably, using the least amount of energy.

If you are wearing a PFD/lifejacket and help is nearby, you can wait for help using the Heat Escape Lessening Position (HELP). Hold the insides of your arms against your sides and place your forearms against your chest. Hold your thighs together and raise your knees toward your chest (Figure 21–5).

Ice Rescue

People needlessly die each year as a result of falling through ice. Unfortunately, some of these incidents also involve well-intentioned responders rushing to someone's aid. Ice rescues are dangerous because if someone has fallen in, this means the ice is unstable in that area. Ice rescues require special training and equipment.

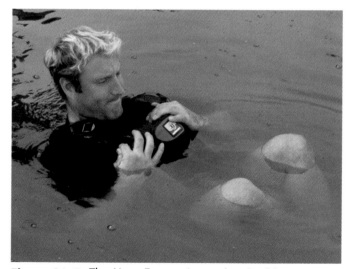

Figure 21–5 The Heat Escape Lessening Position.

Ice is not uniformly thick. Just because ice is safe enough to walk on in one area does not mean it is safe in other areas. While trying to reach the person, you could walk on an undetected thin spot and suddenly fall through the ice.

The safest methods of ice rescue are those that do not require you to make contact with the person. Using a reaching device, such as a stick or pole, is your best initial action to reach someone who is nearby. If the person is farther out on the ice, you should try to throw a line or floatable object to her. If the person is beyond your throwing distance or reach, do not venture onto the ice yourself. Summon necessary personnel, such as fire and rescue personnel, for assistance.

When attempting any ice rescue, you should always have the following:

- *Adequate personnel.* Never attempt a rescue by yourself. You will often need the assistance of several others to pull the patient to safety.

- *Proper clothing.* Items such as wet suits or dry suits are required clothing if you are likely to enter the water.

- *Proper equipment.* PFDs/lifejackets for you and the patient, rope, boat, paddle, and ice pick (screwdriver could substitute) are all necessary items.

- *Appropriate training.* Beyond the basic water rescue skills of throwing and reaching, responders should have the skills needed to operate a rescue boat or ice sled or to move properly over ice toward a patient. These skills can be obtained through specialized ice rescue courses.

MOVING PATIENTS

Three general situations require you to perform an emergency move:

1. *Immediate danger.* This includes danger to you or the patient being rescued from fire, a lack of oxygen, risk of drowning, possible explosion, a collapsing structure, or uncontrolled traffic hazards.

2. *Gaining access to other patients.* A patient with minor injuries may need to be moved quickly to reach other patients who may have life-threatening conditions.

3. *Providing proper care.* Someone with a medical emergency, such as a cardiac arrest or heat stroke, may need to be moved to provide proper care. For example, someone in cardiac arrest needs CPR. It should be performed on a firm, flat surface. If the patient collapses on a bed or in a small bathroom, the surface or space may not be adequate to provide appropriate care. You may have to move the patient to give the proper care.

Usually, when you provide care, you will not face hazards that require moving the patient immediately. In most cases, you can give care where you find the patient. Moving someone needlessly can lead to further injury. For example, moving someone with a closed fracture of the leg without taking the time to splint it could result in an open fracture if the end of the bone tears the skin. Soft tissue damage, damage to nerves, blood loss, and infection could all result unnecessarily. Needless movement of someone with a head or spine injury could cause paralysis or even death.

Some rescue situations bring specialized challenges for gaining access to patients, and these require responders with specialized training and equipment. One such situation is when the patient needing rescue is in a confined space. Confined spaces are particularly challenging because they:

- Are not designed or intended to have people in them

- Have a restricted entrance or exit due to their location, size, or means

- Can present a risk to the health and safety of anyone who enters, including responders, due to one or more of the following factors:

  ■ Their design, construction, location, or atmosphere

  ■ The materials or substances in them

  ■ Work activities being carried out in them

  ■ They present mechanical, process, and/or safety hazards

Before you act, you must consider the limitations of the situation. Consider the following limitations to ensure that you move one or more patients quickly and safely:

- Dangerous conditions at the scene
- The size of the patient
- Your own physical ability
- Whether others can help you
- The patient's condition

Failing to consider these limitations could result in injury. If you become injured, you may be unable to move the patient and may risk making the situation worse. Due to the need to lift and carry a great deal of equipment, back injuries, as well as other musculoskeletal injuries, have a high potential of occurring in an EMS setting. If this occurs at a scene, you will have become part of the problem that arriving personnel with more advanced training will have to deal with. The situation will have become more complicated because now there is one more patient to rescue.

To protect yourself and the patient, follow these guidelines when moving someone:

- Only attempt to move someone you are sure you can comfortably handle.
- Walk carefully, using short steps.
- When possible, move forward rather than backward.
- Look where you are going.
- Support the patient's head and spine.
- Avoid bending or twisting someone with a possible head and/or spine injury.

NOTE:

There are specific ways to deal with confined spaces (e.g., a grain silo, vat, or pipe), and without appropriate training, you are putting yourself at risk. Ensure that the appropriate responders are on the way and manage the scene until they arrive. Only people with specialized training and equipment should enter confined spaces.

Body Mechanics

Some basic principles of body mechanics to be used for all lifts and moves are:

- Use your legs, not your back, to lift—use the muscles of your legs, hips, and buttocks, as well as

your abdomen. Never use the muscles of your back to move or lift a heavy object.

- Keep the weight of the object as close to you as possible—reduce the distance you have to reach.
- Keep your body aligned—imagine a straight line from your shoulders, through your hips down to your feet. These should be stacked on top of each other, and always move them as a unit. This will reduce twisting forces.
- Reduce the height or distance you need to move an object—lift in stages if you need to.
- Keep a normal inward curve in your back and your wrists and knees in normal alignment.

Everyone on the team should use proper body mechanics, which will reduce the risk of injuring everyone else on the team, as well as themselves.

Reaching can also lead to injury of the back ligaments, if done incorrectly. When reaching, keep your back locked (avoid hyperextending it) and never twist your back. You should avoid reaching more than 15 to 20 cm (6 to 8 in.) in front of the body as your muscles in the upper back and shoulders can stay stretched in that position only for just seconds before they become fatigued and the risk of injury increases.

There are many different ways to move someone to safety, but no one way is best. As long as you can move the patient to safety without injuring yourself or causing further injury to the patient, the move is successful.

Moves used by responders include assists, carries, and drags. The most common of these are the:

- Walking assist
- Pack-strap carry
- Two-person seat carry
- Clothes drag
- Blanket drag
- Foot drag
- Extremity lift

All of these moves can be done by one or two people and without equipment. This is important because,

Figure 21–6 A walking assist with one responder.

Figure 21–7 A walking assist with two responders.

with most moves, equipment is not often immediately available and time is critical.

Walking Assist

The most basic move is the walking assist. It is frequently used to help patients who simply need assistance to walk to safety. Either one or two responders can use this method with a conscious patient. To do a walking assist, place the patient's arm across your shoulders and hold it in place with one hand. Support the patient with your other hand around the patient's waist (Figure 21–6). In this way, your body acts as a "crutch," supporting the patient's weight while you both walk. A second responder, if present, can support the patient in the same way from the other side (Figure 21–7).

Pack-Strap Carry

The pack-strap carry can be used on both conscious and unconscious patients. To use it on an unconscious patient requires a second responder to help position the patient on your back. To perform the pack-strap carry, have the patient stand or have a second responder help support the patient. Position yourself with your back to the patient, knees bent, so that your shoulders fit into the patient's armpits. Cross the patient's arms in front of you and grasp the patient's wrists. Lean forward slightly and pull the patient up onto your back. Stand up and walk to safety (Figure 21–8). Depending on the size of the patient, you may be able to hold both of the

patient's wrists with one hand. This leaves your other hand free to help maintain balance, open doors, and remove obstructions.

Two-Person Seat Carry

The two-person seat carry is a method for moving a patient who requires a second responder. To perform the two-person seat carry, put one arm under the patient's thighs and the other across the patient's back. Interlock your arms with those of a second responder under the patient's legs and across the patient's back. The patient is then lifted in the "seat" formed by the responders' arms (Figure 21–9). The move should not be used for someone suspected of having a head and/or spine injury.

Figure 21–8 A pack-strap carry.

Figure 21–9 A two-person seat carry.

Clothes Drag

The clothes drag is an appropriate emergency move for someone suspected of having a head and/or spine injury. This move helps keep the head and neck stabilized. To do a clothes drag, gather the patient's clothing, such as a jacket or shirt, behind the patient's neck. Using the clothing, pull the patient to safety. During the move, the patient's head is cradled by both the clothing and the responder's hands (Figure 21–10). This type of emergency move is exhausting and may result in back strain for the responder, even when done properly.

Blanket Drag

The blanket drag is an appropriate emergency move if you do not have a stretcher. To do a blanket drag, gather half a blanket and place the gathered side alongside the patient. Roll the patient toward you, tuck the blanket under the patient as far as you can, and then roll the patient back onto the blanket. Wrap the blanket around the patient and then drag the patient by pulling the part of the blanket at the patient's head (Figure 21–11).

Foot Drag

To move someone who cannot otherwise be carried or moved, grasp the patient's ankles and pull the patient in a straight line, being careful not to bump the patient's head (Figure 21–12).

Extremity Lift

The extremity lift, also called a fore-and-aft lift, is done with a partner when the patient has no suspected head and/or spine injury and no injuries to the arms or legs (Figure 21–13). This can be used to lift an unconscious patient from the floor to a chair.

1. Crouch at the patient's head. The other responder should kneel at the patient's side, by the knees.

2. Place one hand under each of the patient's shoulders, reaching through to grab the patient's wrists. Ensure that the patient's back is close to your chest.

3. The responder at the knees should slip his hands under the patient's knees.

Figure 21–10 A clothes drag.

Figure 21–11 A blanket drag.

Figure 21–12 A foot drag.

Figure 21–13 An extremity lift.

4. On signal, both responders can then lift and move the patient to the desired location.

Stretchers and Lifting Devices

There are many kinds of stretchers and lifting devices used in the field today. The more common types are:

- Scoop stretcher (clamshell)
- Backboard
- Basket stretcher
- Helicopter stretcher
- Army-type stretcher (furley stretcher)
- Multi-level stretcher (wheeled cot)
- SKED®
- Stair chair

All these devices will carry the patient's entire body.

> **NOTE:**
>
> *All stretchers should be carefully inspected for damage or instability. Rust, cracks, severe discoloration, and bent frames are all signs of damage. Plastic stretchers can be damaged by exposure to prolonged sunlight and to corrosive material.*

Scoop Stretcher

The scoop stretcher, also called a clamshell, is a lifting device suitable for lifting a patient from the ground to another kind of stretcher or a backboard. It is a lifting device only and is not for carrying patients long distances. It has the advantage of allowing patients experiencing trauma to be lifted without moving or rolling them. A disadvantage is that the patient's back cannot be examined unless the patient is rolled.

Backboard

The backboard, also referred to as the spine board or full board, is a lifting device only and is not used to carry patients over long distances. It is constructed of plywood or plastic. The board has holes cut along the sides through which straps may be placed to secure the patient's body to the board. Some boards have a hole at one end in the centre of the board. This is for storage of the board. If possible, avoid placing the patient's head at this end. Most boards are approximately 1.8 metres (6 feet) long. If backboards are used in conjunction with basket stretchers, the board must fit inside the stretcher.

Basket Stretcher

The basket stretcher, also called the Stokes basket, comes in various types and strengths. Traditional basket stretchers are constructed of metal support frames, usually combined with a wire mesh lining. Other basket stretchers have metal frames and high-impact plastic liners. Basket stretchers are commonly used for rescues and as a lifting device.

Follow these guidelines when using a basket stretcher:

- Place blankets under the patient for comfort.

- Place a backboard or litter board on the bottom to make loading and unloading easier.

- If using in combination with a scoop stretcher, the basket stretcher must be able to accommodate the scoop stretcher.

- Secure the patient if the stretcher is to be carried over a long distance or the patient is to be lowered or raised off the ground as in a low- or high-angle rescue.

Helicopter Stretcher

The helicopter stretcher is a flat backboard. Helicopters are equipped with one of these stretchers, and pilots usually know how to use them. The helicopter stretcher is hinged in the middle and folds in half for storage. The responder must ensure that the stretcher is opened and laid with the correct surface up so that it will not unintentionally fold in half during use. The backboard may be secured on top of the helicopter stretcher. Make sure you are aware of the air flight regulations for your area and that the backboard you are using will fit the helicopter stretcher.

Army-Type Stretcher

These stretchers consist of two wooden poles and a canvas or plastic stretcher. The canvas must be checked regularly for tears and rot. If soiled, it can be washed with soap and water. The stretcher is usually stored collapsed. To open, undo the straps and open the stretcher. Once open, the spreader bars should be locked into place. The centre part of the hinge can be further secured using a triangular bandage or tape. The stretcher should be tested prior to loading the patient onto it.

Multi-Level Stretcher

This device is equipped with wheels. It has an adjustable head section and leg section. The stretcher can be lowered or raised using the end or side release. Each side of the stretcher has a safety rail. The stretcher should not be lifted using these bars. This stretcher is commonly used in transportation vehicles such as ambulances.

SKED®

The SKED® is classified as a flexible litter. A flexible litter has no rigid structure of its own. These devices are made of synthetic materials that require some type of spinal immobilization device to provide rigidity. Because they are flexible, they work well when moving patients through narrow passageways. They wrap around the patient like a taco, so the litter is little more than the circumference of the patient's body. Flexible litters also have the distinct advantage of being useable with patients of a variety of sizes, including those for whom a basket stretcher may be restrictive.

Stair Chair

A stair chair is used for transporting a patient in a sitting position. It is used when a wheeled stretcher is deemed to be too long for the rescue or extrication. It is especially useful when there is a small elevator or staircase in which a long stretcher will not fit. The front wheels swivel to manoeuvre around tight corners and landings. It is recommended that three responders be present when using the stair chair to ensure patient safety, two to act as carriers and one to serve as a spotter and watch for potential difficulties. Another benefit of this equipment is that it reduces the risk of back injury to the responders.

Lifting and Moving a Stretcher

When a responder lifts a patient onto a stretcher, it is important to use proper body mechanics and to lift as safely and efficiently as possible. When a stretcher is carried to and loaded into a transport vehicle, the responder should use the following guidelines:

- Use enough helpers.

- Carry the patient feet first.

- Also carry the patient feet first down stairs and steep inclines, as this keeps the abdominal organs away from the diaphragm.

- The stretcher should be placed headfirst into the ambulance.

- Never run with a stretcher.

Positioning a Patient

There are many ways to position a patient on a stretcher. Always follow local protocol.

1

Supine

2

Prone

3

Fowler

4

Semi-Fowler

5

Lateral Recumbent

6

Trendelenburg

There are many different pieces of equipment on the market used to move patients. Use local protocol and manufacturers' directions when using this equipment.

Scoop Stretcher

Multi-level Stretcher

Stair Chair

- Ensure that the appropriate securing devices are in place.

- Use padding if the patient is going to be on the carrying device for a long period of time or the travelling surface is going to be rough.

- Secure the stretcher to the transport vehicle to ensure that it doesn't move during transport.

SUMMARY

Take the time to survey the scene before attempting to gain access to or move a patient. This is especially true in incidents involving hazardous materials. When gaining access, always try the simple approach first, such as checking all doors and windows for easy access into a building or vehicle. Check to see if anyone has keys. If you must forcibly gain access, several basic tools and techniques can be used.

A common mistake to avoid is forcibly gaining access or moving a patient unnecessarily. If you recognize a potentially life-threatening situation that requires a patient to be moved, use one of the techniques described in this chapter. Use the safest and easiest method to rapidly move the patient without causing injury to either yourself or the patient.

In water emergencies, use throwing, reaching, and wading assists to rescue someone without endangering yourself. Enter the water only if you have been trained to do so and have the proper equipment.

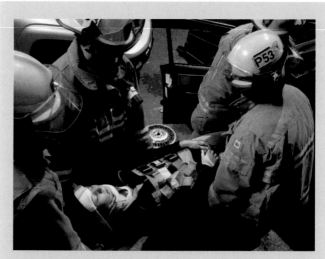

As you extricate the driver, she begins to have a seizure. What do you do?

Multiple Casualty Incidents

A bus is involved in a collision and is severely damaged near the front. The passengers are scared and some are injured. Most are able to exit the bus with little help, but others require assistance. People are starting to crowd around the area and the local fire department is already on the scene. What do you do?

INTRODUCTION

In rush-hour traffic, during a rain storm, the driver of a tractor trailer loses control of the vehicle on a four-lane highway. The rig crosses the centre line, "jackknifes," and slides into an embankment. Numerous cars and a loaded tour bus try frantically to avoid colliding with the tractor trailer. Two cars collide head-on. The bus plunges over an embankment, coming to rest 5 metres (16 feet) below in a ditch. Minor collisions occur farther back from the scene. Many people are injured; some are probably dead.

As a responder, you are likely to be among the first trained individuals nearby or summoned to assist with a serious incident such as this. The task of trying to create order out of chaos will initially fall on you. To respond most effectively to an emergency with multiple people, you need a plan of action. This plan must enable you to rapidly determine what additional resources are needed and how best to use them. During a serious incident, it is not uncommon for you to be on the scene for 15 minutes before any other trained personnel arrive. It could be up to an hour before adequate resources are available to care for the large number of injured people.

An appropriate initial response can eliminate potential problems for arriving personnel and possibly save the lives of several patients. To accomplish this, you must thoroughly understand your plan of action. Your plan must enable you to take charge. This includes making the scene safe for you and others to work, delegating responsibilities to others, managing available resources, identifying and caring for the people most in need of care, and relinquishing command as more highly trained personnel arrive.

MULTIPLE CASUALTY INCIDENTS

As the term implies, a multiple casualty incident (MCI) refers to a situation involving two or more patients. You are most likely to encounter small MCIs involving injury to only a few patients, such as a motor vehicle crash involving the driver and a passenger. But MCIs can also be large-scale events, such as those caused by natural disasters or those from materials/structures made by humans. Examples include:

- Flood
- Fire
- Explosion
- Structure collapse
- Train derailment
- Airliner crash
- Hazardous materials incident
- Earthquake
- Tornado
- Hurricane

Incidents of this magnitude can result in hundreds or even thousands of patients. Whether small or large scale, MCIs can strain the resources of a local community. Coping effectively with an MCI requires a plan that enables you to acquire and manage additional personnel, equipment and supplies.

Organizing Resources

The Incident Command System

Providing appropriate help to one or more patients in an emergency involves organization. Different types of incidents vary in complexity. MCIs can strain the resources of the responding personnel and require additional resources from other areas, some far away. To ensure that the various resources operate in an orderly, united fashion to accomplish a task, the incident command system (ICS) was developed.

The ICS is a management system designed to be used for a wide variety of emergencies. It is especially useful in emergencies involving multiple patients because of its ability to handle several emergency situations at the same time. It is a common system that can be easily understood by different agencies working together at the scene of an emergency.

Originally developed in California to manage the large numbers of firefighters necessary for major brush and forest fires, the ICS has subsequently been modified for use in a variety of MCIs. To understand the ICS, think of it as an organization. An organization is a group of people working together to achieve a common goal. To do this, the organization must clearly define who is in charge, the scope of authority and responsibility, the goal, and the objectives to accomplish the goal. This same approach applies to the ICS. The advantages of the ICS for use in numerous situations include:

• Terms commonly understood by those taking part

• An integrated communications system

• One "boss" with the absolute authority to do what is necessary to accomplish the goal

• One unified command structure with well-established divisions, all working to accomplish the same goal

• Easily managed units normally consisting of not more than four people

The sectors, as designated by command, may include the following (Figure 22–1):

• Triage officer—supervises assessment, tagging, and moving of patients to designated treatment areas

• Treatment officer—sets up a treatment area and supervises treatment, making sure the most seriously injured are transported first

• Transportation officer—arranges for ambulances while also tracking the priority, identity, and destination of all patients leaving the scene

• Staging officer—releases and distributes resources as needed and ensures that there is no transportation gridlock

• Safety officer—maintains scene safety by identifying potential dangers and taking action to prevent them from causing injury to all involved

Using the Incident Command System

A police officer is dispatched to a single motor vehicle collision. Since she is the first responder to arrive at the scene, she assumes the role of incident commander. She surveys the scene to determine the magnitude of the incident. She makes the scene safe for herself, bystanders, and any patients. Once the scene is safe, she approaches the vehicle. The driver has already left the vehicle and is seated on the curb next to the vehicle. The officer determines that the driver is the only injured person and approximates the type of injuries. The officer notifies the dispatcher of the situation, requesting only one ambulance as an additional resource. She gathers information from the patient while providing care until more advanced medical personnel arrive. Once the patient is turned over to the arriving paramedics, the officer reassesses scene safety, checks to make sure nothing else is needed, finishes gathering information, and completes any paperwork.

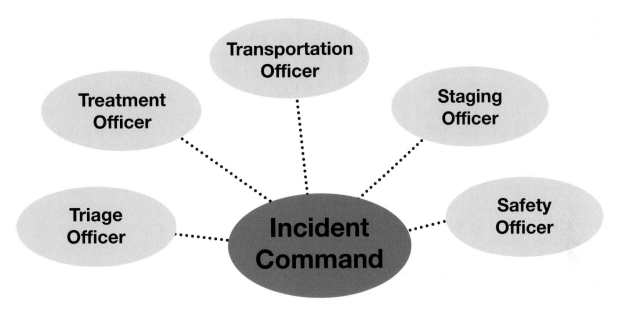

Figure 22–1 Basic structure of an incident command system.

In this situation, the resources needed were minimal. But what if the car had struck a utility pole and knocked down an electrical wire, the injured person had been trapped in a crushed vehicle, or multiple people had been injured? As the incident commander, the police officer would have notified the dispatcher of the situation and requested additional resources. She would have summoned the power company for the downed wire. If a person was trapped in the vehicle, resources such as the fire department or specialized rescue squad personnel would have been sent to the scene.

As these personnel arrive, the police officer could continue to act as the incident commander, or command could be turned over to other, more experienced personnel. These decisions are often based on the type of emergency and on local protocols. If the incident is beyond your scope, you should act as incident commander only until more experienced personnel arrives. At this point, he will assume command.

At other times, you may be responding to a large-scale MCI because it requires additional personnel. Where you are placed and how your services are used will be based on your expertise and the needs at the time. This could include assisting medical personnel, aiding in crowd or traffic control, helping to maintain scene security, or helping to establish temporary shelter. By using the ICS in numerous emergencies, the tasks of reaching, caring for, and transporting patients are performed more effectively, thereby saving more lives. Since there are variations in the ICS throughout the country, you should become familiar with the ICS for your local community.

Caring for the Ill or Injured

Triage

In previous chapters, you learned how to conduct a systematic assessment of a patient by doing a primary and secondary survey. This enabled you to care for life-threatening emergencies before minor injuries. You will recall that the primary survey has three essential steps that involve checking the patient's airway, breathing, and circulation. You will also recall that the second-ary survey has three steps that include interviewing the patient, checking vital signs, and doing a head-to-toe examination.

Although this approach is appropriate for one patient, it is not effective when there are fewer responders than patients. If you took the time to completely conduct each of these steps and to correct all problems that you found, your entire time could be spent with only one patient. A patient who is unconscious and not breathing, simply because the tongue is blocking the airway, could be overlooked and die while your attention is given to caring for someone with a less severe injury, such as a broken arm.

> **NOTE:**
>
> *Pediatric triage may differ in some jurisdictions according to local protocol.*

In an MCI, you must modify your technique for checking patients. This requires you to understand your priorities. It also requires that you accept death and dying because some patients, such as those in cardiac arrest who would normally receive CPR and be a high priority, will be beyond your ability to help in this situation.

To identify which patients require urgent care in an MCI, you use a process known as triage. Triage is an old French term that was first used to refer to the sorting and treatment of those injured in battle. Today, the triage process is used any time there are more patients than responders. Its common definition is the sorting of patients into categories according to the severity of their injuries or illnesses.

The START System

Over the years, a number of systems have been used to triage patients. Most, however, required you to "diag-nose" the exact extent of injury or illness. This was often time-consuming and resulted in delays in assessment and care for people in MCIs. As a result, the START system was created. START stands for Simple Triage And Rapid Treatment. It is a simple way to quickly assess and prioritize patients. The START system requires you to check only three items: breathing, circulation, and level of consciousness. As you check these items, you will classify patients into one of four levels that reflect the severity of injury or illness and need for care. These levels are "minor," "immediate," "delayed," and "dead/non-salvageable."

Using the START system requires the first responders on the scene to clear the area of all those patients with only minor problems. These patients are classified into a category sometimes called the "walking wounded." If someone is able to walk from the site of the incident, allow him to do so. Have these patients walk to a designated area for evaluation by arriving medical personnel. This first action is critical to the success of START. It enables you to move patients to safety, ensures higher-level medical care, and reduces the number of remaining patients that you need to check.

Next, move quickly among the remaining patients, assessing the severity of the problems. As you do so, you are attempting to classify each patient into one of the three remaining categories for care.

The second category is "immediate care." This categorization means that the patient needs immediate transport to a medical facility. An example of an "immediate" patient is one who requires assisted ventilation as she is breathing more than 30 times a minute.

The third category is "delayed care." This category is assigned to a patient who is breathing and has a pulse and level of consciousness within normal limits but who may not be able to move because of a broken leg or back injury.

The final category is "dead/non-salvageable." This category is assigned to those individuals who are obviously dead. Patients who are initially found not breathing and who fail to breathe after attempts are made to open and clear the airway are classified as dead/non-salvageable. This is also true for obvious mortal injury, such as decapitation.

As you classify each patient into one of these four categories, you need to mark the patient in some distinguishing manner so that responders coming

Figure 22–2 Example of a multiple casualty incident tag.

behind you will be able to begin to care for and remove the most critical patients first. This process of labelling patients is easily done with commercial triage markers or multicoloured tape, which should be fastened to the patient in an easily noticeable area, such as around the wrist (Figure 22–2). Colour codes are as follows:

- Minor = green
- Immediate = red
- Delayed = yellow
- Dead/non-salvageable = black or grey

To make this decision, take the following steps:

Check breathing. When you locate a patient, begin by assessing whether he is breathing. If he is not breathing, clear the mouth of any foreign object and make sure the airway is open. If he does not begin breathing on his own, even with the airway open, the patient is classified as "dead/non-salvageable." There is no need to check the pulse. Place a black or grey marker on the patient and move on.

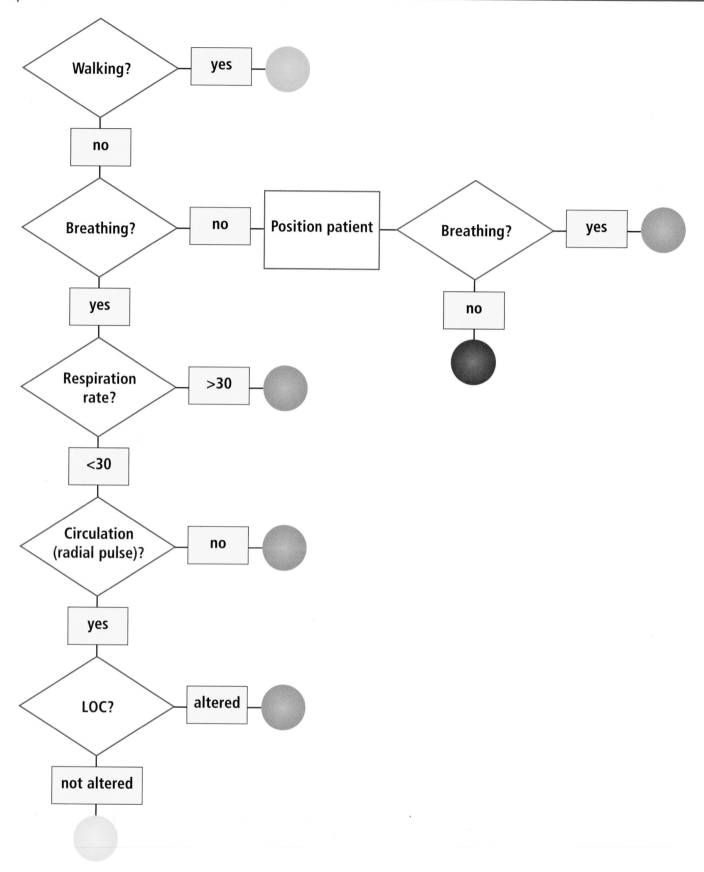

Figure 22–3 The essential steps of the START system.

TABLE 22–1: START CLASSIFICATION SYSTEM

Minor (green)	Delayed (yellow)	Immediate (red)	Dead/non-salvageable (black/grey)
Walking	Breathing normal, radial pulse present, and level of consciousness normal	Breathing more than 30 times a minute	Not breathing
		Breathing normal, but radial pulse absent	
		Breathing normal, radial pulse present, but level of consciousness abnormal	

On the other hand, if the patient does begin to breathe on his own when you open the airway, this patient should be classified as needing "immediate" care. Any individual who needs help maintaining an open airway is a high priority. Position the patient in a way that will maintain an open airway, place a red tag on the patient, and move on to the next patient. Once triage of all patients is complete, you may be able to come back and assist with their care.

If the patient is breathing when you arrive, you must check the rate of the patient's breathing. Someone breathing more than 30 times a minute should be classified "immediate." A patient breathing less than 30 times a minute should be further evaluated. This requires you to move to the next check—circulation.

Check circulation. The next step is to evaluate the breathing patient's pulse. You do this by checking the radial pulse. You are only checking for the presence of the radial pulse. If you cannot find the radial pulse in either arm, then the patient's blood pressure is substantially low. Control any severe bleeding by using direct pressure and applying a pressure bandage. Classify the patient as one requiring "immediate" care and move on to the next patient. If the pulse is present and no severe bleeding is evident, conduct the final check—level of consciousness.

Check level of consciousness. The final step is to assess the patient's level of consciousness. At this point, you know the following about the patient:

- Breathing is normal (less than 30 times per minute).

- Radial pulse is present. (Severe bleeding may or may not be present.)

This final check will serve to classify this patient. You determine the patient's level of consciousness by using the AVPU scale. You give a patient who is alert and responds appropriately to verbal stimuli a final classification of "delayed." This patient has some injury that prevents him from moving to safety, but his present condition is not life-threatening. Someone who remains unconscious and responds only to painful stimuli or responds inappropriately to verbal stimuli is classified as "immediate."

By using the START system, you will be able to move quickly among patients, assessing and classifying them (Figure 22–3). Remember, your role is not to provide extensive care for the patient. Instead, you are expected to get to as many patients as possible. You should not at any time stop triaging patients to begin CPR on one of them. This patient is dead, and if you start CPR, you will need to continue. If you do, others who might have lived if you had done your job properly could now die as a result of delay. The likelihood that someone in a trauma situation in cardiac arrest will survive is extremely rare. Table 22–1 provides a simple overview of the START classification system.

SUMMARY

MCIs can be small- or large-scale operations. They can range from two patients injured in a motor vehicle collision to hundreds injured in the collapse of a structure. Coping effectively with the magnitude of the problem requires an organized approach. The ICS provides this approach. The ICS provides for efficient use of resources, such as personnel, equipment, and supplies. When the ICS is used with an effective triage system such as START, the lives of many patients can be saved because responders are able to reach, sort, and care for patients in the most efficient manner.

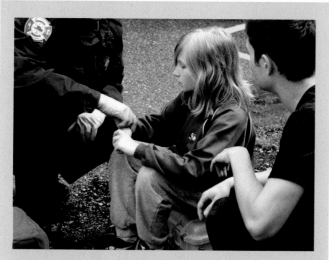

A young man is yelling at you to help his sister who is having difficulty breathing. He says she is asthmatic and does not have her puffer. What do you do?

Chapter 23

Transportation

You are on the scene of a motor vehicle collision. One of the people injured has a head and spine injury and will need to be transported to a nearby hospital. Helicopter evacuation has been requested. What do you do?

INTRODUCTION

As an emergency medical responder (EMR), your responsibilities are not necessarily completed after you have provided assessment and treatment at the scene. You may be required to prepare and transport the patient to a hospital or medical facility.

Modern emergency vehicles are more than just vehicles for transporting someone to the hospital. They are well-equipped and efficiently organized vehicles or aircraft with advanced communications and technology that can bring needed medical supplies, personnel, and advanced life support (ALS) care to the scene.

TRANSPORTATION

Emergency Vehicle Maintenance and Safety Check

Completing an ambulance equipment and supply checklist at the beginning of every work shift is important for safety, patient care, and risk management issues and helps ensure the appropriate functioning of the vehicle for use in emergency and non-emergency responses. Some equipment on the ambulance (e.g., AEDs) requires routine maintenance and testing to ensure safe and effective operation when needed (Figure 23–1). See Appendix B: Sample Ambulance Equipment List.

The vehicle and equipment must be disinfected and cleaned at times, both inside and out, to ensure that pathogens have been removed and that the vehicle represents a professional appearance. The procedure for vehicle maintenance and routine care varies by jurisdiction. The procedure for vehicle checks is often legislated by a governmental body, but specific EMS services may develop their own equipment checklists.

You should follow your operational guidelines for the safe and effective procedures for checking vehicles, equipment, and supplies. It is important to note and record any problems or deficiencies found when checking the emergency vehicle. Place any vehicle or piece of equipment out of service if an immediate safety issue arises.

Figure 23–1 Equipment on the ambulance requires routine maintenance and testing to ensure effective operation.

Safe Vehicle Operations

Safe vehicle operation is important for the safety of patients being rescued, the EMR crew, and the public in the vicinity of an emergency response. It is encouraged that all EMR agencies, where there is a requirement to transport patients, require personnel to complete an emergency driving course and maintain that certification throughout their career. Never drive a private vehicle as if it were an emergency vehicle. Even if you have lights and sirens, people do not always see you, hear you, or yield the right-of-way. People hurrying to an emergency or a hospital sometimes cause collisions because they fail to drive safely.

When operating an emergency vehicle, follow these guidelines:

- Follow all laws and acts with respect to the operation of an emergency vehicle in your province or territory.

- Follow all operational guidelines for your jurisdiction.

- Be tolerant and observant of other motorists and pedestrians.

- Always use your seat belts and restraining devices.

- Be familiar with the characteristics of the emergency vehicle.
- Be alert to changes in weather and road terrain and conditions.
- Exercise caution in the use of audible and visible warning devices.
- Drive within the speed limit, except in circumstances allowed by law.
- Select the fastest and most appropriate route to and from the scene.
- Maintain a safe following distance.
- Drive with due regard for the safety of others.
- If possible, drive in a manner that allows the patient comfort.
- Always drive in a manner consistent with managing acceptable levels of risk.

In addition to the size and weight of the emergency vehicle and driver's experience level, factors that influence safe operation include:

- Attitude
- Environmental conditions
- Appropriate use of warning devices
- Proceeding safely through intersections
- Parking at the emergency scene
- Operating with due regard for the safety of all others

Attitude

Attitude is the mental framework that structures your day-to-day driving performance. It is the way you see yourself as a driver and how you view other drivers. Attitudes are influenced by experiences, emotions, values, feelings, prejudices, and personality. Being a safe driver requires an open mind, a willingness to learn, and a desire to improve.

Safe drivers are courteous and considerate. They are willing to yield the right-of-way and they keep a constant check on traffic and adapt to changing conditions. A positive attitude will help you drive amicably with others and help maintain the safe operation of your vehicle.

Environmental Conditions

Environmental conditions can pose significant dangers to EMRs when responding to calls. Factors that can affect safe operation include road and weather conditions, such as fog and heavy rain that decrease visibility, and slippery conditions caused by snow, ice, or water that can cause the vehicle to hydroplane. When hazardous environmental conditions are present, the driver should proceed at safe speeds appropriate to the conditions.

Appropriate Use of Warning Devices

When responding to an emergency call, the driver must use audible and visual warning devices according to local protocols and based on provincial/territorial motor vehicle laws. Use of warning devices while transporting someone should be based on assessment of the patient and appropriate protocol for treatment and transportation. When responding to or from a call using warning devices, keep in mind that motorists who drive with car windows rolled up or who are using a radio, air conditioning, or heating system may not be able to hear the warning devices. It is important that you proceed with caution and never assume that the warning devices provide an absolute right-of-way to proceed. When backing up, take extra caution to ensure that there is nothing in your path and use backup signals if available.

Proceeding Safely Through Intersections

Most provinces and territories require all emergency vehicles to come to a complete stop at all controlled intersections (i.e., red light, stop sign) and proceed through the intersection when safe to do so. Take precautions when proceeding through controlled intersections to gain the attention of surrounding motorists such as:

- Changing the mode of the siren
- Using air horns
- Using legislated sirens

Parking at the Emergency Scene

When parking the emergency vehicle at the scene, consider any hazards such as leaking fuel, hazardous materials, or leaking gas. If any of these conditions are present, position the vehicle upwind and at a safe distance. In addition, position the vehicle so that it protects you and the patient from other motorists and hazards. When parking or positioning your vehicle, keep the following in mind:

- Vehicle exhaust fumes
- Downed electrical wires
- Poor lighting
- Blocking extrication vehicles and equipment
- The possibility of collapse of surrounding buildings due to fire or explosion

Operating With Due Regard for the Safety of All Others

Most provinces and territories allow privileges for drivers of emergency vehicles, such as driving slightly above the speed limit and proceeding through controlled intersections (after a complete stop) during an emergency response.

However, these privileges must take into consideration the safety of others. "Due regard for the safety of all others" carries legal responsibility and can result in liability for you and the agency you represent if damage, injury, or death results from its failure. As an EMR, you must be familiar with and aware of local and provincial/territorial laws and regulations pertaining to the operation of an emergency vehicle.

Air Medical Transportation

In certain situations, it is sometimes best for the patient to be transported to the medical facility by a helicopter or a fixed-wing aircraft. This type of transport enables severely injured or ill patients to be transported quickly to specialty centres and large treatment facilities. Geography and other circumstances play a large role in this type of transport decision, and emergency personnel should follow local and provincial/territorial protocols.

Air ambulance services typically use fixed-wing and/or rotary-wing (helicopter) aircraft throughout the country. Fixed-wing aircraft are not usually as high profile as helicopters but are particularly useful for long-distance (i.e., greater than 200 km) and inter-hospital transfers of patients or vital organs. Fixed-wing aircraft can also operate in weather conditions that may restrict rotary-wing aircraft.

Landing Site Preparation

A helicopter landing zone should be approximately 46 x 46 metres (151 x 151 feet). It should have no vertical structures that can impair landing or takeoff and should be relatively flat and free of high grass, crops, or other factors that can conceal uneven terrain or hinder access. The landing site should also be free of debris that could injure people or damage structures or the aircraft. Rescue personnel close to the landing site should wear protective eyewear and helmets. Given the time of day, the landing site may need lighting such as portable lights and traffic cones with reflectors or may require positioning of the emergency vehicles, with warning lights on, around the perimeter of the landing zone. If white lights are used, point them toward the centre of the landing zone and not directly at the aircraft. If conditions are very dry, you may need to wet the landing zone to prevent the pilot and drivers of vehicles on the ground from being blinded by clouds of dust. It may also be helpful to use radio communications with the pilot to advise her of conditions such as wind direction or any hazards or obstructions of which she needs to be aware. In some cases, when the helicopter is landing, it may be appropriate for you to use hand signals to guide the pilot.

Ground Safety Precautions

Keep the landing zone clear during takeoffs and landings. Maintain a distance of 60 metres (200 feet). In addition, adhere to the following guidelines:

- Never allow ground personnel to approach the helicopter unless requested to do so by the pilot or flight crew.
- Stay in view of the flight crew at all times.
- Stay away from propellers.

- Allow only necessary personnel to help load or unload patients.

- Secure any loose objects or clothing that could be blown by rotor or downwash (e.g., stretcher, sheets, or blankets).

- Do not allow smoking.

- After the aircraft is parked, move to the front, beyond the perimeter of the rotor blades, and wait for a signal from the pilot to approach.

- Approach the helicopter in a crouched position, staying within view of the pilot or other crew members (Figure 23–2).

- Never approach the aircraft (rotary or fixed wing) from the rear (Figure 23–3). The tail rotors on most aircraft are near the ground and spin at high rpm, which makes them virtually invisible. Tail rotor injuries are often fatal.

- Carry long objects horizontally and no higher than waist height.

- Depart the helicopter from the front and within view of the pilot.

Medical Evacuation From a Ship

A helicopter should not be requested for evacuation from a ship unless the patient is in serious condition. In many cases, the decision to use aeromedical evacuation is made in consultation with the medical advisor, based on the medical information provided by the attendant.

Preparing the Patient for Transfer

To prepare a patient for transfer, follow these steps:

- Ensure that the patient's airway, breathing, and circulation are under control. If indicated, strap the patient in a stretcher to prevent her from slipping or falling out.

- Place the patient's medical records (if any) with all necessary papers (including passport, if available) in a plastic envelope to be sent along with her.

- Add notes of any treatment given.

- If possible, ensure that the patient is wearing a PFD/lifejacket before moving her to the stretcher.

- Perform a concise but thorough assessment and relay all pertinent information directly to one of the flight crew members.

Figure 23–2 Approach a helicopter in a crouched position.

Figure 23–3 Never approach an aircraft from the rear. Approach only upon direction of the flight crew or pilot. Ensure the pilot can see you at all times.

- Describe any bandaged or covered injury, or any physical finding, to the flight medical crew, along with a concise history of the event.

Ship-to-Ship Transfer

Ship-to-ship transfer involves difficult manoeuvring for two vessels. It is a seamanship problem demanding high standards of competence for its safe and efficient performance. Light (unloaded) ships must be approached slowly and with caution. Ships with the higher freeboard should provide the illumination and boarding facilities. The transfer should be performed quickly, and ships should not linger alongside for any reason.

SUMMARY

Your job does not necessarily end after you have assessed and cared for a patient at the emergency scene. In some circumstances, you may be required to transport the patient to a medical facility or assist with air medical transportation or medical evacuation from a ship. This responsibility includes maintaining

and safely operating an emergency vehicle as well as understanding how to prepare a landing zone for an air ambulance in any type of emergency situation.

The helicopter is on its way and you are told to get the landing zone ready. What do you do?

Chapter *24*

Marine Environment

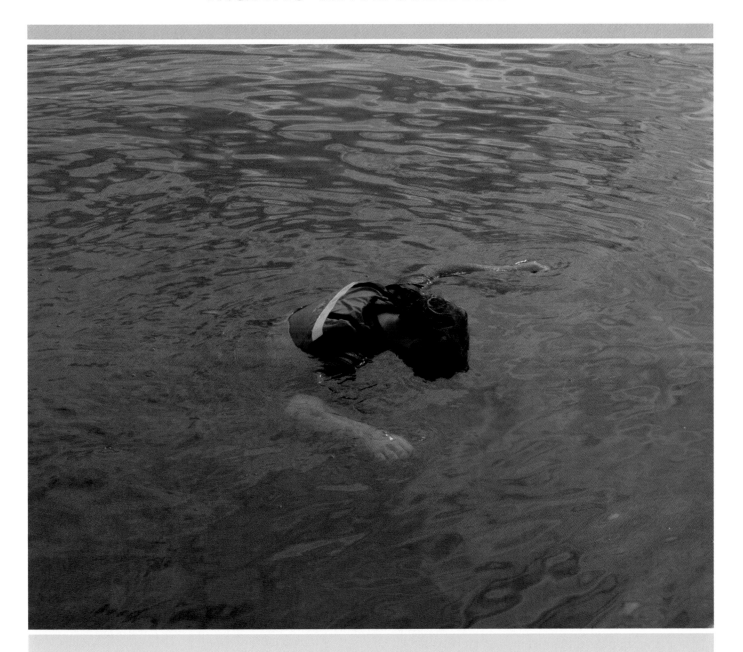

One of your crew members has fallen overboard into frigid waters. It has only been a minute or two since he went in the water but he is quickly becoming less and less responsive. What do you do?

INTRODUCTION

As a marine advanced first aid attendant, you are required to hold a marine first aid certificate specified by Transport Canada, Marine Safety. This chapter references the need for specialized training for those responsible for the medical care of seafarers, particularly in oxygen administration, airway adjuncts, drug administration, Workplace Hazardous Materials Information System (WHMIS), and confined space entry. Although this chapter outlines procedures intended for those with specialized training, as a marine first aid attendant you may be requested to gather supplies and/or assist a ship's doctor or more advanced medical personnel with procedures. This information is being provided to familiarize you with the equipment and safety precautions required for each procedure.

NOTE:

Any procedure described in this chapter should be applied by the first aid attendant under appropriate supervision in accordance with professional standards of care used with regard to unique circumstances that apply to each situation.

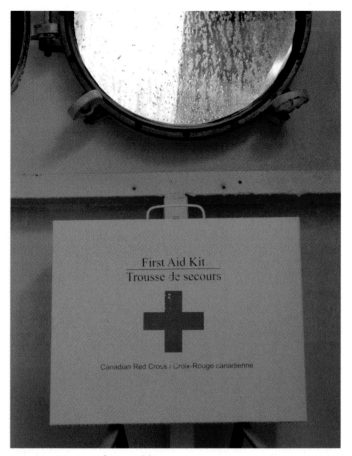

Figure 24–1 A first aid kit.

Preparing to Respond

First Aid Kits, Supplies, and Equipment

As a marine first aid attendant, it is important for you to be aware of the location of your ship's:

• First aid station(s), which are found in the wheelhouse, engine room, galley, and in lifesaving equipment such as lifeboats

• First aid kits (Figure 24–1) and equipment

• Medical supplies

You should also be familiar with the contents and proper use of the supplies contained in each kit. First aid kit contents for vessels travelling in international waters are outlined in Table 24–1, whereas Table 24–2 outlines the kit contents for each vessel type when travelling in Canadian waters, as per the current version of the *Canadian Labour Code: Marine Occupational Safety and Health Regulations*. Survival crafts, such as lifeboats, require certain minimum kit contents as outlined in Table 24–3.

First aid attendants should also understand the importance of checking the expiry date of all first aid materials, having reliable supplies available, routinely checking the first aid stations, and ensuring that the first aid station and its contents are in a clean, dry, and serviceable condition. Throughout this chapter, specific equipment lists have been provided where appropriate.

NOTE:

Unless there is a person qualified on board the ship, such as a registered nurse or doctor, the ship captain is ultimately responsible for the administration of medicine. The ship captain is normally the custodian of the medical chest on board any ship; however, the decision whether to administer the medicine is made after consulting with the medical advisor. Also, the captain must maintain a log book of all medicine administered during the voyage and for which type of illnesses. An official entry in the ship's log book must also be made.

TABLE 24–1: INTERNATIONAL FIRST AID KIT CONTENTS[31]

Category	Recommended Item	Quantity per 10 crew
1	**RESUSCITATION EQUIPMENT**	
Equipment for the administration of oxygen	Portable oxygen set, complete, containing:	1
	1 oxygen cylinder (D: 425 litres or E: 680 litres)	1
	1 spare oxygen cylinder (D: 425 litres or E: 680 litres)	1
	Pressure regulator and flowmeter, with tubes such that ship's industrial oxygen can also be used	1
	3 disposable face masks of choice including resuscitation mask and non-rebreather mask	3
Oropharyngeal airway (OPA)	Sizes medium and large	2
Suction device	Manual suction to clear upper airways, including 2 catheters	1
Bag-valve-mask (BVM) resuscitator	BVM supplied with large, medium and small masks	1
Barrier devices for mouth-to-mouth resuscitation	Pocket mask with one-way valve	1
2	**DRESSING MATERIAL AND SUTURING EQUIPMENT**	
Adhesive bandages	Assorted sizes, water-resistant	200
Sterile gauze compress	Gauze compress, 5 x 5 cm, sterile	100
	Gauze compress, 10 x 10 cm, sterile	100
Gauze roll	Gauze roll, 5 cm and 90 cm (or 60 cm) x 100 m, non sterile	1
Gauze dressing with non-adherent surface	Non-adherent gauze dressing, 10 cm x 10 cm, sterile	100
Vaseline® gauze	Paraffin gauze dressing, 10 x 10 cm, sterile	50
Elastic bandage	Elastic fixation bandage, 6 cm x 4 m	3
Sterile pressure bandage	Sizes small/medium/large	5
Tubular gauze for finger bandage	Tubular gauze bandage for finger bandage with applicator, 5 m	1

Adhesive elastic bandage	Adhesive elastic bandage, 6 cm x 4 m	10
Triangular bandages	Triangular bandages	5
Sterile sheet for burns	Sterile sheet for burns	1
Adhesive sutures (or zinc oxide bandages)	Adhesive tape, waterproof, skin-friendly, 5 x 1.25 cm	10
Q-tips®	Q-tips® (wooden)	100
Safety pins	Safety pins (stainless steel) 12 pcs	50
Butterfly sutures	Butterfly sutures, skin closures, sterile	20
Skin adhesive	2-octyl cyanoacrylate liquid, 0.5 mL	2
Suturing equipment	Sutures, absorbable with curved non-traumatic needles, 1-O, 3-O, & 4-O (or 5-O)	10 each
Gloves (latex free)	Disposable examination gloves	50
	Surgical gloves sizes 6.5, 7.5, 8.5, sterile, in pairs	3 of each size
3	**INSTRUMENTS**	
Disposable scalpels	Scalpel, sterile, disposable	20
Stainless steel instrument box	Instrument box (stainless steel)	1
Scissors	Operating scissors, straight (stainless steel)	1
	Bandage scissors (stainless steel)	1
Forceps	Splinter forceps, pointed (stainless steel)	3
	Teeth tissue forceps (stainless steel)	1
Needle holder	Needle holder, 80 mm straight	1
Hemostatic clamps	Hemostatic clamp, 125 mm (stainless steel)	3
Disposable razors	Razor, disposable	50
4	**EXAMINATION AND MONITORING EQUIPMENT**	
Disposable tongue depressors	Tongue depressors, disposable	100
Reactive strips for urine analysis	Reactive strips for urine analysis (blood/glucose/protein/nitrite/leukocytes)	100
Microscope slides	Microscope slides	100
Stethoscope	Stethoscope	1

Blood pressure cuff	Blood pressure cuff, preferably automatic	1
Standard thermometer	Digital if possible	1
Rectal thermometer	Thermometer, digital if possible	1
Hypothermic thermometer	Thermometer 32°–34°C, digital if possible	1
Penlight	Penlight plus blue cover	1

5	**EQUIPMENT FOR INJECTION, INFUSION, AND CATHETERIZATION**	
Equipment for injection	Syringes, Luer connection, 2 mL, sterile disposable	50
	Syringes, Luer connection, 5 mL, sterile, disposable	50
	Hypodermic subcutaneous needle, Luer connection, 16 x 0.5 mm, sterile, disposable	20
	Hypodermic intramuscular needle, Luer connection, 40 x 0.8 mm, sterile, disposable	20
	Needles, 19 gauge blunt, "drawing up" type	20
Equipment for infusion	Intravenous, infusion cannula 16 gauge (1.2 mm) and 22 gauge (0.8 mm), Luer-lock connection, sterile, non-recap type	10 each
	Intravenous giving set, Luer-lock connection, sterile	3
	Tourniquet, blood-taking type, to be used with intravenous infusion cannula	1
Bladder drainage equipment	Penile sheath set with condom catheter (Texas Catheter™), tube, and bag	2
	Short-term urine catheter with Soft Eye™ straight tip Thieman No. 12 and No. 16 or equivalent (Foley), sterile, individually packed, prelubricated or with additional lidocaine/chlorhexidine lubricant	2
	Urine collecting bag and tube	2

6	**GENERAL MEDICAL AND NURSING EQUIPMENT**	
Eye protection	Plastic goggles or full-face masks	2
Plastic apron	Disposable	20
Kidney dish (basin)	Kidney dish, stainless steel, 825 mL	2
Plastic backed towels	Towels, plastic backed, absorbent, 600 x 500 mm	10
Safety box (sharps container)	Safety box for sharps disposal, 5 L	1

Masks	Masks, duckbill type, disposable	50
Tape measure	Tape measure, vinyl coated, 1.5 m	1
Draw sheets	Draw sheet, plastic 90 x 180 cm	2
Bedpan	Bedpan, stainless steel	1
Hot-water bottle	Hot-water bag	1
Urine bottle	Urinal, male (plastic)	1
Ice bag	Cold pack	1
Emergency blanket (aluminum foil blanket)	Aluminum foil blanket	1
Condoms	Male condoms	100
Wash bottle	Plastic wash bottle, 250 mL	1
Plastic bottle	Bottle, 1 litre, plastic with screw top	3
Dressing tray	Stainless steel dressing tray, 300 x 200 x 30 mm	1
Bowl	Bowl, stainless steel, 180 mL	3
Specimen jars	Jars, plastic, with lids and labels, 100 mL	10
Plaster-of-Paris bandage	Bandages, POP, 5 cm and 10 cm x 2.7 m	12 each
Stockinet	Sizes for arm and leg splints, 10 m roll	1 each
Cotton wool	Cotton wool roll, 500 g	10
Alcohol swabs	70% alcohol swabs for skin cleansing prior to injection	200
Nail brush	Nail brush	1
7 IMMOBILIZATION AND TRANSPORTATION EQUIPMENT		
Malleable splints	Malleable finger splint Malleable forearm/hand splint	1 of each

TABLE 24–2: FIRST AID KIT CONTENTS AS PER THE CANADA LABOUR CODE[32]

ITEM SUPPLIES AND EQUIPMENT	TYPE OF FIRST AID KIT				
	ON A SHIP				AT A DETACHED WORK PLACE
	With 2–5 employees	With 6–19 employees	With 20–49 employees	With 50+ employees	
	Quantity per Type of First Aid Kit				
Antiseptic-wound solution, 60 mL or antiseptic swabs (10-pack)	1	2	3	6	1
Applicator—disposable (10-pack) (not needed if antiseptic swabs used)	1	2	4	8	—
Bag—disposable, waterproof, emesis	1	2	2	4	—
Adhesive bandages	12	100	200	400	6
Gauze rolls, 2.5 cm x 4.5 m (not needed if ties attached to dressing)	2	6	8	12	—
Triangular bandages (with 2 safety pins)	2	4	6	8	1
Container—First Aid Kit	1	1	1	1	1
Gauze compress, 7.5 x 12 cm, sterile	2	4	8	12	—
Gauze dressing, 7.5 x 7.5 cm, sterile	4	8	12	18	2
Forceps (splinter)	1	1	1	1	—
First Aid manual, English — current edition	1	1	1	1	—
First Aid manual, French — current edition	1	1	1	1	—
Pad with shield or tape for eye	1	1	2	4	1
Record—First Aid	1	1	1	1	1
Scissors — 10 cm	—	1	1	1	—
Roll of waterproof adhesive tape, 1.2 cm x 4.6 m (not needed if ties attached to dressings)	1	1	2	3	—
Antipruritic lotion, 30 mL or swabs (10-pack)	1	1	1	2	—
Elastic bandage, 7.5 cm x 5 m	—	—	1	2	—
Emergency blanket (aluminum foil blanket)	—	—	—	—	1

	1	1	1	2	—
Dressing-burn, sterile, 10 x 10 cm	1	1	1	2	—
Hand cleanser or cleaning towelettes, 1 pack	1	1	1	1	—
Splint set with padding	—	1	1	1	—
Stretcher	—	—	1	1	—

TABLE 24–3: MINIMUM FIRST AID KIT CONTENTS ON SURVIVAL CRAFTS (INCLUDING LIFEBOATS AND RAFTS)[33]

Item Supplies and Equipment	Quantity
Adhesive bandages, 7.5 x 2.2 cm (individually wrapped)	32
Gauze rolls, 5 cm x 4.6 m	4
Compress bandages, 10 x 10 cm with 90-cm gauze tabs	8
Sterile abdominal pads, 15.2 x 20.3 cm	2
Triangular bandages	6
Sterile eye pads, 4.69 x 6.98 cm	10
Extra-ocular ophthalmic irrigating solution in an unbreakable bottle that shows a drug identification number and an expiry date	120 mL
Unbreakable plastic eyewash cup	1
Wire splint, 9.5 x 60 cm	1
Individual packs of ammonia inhalant	20
Pads impregnated with povidone and iodine that show an expiry date	20
Pocket guide to Emergency First Aid, in English and French, published by the Canadian Red Cross or St. John Ambulance	1
Waterproof contents list and instruction sheet in English and French	1
Safety pins	6
Bandage scissors (stainless steel)	1
Roll of waterproof adhesive tape, 2.5 cm x 4.5 m	1

The first aid kit shall be placed in a container that is:

• Watertight

• Resealable

• Fitted with a gasket to ensure a tight seal

• Made of a rigid plastic that is capable of withstanding temperatures of -30°C, such as acrylonitrile butadienestyrene (ABS) or high-impact polystyrene (HIPS)

AIRWAY ADJUNCTS

Endotracheal Intubation

Advanced medical personnel prefer endotracheal intubation as the advanced technique for airway management for people who are unable to maintain an open airway. Endotracheal (ET) intubation provides a definitive means to control a person's airway. Intubation with a cuffed ET tube helps ensure that the airway remains open by preventing aspiration. Once an ET tube is placed properly within the trachea, it is possible to provide controlled ventilation with 100% oxygen without concern for pushing air into the stomach.

Indications for ET intubation include situations when:

- The responder is unable to ventilate an unconscious person with conventional methods (e.g., mouth-to-mask, BVM)

- The person is unable to protect his own airway due to coma or respiratory or cardiac arrest

- Prolonged resuscitation is necessary

In addition, ET intubation provides the following advantages:

- It isolates the airway, preventing aspiration of material, such as vomit, into the lower airway.

- It facilitates ventilation and oxygenation of the body.

- It facilitates suctioning of the trachea and bronchi.

- It prevents wasted ventilation and gastric distention during positive-pressure ventilation.

- It provides a route for the administration of some medications.

Figure 24–2 Laryngoscope with blades.

Although ET intubation provides many advantages, it is a technically challenging procedure that poses risks and potential complications that can be considered life-threatening. It is important to note that the priority for a nonbreathing person is ventilation, not intubation.

Preparing the Equipment

One of the first steps in ET intubation is to make careful preparations. To perform ET intubation, you may be requested to gather and prepare the intubation equipment outlined in Table 24–4.

A laryngoscope is an instrument used to see the vocal cords for ET tube placement (Figure 24–2). It consists of two parts: a handle (which contains the batteries) and a lighted blade. Two to three blades should be available to allow for differences in size and anatomy of different people. The blade has a notch that attaches to a locking bar on the laryngoscope handle. Locking the blade in

TABLE 24–4: EQUIPMENT NEEDED FOR ENDOTRACHEAL INTUBATION

• Gloves	• Water-soluble lubricant	• 10 mL syringe
• Goggles	• Suction unit	• Stylet
• Laryngoscope blades and handle	• BVM	• Assorted endotracheal tubes
• Towel	• Tape and/or commercial securing device	• Stethoscope

Figure 24–3 ET tube and syringe.

Figure 24–4 A bag-valve-mask (BVM).

place causes a light to turn on, allowing you to see the vocal cords. Check the light. It should be bright white and steady.

ET tubes are available in several sizes. Sizes, in millimetres, are determined by the internal diameter of the tube (Figure 24–3). You will need two to three cuffed ET tubes in different sizes. A 7.5 mm tube usually fits an adult.

The ET tube cuff holds about 10–20 mL of air. Test the cuff for leaks prior to intubation attempts.

A stylet is used to provide stiffness to the ET tube during insertion. This allows the tube to be directed toward the vocal cords. Stylets are malleable metal rods that are inserted into the ET tube and moulded to the desired shaped curve. To place a stylet into the ET tube, first lubricate it with water-soluble lubricant. Then, insert the stylet into the ET tube, ensuring that it does not extend beyond the end of the tube.

> **NOTE:**
>
> *The ship medic, nurse, or doctor may be required to perform airway intervention. The information on the techniques and procedures for intubation is intended as a basic overview only. These skills require specialized training and are intended for those who provide advanced medical care.*

Intubating the Person

In preparation for ET intubation, place the person in the sniffing position (the head backward as if the person's nose is pointing up sniffing the air). This provides the best alignment for directly seeing the larynx (vocal cords). The tube should be lubricated, and a stethoscope, stylet, and suction equipment should be readily available. As in all advanced airway procedures, you should ventilate the person's lungs with 100% oxygen for one to two minutes before intubation using a BVM (Figure 24–4) and supplemental oxygen.

To ventilate the person using ET intubation, begin by holding the laryngoscope in the left hand. Insert the blade into the right side of the mouth, displacing the tongue to the left. Advance the ET tube through the corner of the mouth, and under direct vision, through the vocal cords. First, inflate the cuff with 10 to 20 mL of air and then ventilate the person's lungs with a BVM. While ventilating the person, confirm ET placement by listening to the abdomen and chest with a stethoscope. Finally, secure the ET tube to the person's head and face with tape or a commercially available device designed for this use, and provide ventilatory support with supplemental oxygen.

ET Tube Removal

If the person begins to breathe on his own, the ET tube may need to be removed. To accomplish removal, first suction the person's mouth, nose, and back of the throat. Then, deflate the cuff of the ET tube. If the person is conscious, instruct the person to take a deep breath. Have them blow out while you withdraw the tube. Be prepared to suction the person's mouth in case of vomiting.

TOXICOLOGICAL HAZARDS ON BOARD A SHIP

Workplace Hazardous Materials Information System (WHMIS)

Many workers are exposed to chemical hazards in the workplace. To help protect employees, the federal, provincial, and territorial governments have legislated WHMIS, a nationwide class identification system that provides Canadian workers and employers with information on the hazardous materials they use on the job. WHMIS regulations require employers to (1) clearly label hazardous materials, including all toxic substances, and (2) inform employees about risks and precautions.

WHMIS uses the following three main approaches to help identify and handle hazardous materials safely:

1. Labels (risks, precautionary measures, and first aid to be given in case of exposure or poisoning)

2. Material Safety Data Sheets (MSDSs)

3. Worker education

To minimize safety and health risks, workers should observe all warning labels, tags, and placards in the workplace and follow the required precautions. When both employer and employee follow these government guidelines, hazardous materials injuries in the workplace can be prevented.

Material Safety Data Sheets (MSDSs)

Material Safety Data Sheets are documents containing important technical information for workers on the work site. An MSDS must be available for every hazardous material on the work site.

WHMIS will be changing to an international class identification system called the Globally Harmonized System (GHS) of Classification and Labelling of Chemicals. GHS provides employers and workers with information about the hazardous materials they work with. The GHS was initiated at the Rio Earth Summit in 1992, when the United Nations Conference on Environment and Development agreed to develop "a globally harmonized hazard classification and compatible labelling system, including Material Safety Data Sheets and easily understandable symbols." This harmonization is intended to better protect both people and the environment.[34] The GHS will introduce some new terminology, including Safety Data Sheets (SDSs) instead of Material Safety Data Sheets (MSDSs), and pictograms, which are the hazard symbols on labels.[35] Health Canada is working on implementing the GHS in Canada.

The employer must be aware of the following nine main sections:

1. Product information and use

2. Hazardous ingredients

3. Physical data

4. Fire and explosion data

5. Reactivity data

6. Toxicological properties

7. Preventive measures

8. First aid measures

9. Preparation information

NOTE:

Inhalation is the most common method of poisoning in the shipping industry. The toxic substance may consist of vapour, gas, mist, spray dust, or fumes.

It is recommended that copies of all relevant MSDSs be kept in a location where the first aid attendant will have ready access to the information. For worker reference, appropriate MSDSs must also be available at all locations where the products are used.

Potentially Toxic Substances

Toxic substances can cause death, illness, or serious injury. They can be harmful when they are swallowed or inhaled or come into contact with skin. Toxic substances can be gases, solids, or liquids.

Carbon monoxide gas can occur in hold fires, as the product of an explosion, in the waste gases of petroleum and oil-driven engines, and when refrigerated meat cargoes decompose. Refrigerant gases such as ammonia vapour, carbon dioxide, or freon, will displace oxygen, making the air unsafe to breathe. In the presence of an open flame, the properties of freon change, producing a toxic substance. Certain refrigerated cargoes, including fruit, vegetables, and cheese, generate carbon dioxide during normal storage. With failure of a refrigerating plant, food cargoes, especially meat, may generate poisonous and inflammable cargo space. This can be particularly dangerous if the cargo space is flooded. Carbon monoxide, ammonia, hydrogen sulphide, and hydrogen may be generated in addition to carbon dioxide. In any great concentration, these gases are extremely poisonous, and some are explosive.

NOTE:
Never enter a confined space without the authorization of the master or a responsible officer.

Storage of Dangerous Goods on Board

Every hazardous substance stored, handled, or used in a workplace must be managed to ensure that the potential hazard to workers is minimal. This is accomplished by clearly marking and labelling packages and by placing warning placards on containers and transport units as indicated by national and international regulations.

Figure 24–5 A survival rescue craft.

Confined Space: Characteristics and Dangers

Crew members entering confined spaces where air cannot support life risk injury or even death. Such spaces may lack oxygen content; some may even contain asphyxiating or toxic gases. Pump rooms or tanks that previously contained petroleum or chemicals are a particular risk for toxic gases. Rusting, fire, and bacteria present in any enclosed space can also use up and deplete oxygen content.

Only specially trained personnel are permitted to work in a confined space. When respiratory protection is required, workers in a confined space must wear a safety or body harness securely attached to a lifeline. A safety watch must be stationed outside the confined space to provide constant watch and maintain communication with the worker inside. The safety watch must activate a suitable alarm if a rescue in a confined space becomes necessary.

MEDICAL CARE OF RESCUED PERSONS

Immediate Care of Survivors

Survival in a rescue craft (lifeboat or raft) is one of the most strenuous ordeals a person can face (Figure 24–5). Survivors must be cared for as soon as possible.

Rescued survivors may be found suffering from various injuries and conditions, including the following:

- Drowning

- Hypothermia and other cold-related injuries

- Emotional conditions

- Seasickness

- Sunburn

- Heat exposure (heat cramps, heat exhaustion, and heat stroke)

- Contamination with oil

- Dehydration and malnutrition

- Immersion foot (trench foot)

Emergency Care on a Survival Craft and on Board a Rescue Vessel

A medical survival kit and supplies may not always be available on a survival craft. Therefore, always establish a plan of action when caring for people in any emergency.

1. **Persons Rescued From a Drowning Incident**

   When rescued from a drowning incident, the person survives submersion, although sometimes only temporarily. The process of drowning begins when small amounts of water are inhaled into the lungs. As a result, the person may eventually suffocate and become unconscious. In some cases, those rescued promptly from the water recover immediately. In other cases, however, your ABC check may reveal that treatment may consist of immediate resuscitation. You should attempt to resuscitate the person even if she has been submerged for a prolonged period. People have been successfully resuscitated even after having been submerged for longer than 30 minutes in cold water.

2. **Generalized Hypothermia Due to Immersion or Other Cold-Related Injuries**

   (See Chapter 18: Heat- and Cold-Related Emergencies)

3. **Emotional Conditions**

   People who have abandoned ship or have experienced a traumatic situation have faced an emotional crisis. Provide emotional support by listening. Some survivors may require further crisis intervention. To ensure that you are prepared to deal with cases of crisis intervention, you should develop a local contact as a resource. To find local crisis intervention resources, speak to your Instructor or contact the local crisis intervention help line.

4. **Seasickness**

   Seasickness (motion sickness) is an acute illness largely due to the motion of the ship or vessel. Signs and symptoms vary but include the following:

   - Loss of appetite

   - Headaches

   - Nausea

   - Cold sweat

   - Dizziness

   - Abdominal cramps

   - Vomiting

   - Exhaustion

   - Dry mouth

Persons who are not accustomed to the sea are most susceptible; but even experienced seafarers may be affected in rough conditions (Figure 24–6).

- In mild cases, the condition will gradually wear off, perhaps during sleep, and no specific treatment may be necessary.

- Keep the person quiet and warm.

- Provide dry foods in small portions, such as crackers or toast, to help settle the person's stomach.

Figure 24–6 Vomiting is a symptom of seasickness and can affect even experienced seafarers.

- Cracked ice may help relieve the person's thirst.

- More severe cases of prolonged vomiting may be managed with over-the-counter preventive medications in dosages recommended by the manufacturer. It is very important to note the contraindications and side effects of these medications before drug administration (see the Pharmacology section in this chapter).

NOTE:

Ginger tablets help settle the stomach.

---

5. **Sunburn**

   (See Chapter 12: Soft Tissue Injuries)

6. **Heat Exposure: Heat Cramps, Heat Exhaustion, and Heat Stroke**

   (See Chapter 18: Heat- and Cold-Related Emergencies)

7. **Contamination With Oil**

   Survivors of shipwreck are sometimes covered in oil. If a person has suffered oil contamination, do the following:

   - Clean the skin only after the person is warm and comfortable (clean the areas around the mouth and eyes immediately).

   - Wipe the skin with a soft cloth or strong paper towels. You can also have the person take a warm shower using regular hair shampoo and body soap. If the person has any signs of burns, do not wipe that area directly.

NOTE:

Contamination with oil can lead to breathing difficulties, if inhaled, or nausea and vomiting, if ingested.

---

8. **Dehydration and Malnutrition**

   Survivors who have been adrift for several days may be found suffering from dehydration. If they have been adrift for several weeks, malnutrition may also have developed.

   - Remember to give food and water in small amounts at first to avoid reversing dehydration or malnutrition too rapidly.

- You should seek radio medical advice on how to treat the person.

  - Initially, a diet of nourishing liquids (sugar and water combination, milk, or soup) will help satisfy nutritional requirements.

  - This diet should continue until the survivor can be transferred to medical care ashore.

9. **Immersion Foot (Trench Foot)**

   Immersion foot is caused by exposure of the lower extremities to water above freezing temperatures, but usually below 10°C (50°F) for more than 12 hours. It typically occurs in shipwrecked sailors who have survived but who are, for the most part, inactive, in lifeboats or rafts in adverse weather conditions and with wet and constrictive clothing, and who have a poor diet.

Preventing Immersion Foot

- Keep your feet clean and dry.
- Wear proper-fitting boots.
- Wear wool or synthetic socks.
- Sleep in dry socks or barefoot.
- Dry and massage your feet twice a day.

Signs and Symptoms of Immersion Foot

Initial signs and symptoms include (Figure 24–7):

- Swollen, cold, waxy feet
- Peeling skin
- Reduced sensitivity to touch
- Wooden feeling in feet
- Delayed capillary refill time (nail beds stay white after you squeeze them)

After the foot warms up:

- Warm, dry, red skin
- Blisters
- Pain
- Tingling or itching
- Increased sensitivity to cold

Care for Immersion Foot

When caring for immersion foot, handle the area

Figure 24–7 A sign of immersion foot includes swollen, waxy feet.

gently and warm it slowly. Raise the foot (or feet) and continue to monitor the person as well as the affected area.

RADIO MEDICAL ADVICE

As a general rule, procedures beyond your training and ability as a marine first aid attendant should not be attempted. However, you should be aware that medical advice is available, especially in cases in which more advanced medical procedures are required. Medical advice can be accessed through a doctor by:

• Cellphone;

• Direct radiotelephone contact with a shore radio station using a prearranged radio frequency (e.g., Rescue Coordination Centre [RCC]/Maritime Rescue Sub-Centres [MRSC] or the Marine Communications and Traffic Services Centre [MCTS]). You should request to speak to a doctor; or

• Contacting a nearby port or nearby ship with a doctor on board. The advice received from a medical advisor will depend on the severity of the situation and the appropriate supplies and medical personnel available on board the ship. You should prepare for the medical advice by having the list of medications and supplies carried on hand during the call.

Preparing Information for Radio Medical Advice

When seeking radio medical advice, provide as much information as possible to the medical advisor. Remember to repeat the information back to the advisor to ensure that the information exchanged is accu-

rate. You may want to record the exchange on tape to help clarify any written notes.

Prior to seeking radio medical advice, you should prepare key information about your ship, the ill or injured person, and treatment rendered (Table 24–5).

Radiotelephone Procedures

Transport Canada provides a reference regarding radiotelephone procedures (TP 9878E: Safety and Distress Radiotelephone Procedures), which should be displayed next to your vessel's radiotelephone. The procedures in this reference advise that safety and distress radio messages should be made on Channel 16 (156.8 MHz) or on frequency 2,182 kHz, MF.

> **NOTE:**
>
> *For medical-legal purposes, remember to transcribe your notes regarding the instructions given and the medical actions taken on to the person's and ship's records. Always keep a copy of the records on board.*

The normal procedure to obtain radio medical advice is as follows:

1. Make contact with the shore radio station and request medical advice (Figure 24–8).

2. Give the doctor all the information you can so that a medical assessment of the situation can be made.

3. The doctor will give advice on the immediate care of the person.

> **NOTE:**
>
> *The phonetic alphabet (see Appendix C) may be useful in conveying information such as call signs or to clarify a person's medical condition or the name of a medication.*

4. After the link call is over, the doctor will advise the Search and Rescue (SAR) authority or coast guard service (e.g., RCC) on the best method of evacuation.

5. If helicopter evacuation is determined desirable, the coast guard will keep in touch with the ship.

TABLE 24–5: FORMS TO BE USED IN COMMUNICATING TO A DOCTOR INFORMATION ABOUT A PERSON'S ILLNESS (PART A) OR INJURY (PART B)[36]

(A) IN THE CASE OF ILLNESS

1. *Routine information about the ship*

    1.1   Name of ship

    1.2   Call sign

    1.3   Date and time (GMT)

    1.4   Course, speed, position, and cargo

    1.5.1   Port of destination _____

    which is _____ hours/days away

    1.5.2   Nearest port _____

    which is _____ hours/days away

    1.5.3   Alternative port _____

    which is _____ hours/days away

    1.6   Local weather (if relevant)

2. *Routine information about the person*

    2.1   Surname

    2.2   Other names

    2.3   Rank

    2.4   Job on board (specify kind of work, not just the trade)

    2.5   Age and sex

3. *Details of illness*

    3.1   When did the illness first begin?

    3.2   Has the illness occurred before? If so, when?

    3.3   How did the illness begin (suddenly, slowly, etc.).

    3.4   What did the person first complain of?

    3.5   List all the person's complaints and symptoms.

    3.6   Describe the course of the present illness from the start of the illness to the present time.

    3.7   Give details of past illnesses/injuries/operations.

    3.8   List serious illnesses of parents, brothers, sisters, if known (family history).

    3.9   List social pursuits and previous occupations, including hobbies (social and occupational history).

3.10   List all medicines/tablets/drugs that the person was taking *before the present illness began* and indicate the dose(s) and frequency of administration.

3.11   Does the person smoke? If so, how much and how often?

3.12   Does the person drink alcohol? If so, how much (on how many days a week, on average, and how many drinks a day, on average)?

3.13   Does the person take any herbal or folk medicines? If so, how are they taken?

3.14   Does the person use recreational drugs? If so, how are they taken?

4. *Results of examination of person*

4.1   Note temperature, pulse, blood pressure, and respiration.

4.2   Describe the general appearance of the person (healthy, obviously ill, pale, etc.)

4.3   Describe the appearance of affected parts of the body (consider faxing or emailing a digital photograph).

4.4   Describe your observations about the affected parts of the body (swelling, tenderness, lack of movement, etc.).

4.5.1   What tests have you done (urine, blood, other) and what were the results?

4.5.2   Give the results, if available, of any previous blood tests, X-rays, or other investigations.

5. *Diagnosis*

5.1   What is your diagnosis?

6. *Treatment*

6.1   Describe care you have administered since the illness began.

6.2   List ALL medicines/tablets/drugs that the person has taken or been given, and indicate the dose(s), the number of times given, and frequency of administration.

6.3   How has the person responded to the treatment?

7. *Problems*

7.1   What problems are worrying you now?

7.2   What do you need advice about?

8. *Other comments*

9. *Comments by the doctor*

(B) IN THE CASE OF INJURY

1. *Routine information about the ship*

1.1   Name of ship

1.2   Call sign

1.3   Date and time (GMT)

1.4   Course, speed, position, and cargo

1.5.1   Port of destination _____

         which is _____ hours/days away

1.5.2   Nearest port _____

         which is_____hours/days away

1.5.3   Alternative port _____

         which is _____ hours/days away

1.6   Local weather (if relevant)

2.   *Routine information about the person*

2.1   Surname

2.2   Other names

2.3   Rank

2.4   Job on board (specify kind of work, not just the trade)

2.5   Age and sex

3.   *History of the injury or injuries*

3.1   Exactly how did the injury or injuries occur?

3.2   Did the person lose any blood? If so, how much?

3.3   When did the injury or injuries occur?

3.4   How long before the incident did the person last eat or drink?

3.5   What does the person complain of? (List the complaints in order of importance or severity.)

3.6   List all past illnesses/injuries/operations.

3.7   List all medicines/tablets/drugs that the person was taking *before the present injury or injuries occurred*, indicate the dose(s) and frequency of administration.

3.8   Has the person been taking any alcohol?

3.9   Do you think the person might have taken narcotic drugs, amphetamine, etc?

3.10   Does the person remember everything that happened? If not, how long before the accident is his last clear memory?

3.11   Did the person lose consciousness, even for a very short time? If so, for how long and when in relation to the injury?

4. *Results of examination of person*

    4.1   Note temperature, pulse, blood pressure, and respiration.

    4.2   Describe the general condition of the person.

    4.3   List what you believe to be the person's injuries in order of importance and severity.

    4.5.1   What tests have you done (urine, blood, other) and what were the results?

    4.5.2   Give the results, if available, of any previous blood tests, X-rays, or other investigations.

5. *Treatment*

    5.1   Describe care you have administered since the injury or injuries occurred.

    5.2   List ALL medicines/tablets/drugs that the person has taken or been given, and indicate the dose(s), the number of times given, and frequency of administration.

    5.3   How has the person responded to the treatment?

6. *Problems*

    6.1   What problems are worrying you now?

    6.2   What do you need advice about?

7. *Other comments*

8. *Comments by the doctor*

Figure 24–8 Obtaining radio medical advice.

Communication With Doctors

A written letter or form should always accompany any person seeing a doctor. A clearly written communication in a foreign language is sometimes better understood than a spoken one (see Table 24–6).

TRANSFER AND TRANSPORT

Medical Evacuation From a Ship

People who require rapid transport to a hospital facility due to severe trauma or medical emergency are indications for medical evacuation from a ship.

Evacuation by Helicopter

Once helicopter evacuation is determined to be necessary, the following measures should be taken:

TABLE 24–6: MEDICAL REPORT FORMS FOR SEAFARERS[37]

Ship Master's Report Form

Date of report _____

* *

Ship's Identity and Navigation Status

Name _____

Owner _____

Name and address of on-shore agent _____

_____

Position (latitude, longitude) at onset of illness _____

Destination and ETA (expected time of arrival) _____

_____

* *

The Person and the Medical Problem

Surname and first name _____

Sex _____ Male ☐ Female ☐

Date of birth (dd-mm-yyyy) _____

Nationality _____

Seafarer registration number _____

Shipboard job title _____

Hour and date when taken off work _____

Hour and date when returned to work _____

* *

Injury or Illness

Hour and date of injury or onset of illness _____

Hour and date of first examination or treatment _____

Location on ship where injury occurred _____

Circumstances of injury _____

_____

Symptoms _____

Findings of physical examination _____

_____

Findings of X-ray or laboratory tests _____

Overall clinical impression before treatment _____

_____

Treatment given on board _____

_____

Overall clinical impression after treatment _____

_____

* *

Telemedical Consultation (on-line medical control)

Hour and date of initial contact _____

Mode of communication (radio, telephone, fax, other) _____

Surname and first name of telemedical consultant _____

Details of telemedical advice given _____

_____

* *

N.B. Attach all relevant medical reports to this report form.

Person Health Status Form

(To accompany person being evacuated)

Surname and first name _____

Age (years) _____

Sex _____

Time (hour) and date _____

Vital signs _____

        Blood pressure (systolic/diastolic) _____

        Pulse (beats/min) _____

        Body temperature (oral), note F or C _____

Presenting medical problem: symptoms, site(s) of pain or injury, time of onset, duration of problem, contributing factors _____

_____

_____

Treatment given (medication, dressings, etc.) _____

_____

Telemedical advice (on-line medical control) received _____

_____

Other current medical problems _____

_____

Past history of significant medical problems _____

_____

Current medication being taken (generic and brand names; dosage; time of last dose)

_____

- Give the ship's position, description, and details of the person's condition.

- Advise the bridge and engine room watches that someone should maintain direct communication with the helicopter.

- If direct communication with the helicopter cannot be made, send a message via a shore radio station or coast guard station (on 2,182 kHz, MF or on VHF) and follow all instructions provided.

- Clear as large an area as possible on the deck and mark the area in white with a large letter "H" to identify the "hoist area." If possible, whip and wire aerials in and around the area should be taken down.

- Ensure that all loose articles are securely tied.

- In heavy shipping areas, it is helpful to identify the ship to the flight crew with a signal (orange-coloured smoke, for example, which is often used in lifeboats).

- Never hook the hoist cable of the helicopter to any part of the ship.

- A helicopter can build up a significant charge of static electricity, so the winch wire should be handled only by personnel wearing rubber gloves.

- If the hoist is being carried out at night, point search lights vertically upward as aid in locating the ship. Light the pick-up area as much as possible. Be sure not to blind the pilot by shining any lights directly on the helicopter.

- Obey the helicopter crew instructions at all times.

NOTE:

See Chapter 23 for information on preparing a person for transfer, and ship-to-ship transfer.

PHARMACOLOGY

Medications and Health Supplies Carried on Board

In the *International Medical Guide for Ships, 3rd Edition* (2007), the World Health Organization (WHO) recommends a list of medications and health supplies to be carried on board for the ship's medicine chest (see Table 24–7). The quantities of medications recommended depend on the:

- Type of vessel

- Length of time the vessel may be away from port or port of call

- Size of the crew complement

Medical supplies and medications are most likely located in the ship's sick bay (ship's hospital). Cabinets and drawers in the sick bay should hold a working quantity of the recommended medications and should be clearly labelled. The contents of the ship's medicine chest should be inspected annually by a pharmacist.

NOTE:

Drug administration requires specialized training and is intended for those who provide advanced medical care. The following section, which describes medications found on ships, and their side effects, is intended to provide a basic overview only.

Drugs Requiring Medical Advice

Safe drug therapy requires clear communication between the ill or injured person and medical professionals. In some situations, first aid attendants must access radio medical advice before administering medication (see "Radio Medical Advice" in this chapter). For example, nitroglycerin spray (Figure 24–9) is a medication restricted to "on the advice of a doctor" in DFO/5758. The *International Medical Guide for Ships, 3rd Edition* (2007) gives advice on other specific

Figure 24–9 Nitroglycerin spray is one of the medications requiring medical advice.

medications, with precautions stating, "Give only on radio medical advice from a doctor"; "Should the patient be allergic to the drug, radio medical advice should be obtained for an alternative anti-infective treatment"; or "Do not administer this drug before obtaining radio medical advice." In a marine environment, refer to the drug guide stored on your ship or check with local standards and protocols for clarification. For some medications, first aid attendants are likely to assist a person in taking medications from his own supply. Assisting a person with his medications includes:

- Finding the medication bottle

- Getting water for pills

- Helping the person hold a glass or read a label

Use (Indications) and Precautions (Contraindications and Side Effects)

Indications, side effects, and contraindications are essential characteristics of each medication. The name, strength, dose, and directions are printed on the label of each drug container. In a marine environment, the *International Medical Guide for Ships, 3rd Edition* (2007) provides a drug guide in the following format for each medicine: dosage, indications, contraindications, and side effects.

Before taking a medication, read the precaution(s) (contraindications and side effects) and note(s) relating to

---

NOTE:

The marine first aid attendant cannot give medications directly to the person.

---

each drug. If a side effect from a drug is pronounced, seek medical advice regarding appropriate care for the person.

The process for drug administration includes:

- Assessing a person, both before and after a medication is taken

- Knowing the drug use

- Knowing the precautions of the drug

- Obtaining authorization to administer the drug

Assess signs and symptoms as well as vital signs, and find out if the person has allergies, medical conditions, and medications. This is to determine if the person has a condition for which a medication might be helpful. The first aid attendant may also find situations in which the person cannot take the medication (precautions, e.g., no nitroglycerin if the person has taken an erectile dysfunction drug such as Viagra® or Levitra® in the past 24 hours or Cialis® in the past 48 hours). Once you determine that an intervention with a medication may be required, you should obtain authorization for administering the drug by contacting a medical advisor for direction.

TABLE 24–7: WORLD HEALTH ORGANIZATION (WHO) LIST OF MEDICINES RECOMMENDED FOR THE SHIP'S MEDICINE CHEST[38]

Generic name	Acetylsalicylic acid
Dosage form, strength	tablet 300 mg
Indications (on board ship)	high dose (600–900 mg); to reduce pain, fever, inflammation
	low dose (100–150 mg) to inhibit formation of blood clots in angina pectoris, myocardial infarction, stroke
Contraindications	peptic ulcer, history of gastrointestinal bleeding, hemophilia, fever in people under 18, trauma
Unwanted effects	indigestion
	gastric bleeding
	increased bleeding during surgery

Generic name	Aciclovir
Dosage form, strength	tablet 400 mg
Indications (on board ship)	treatment of primary or recurrent herpes simplex virus infection
	may be useful for severe varicella and herpes zoster (doctor should be consulted)
Contraindications	ND
Unwanted effects	ND

Generic name	Adrenaline
Dosage form, strength	ampoule 1 mL = 1 mg
Indications (on board ship)	to raise blood pressure in anaphylaxis
	to dilate airways in severe asthma or anaphylaxis
Contraindications	none in emergencies
Unwanted effects	palpitations
	cardiac dysrhythmia
	hypertension
	chest pain
	headache
	restlessness

Generic name	Amethocaine 0.5% eye drops
Dosage form, strength	single-use vial 1 mL
Indications (on board ship)	for eye examination and procedures
Contraindications	ND
Unwanted effects	transitory burning sensation soon after application

Generic name	Amoxicillin + Clavulanate
Dosage form, strength	tablet 875 mg + 125 mg
Indications (on board ship)	to treat infections responsive to this antibiotic
Contraindications	allergy to penicillin and beta-lactam antibiotics
	glandular fever (infectious mononucleosis)
	liver disease
Unwanted effects	diarrhea
	hepatitis due to clavulanate is rare but may be serious

Generic name	Artemether
Dosage form, strength	ampoule 1 mL = 80 mg
Indications (on board ship)	treatment of severe malaria
Contraindications	ND
Unwanted effects	pain at injection site

slow pulse rate

seizures

Generic name	Artemether + Lumefantrine
Dosage form, strength	tablet 20 mg + 120 mg
Indications (on board ship)	treatment of malaria
Contraindications	not to be used in women in early pregnancy without medical advice
Unwanted effects	headache
	dizziness
	sleep disorder
	palpitations
	anorexia
	nausea
	vomiting
	diarrhea
	itch
	rash
	arthralgia (joint pain)
	myalgia (muscle pain)
	weakness
	fatigue

Generic name	Atropine
Dosage form, strength	ampoule 1.2 mg/mL
Indications (on board ship)	to treat slow heart rate in myocardial infarction
	to treat organophosphate insecticide poisoning
Contraindications	none in emergencies
Unwanted effects	dry mouth
	blurred vision
	urinary retention
	hallucinations and psychosis (with very large doses)

Generic name	Azithromycin
Dosage form, strength	tablet 500 mg
Indications (on board ship)	to treat infections responsive to this antibiotic
Contraindications	allergy to erythromycin or similar (macrolide) antibiotics
Unwanted effects	diarrhea
	vomiting
	stomach pain

Generic name	Ceftriaxone
Dosage form, strength	ampoule 1 g powder for injection (dissolve in water for injection)
Indications (on board ship)	to treat infections responsive to this antibiotic
Contraindications	allergy to cephalosporin or penicillin antibiotics
Unwanted effects	diarrhea
	pain at injection site
	formation of biliary sludge and kidney stones
Generic name	Cetirizine
Dosage form, strength	tablet 10 mg
Indications (on board ship)	to treat allergy symptoms in hay fever, hives, allergic dermatitis, etc.
Contraindications	allergy to cetirizine
Unwanted effects	drowsiness (in 10–15% of cases)
	dry mouth
	headache
	nausea
Generic name	Charcoal, activated
Dosage form, strength	50 g in 300 mL purified water
Indications (on board ship)	to absorb ingested poisons
Contraindications	bowel obstruction
Unwanted effects	abdominal pain
	vomiting
	constipation
Generic name	Ciprofloxacin
Dosage form, strength	tablet 250 mg
Indications (on board ship)	to treat infections responsive to this antibiotic
Contraindications	allergy to quinolones
Unwanted effects	vomiting
	diarrhea
	depression
	ankle pain
	makes sunburn worse
	may increase the effect of caffeine, with headache, palpitations, and nausea
Generic name	Cloves, oil of
Dosage form, strength	oil
Indications (on board ship)	toothache
Contraindications	ND

Unwanted effects	irritation of the mucous membranes
Generic name	Dexamethasone
Dosage form, strength	ampoule 4 mg/mL
Indications (on board ship)	to treat life-threatening and severe asthma
	to treat anaphylaxis
	to treat severe allergic reactions
Contraindications	none in emergencies
Unwanted effects	with repeated doses exacerbates peptic ulcer
	euphoria or depression
	exacerbates diabetes mellitus
Generic name	Diazepam
Dosage form, strength	tablet 5 mg
Indications (on board ship)	to treat alcohol withdrawal
Contraindications	severe respiratory disease
	opioid intoxication
	severe liver disease
	myasthenia gravis
Unwanted effects	drowsiness
	confusion
Generic name	Docusate + Senna (or equivalent)
Dosage form, strength	tablet 50 mg + 8 mg
Indications (on board ship)	to avoid straining in people with anal fissure and hemorrhoids
	to prevent constipation caused by opioid use
Contraindications	suspected bowel obstruction
	inflammatory bowel disease
	appendicitis
Unwanted effects	flatulence
	abdominal cramps (rare)
	diarrhea
Generic name	Doxycycline
Dosage form, strength	tablet 100 mg
Indications (on board ship)	as recommended in IMGS3 for the specific infection
Contraindications	allergy to tetracyclines
	severe liver disease
	not to be used in children under eight years of age or pregnant women
Unwanted effects	vomiting

diarrhea

makes sunburn worse

ulceration of the esophagus (rare)

Generic name	Ethanol 70%, hand cleanser gel
Dosage form, strength	gel
Indications (on board ship)	an alternative to handwashing when hands are not obviously soiled
Contraindications	soiled hands
Unwanted effects	dryness, but less than with soap and water

Generic name	Ethanol 70%, liquid
Dosage form, strength	liquid
Indications (on board ship)	to disinfect instruments and surfaces
Contraindications	ND
Unwanted effects	ND

Generic name	Fluorescein 1%, strips
Dosage form, strength	ND
Indications (on board ship)	to detect damage to cornea: damaged area stains yellow/green
Contraindications	ND
Unwanted effects	ND

Generic name	Furosemide
Dosage form, strength	ampoule 4 mL = 40 mg
Indications (on board ship)	to treat severe fluid retention in lungs (pulmonary edema) due to cardiac failure
Contraindications	none in an emergency
Unwanted effects	dehydration
	loss of potassium
	hearing loss if given too quickly IV

Generic name	Glucagon, ready to use
Dosage form, strength	ampoule 1 mg
Indications (on board ship)	to treat low blood sugar (hypoglycemia) due to insulin when oral intake is impossible and intravenous glucose cannot be given
Contraindications	ND
Unwanted effects	ND

Generic name	Haloperidol
Dosage form, strength	ampoule 1 mL = 5 mg
Indications (on board ship)	to treat psychotic hallucinations and delusions
	to treat severe agitation and aggressiveness

Contraindications	coma of whatever cause
	severe alcohol intoxication
Unwanted effects	drowsiness
	low blood pressure
	confusion
	dry mouth
	urine retention

Generic name	Hydrocortisone 1% cream
Dosage form, strength	cream
Indications (on board ship)	to treat allergy and some other inflammatory skin conditions
Contraindications	open wounds or skin infections caused by bacteria, viruses or fungi
Unwanted effects	minimal with short-term use
	thinning of skin with long-term use

Generic name	Ibuprofen
Dosage form, strength	coated tablet 400 mg
Indications (on board ship)	to treat inflammation
	to reduce mild-to-moderate pain, especially if associated with inflammation
Contraindications	peptic ulcer
	gastrointestinal bleeding
	kidney failure
	liver failure
	history of exacerbation of asthma after taking aspirin
Unwanted effects	stomach pain
	vomiting
	diarrhea
	headache
	edema
	hypertension

Generic name	Isosorbide dinitrate
Dosage form, strength	tablet 5 mg
Indications (on board ship)	to treat angina pectoris
	to treat myocardial infarction
Contraindications	hypotension
	known heart valve disease
	head injury
	treatment with sildenafil (Viagra®) and similar drugs

Unwanted effects	headache
	flushing
	dizziness or fainting
	palpitations
Generic name	Lidocaine 1% (without adrenaline)
Dosage form, strength	ampoule 5 mL
Indications (on board ship)	for local anaesthesia when suturing wounds or performing minor surgery
Contraindications	allergy to local anaesthetics
Unwanted effects	stinging on injection
Generic name	Loperamide
Dosage form, strength	tablet 2 mg
Indications (on board ship)	to treat symptoms of diarrhea
Contraindications	bowel obstruction
	dysentery
	acute ulcerative colitis
Unwanted effects	abdominal pain
	bloating
	constipation
Generic name	Mebendazole
Dosage form, strength	tablet 100 mg
Indications (on board ship)	to treat intestinal worm infections
	not effective for tapeworm infection or hydatid disease
Contraindications	allergy to mebendazole
Unwanted effects	diarrhea
	stomach pain
Generic name	Metoprolol
Dosage form, strength	tablet 100 mg
Indications (on board ship)	to treat hypertension
	to treat atrial fibrillation
	to treat angina pectoris
	to prevent migraine
Contraindications ·	asthma
	shock
	heart rate less than 50 beats/min
	cardiac failure
Unwanted effects	tiredness

light-headedness

cold hands and feet

slow heart rate

shortness of breath

wheezing

fainting due to low blood pressure

Generic name	Metronidazole
Dosage form, strength	tablet 500 mg
Indications (on board ship)	to treat infections responsive to this antibiotic
Contraindications	allergy to metronidazole
Unwanted effects	metallic taste in the mouth
	nausea
	vomiting
	diarrhea
	nerve damage (rare)

Generic name	Miconazole 2% cream
Dosage form, strength	cream
Indications (on board ship)	to treat fungal skin infections
Contraindications	allergy to miconazole
Unwanted effects	ND

Generic name	Midazolam
Dosage form, strength	ampoule 1 mL = 5 mg
Indications (on board ship)	to terminate epileptic seizures
Contraindications	ND
Unwanted effects	sedation

Generic name	Misoprostol
Dosage form, strength	tablet 200 mg
Indications (on board ship)	to prevent post-partum hemorrhage
Contraindications	none if given according to IMGS3 recommendations
Unwanted effects	diarrhea

Generic name	Morphine (injectable)
Dosage form, strength	ampoule 1 mL = 10 mg
Indications (on board ship)	to reduce severe pain
	to reduce pain not relieved by other analgesics
Contraindications	coma, unless the person is dying of a clearly documented illness, such as cancer

	severe liver disease
	asthma
	severe respiratory disease except pneumonia or pleurisy associated with severe pain
	to be used with caution in people known to have epilepsy, head injury, acute alcohol intoxication, withdrawal, shock (of whatever cause)
Unwanted effects	sedation
	confusion
	nausea
	vomiting
	low blood pressure
	respiratory depression
	small pupils
	constipation

Generic name	Morphine (oral)
Dosage form, strength	liquid 1 mg/mL
Indications (on board ship)	to reduce severe pain likely to last several days in people able to eat and drink
Contraindications	as for morphine given by injection
Unwanted effects	as for morphine given by injection

Generic name	Naloxone
Dosage form, strength	ampoule 1 mL = 0.4 mg
Indications (on board ship)	to reverse effects of opioids, especially in cases of overdose
Contraindications	ND
Unwanted effects	ND

Generic name	Omeprazole
Dosage form, strength	tablet 20 mg
Indications (on board ship)	to treat gastro-esophageal reflux
	to treat peptic ulcer disease
Contraindications	ND
Unwanted effects	nausea
	diarrhea

Generic name	Ondansetron
Dosage form, strength	tablet 4 mg
Indications (on board ship)	to prevent vomiting
	to prevent seasickness

Contraindications	ND
Unwanted effects	headache
	fatigue
	constipation

Generic name	Oral rehydration salts
Dosage form, strength	sachets of powder for reconstitution
Indications (on board ship)	to prevent or treat dehydration, especially due to diarrhea
Contraindications	ND
Unwanted effects	vomiting

Generic name	Oxymetazoline 0.5% (or equivalent)
Dosage form, strength	drops
Indications (on board ship)	to treat nasal obstruction due to allergies or viral infection
	to improve sinus drainage in sinusitis
Contraindications	use of anti-depressants
Unwanted effects	stinging or burning in nose or throat
	dry nasal mucosa
	rebound obstruction

Generic name	Paracetamol (acetaminophen)
Dosage form, strength	tablet 500 mg
Indications (on board ship)	to reduce pain and fever (but not inflammation)
Contraindications	liver disease
Unwanted effects	rare at normal doses

Generic name	Permethrin 1% lotion
Dosage form, strength	lotion
Indications (on board ship)	to eliminate hair, pubic, and body lice
Contraindications	ND
Unwanted effects	increased likelihood of skin irritation in cases of scabies

Generic name	Permethrin 5% lotion
Dosage form, strength	lotion
Indications (on board ship)	to treat scabies
Contraindications	ND
Unwanted effects	increased likelihood of skin irritation

Generic name	Povidone iodine ointment 10% and solution 10%
Dosage form, strength	ointment, liquid
Indications (on board ship)	to disinfect skin and wounds

Contraindications	allergy to iodine
Unwanted effects	skin irritation

Generic name	Prednisone
Dosage form, strength	tablet 25 mg
Indications (on board ship)	to treat severe asthma
	to treat other inflammatory conditions (on medical advice)
Contraindications	ND
Unwanted effects	exacerbates diabetes mellitus, depression or euphoria

Generic name	Salbutamol aerosol
Dosage form, strength	inhaler 0.1 mg/dose with volume spacer
Indications (on board ship)	to treat asthma
	to treat chronic bronchitis
	to treat emphysema
	to treat other lung diseases
Contraindications	ND
Unwanted effects	dry mouth
	throat irritation
	tremor
	nervousness
	dizziness
	excitement
	rapid heartbeat
	headache

Generic name	Sodium chloride 0.9% infusion
Dosage form, strength	plastic bottle 1 litre
Indications (on board ship)	for fluid replacement
Contraindications	ND
Unwanted effects	cardiac overload and pulmonary edema if large doses are administered at a high flow rate

Generic name	Tetracycline 1% ointment
Dosage form, strength	ointment
Indications (on board ship)	to treat minor eye infections
	to prevent infection following damage to the cornea
Contraindications	allergy to tetracyclines
Unwanted effects	ND

Generic name	Vitamin K
Dosage form, strength	ampoule 1 mL = 10 mg
Indications (on board ship)	to reverse excessive or unwanted effect of warfarin or related drugs
Contraindications	ND
Unwanted effects	pain at the injection site if given IM
	anaphylaxis, if given IV

Generic name	Water for injection
Dosage form, strength	ampoule 5 mL
Indications (on board ship)	reconstitution of injectable drugs provided as powders
Contraindications	ND
Unwanted effects	ND

Generic name	Zidovudine + Lamivudine
Dosage form, strength	tablet 300 mg + 150 mg
Indications (on board ship)	prophylaxis against HIV infection after needle-stick injury
Contraindications	allergy to either component
	pre-existing HIV infection
Unwanted effects	Common: headache, fatigue and malaise, insomnia, nausea, vomiting, diarrhea or constipation, cough, loss of appetite, muscle soreness or weakness
	Uncommon but potentially serious: low white blood cell count, anemia, hepatitis, severe muscle weakness, pancreatitis

Generic name	Zinc oxide
Dosage form, strength	paste or ointment 20%
Indications (on board ship)	protection of irritated skin
Contraindications	ND
Unwanted effects	soiling of clothes

Notes: • Medicines are listed in alphabetical order based on their generic name.

• The choice of medications recommended in this table is based on effect, unwanted effects, route of administration, shelf life, worldwide availability, price, storage conditions, and the medical skills officers on board are presumed to possess.

• A doctor needs to give permission to administer these medications, and will recommend dosages and frequency depending on the seriousness of the person's symptoms.
ND = not determined

SUMMARY

Providing care on a ship brings special challenges, and marine first aid attendants require specialized training for the medical care of seafarers. This care covers a range of skills, in particular for administering oxygen, using airway adjuncts such as endotracheal intubation, administering medications, understanding hazardous materials, and working in confined spaces. It is important to be familiar with the equipment and safety precautions required for these specialized procedures.

You may be called upon to provide care for a rescued person who has suffered a drowning incident, hypothermia, or other illness or injury. Providing first aid treatment on a survival craft can present situations not encountered on land. You may also need to know how to radio for medical help or prepare someone for transfer to another ship or a helicopter.

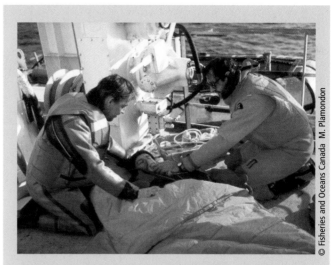

Once back on board he is sluggish and is having problems taking a deep breath without coughing. What do you do?

Chapter 25

Workplace

You are at a demolition site, where your crew has been working for the past three weeks. You hear yelling. Your supervisor runs up to you, shouting for you to come quickly—there's an emergency. The crew had been setting off explosives, but one of the explosives detonated early. A section of the building collapsed, crushing the legs of one of your co-workers. What do you do?

INTRODUCTION

Some of the most serious injuries occur at workplaces because of the equipment involved and/or the nature of the work being performed. Emergencies happen in all kinds of workplace settings—industrial work sites, agricultural operations, construction sites, remote locations such as in forestry and mining industries, and even office environments. Most workplaces are required by law to have first aid attendants. When you are employed as a workplace first aid attendant, you have the duty to act. Regulations require you to provide care to the level of your training and to document all incidents appropriately.

Your knowledge of what to do and your ability to react quickly can make a difference for an ill or injured employee. Applying your knowledge and expertise will help promote a safe and healthy workplace.

ROLES AND RESPONSIBILITIES OF THE FIRST AID ATTENDANT

Workplace first aid is first aid performed in the workplace by a designated person, the first aid attendant. The first aid attendant must be familiar with workplace occupational health and safety regulations in his jurisdiction and be an employee with a recognized first aid certificate in good standing from a recognized training agency. The first aid attendant is an essential part of first aid services in the workplace under health and safety regulations.

The first aid attendant must:

• Maintain his knowledge and skills.

• Be prepared to respond both alone and as part of a first aid team.

• Provide all care in a professional manner.

• Provide care within the scope of his training.

• Document thoroughly any first aid-related actions and process paperwork according to legislative requirements (Figure 25–1).

• Report to the supervisor and joint health and safety committee as required.

• Conduct follow-up with the ill or injured person approximately three days after the person returns to work.

• Be familiar with specific elements of the particular work site, including:

■ The first aid room, rescue vehicles, and first aid equipment

■ Work site entry and exit areas

■ Specific hazards and precautions related to the work site

■ Legislative regulations

■ Means of communication (e.g., radio system, satellite phone)

■ Emergency phone numbers

RESPONSIBILITIES OF THE EMPLOYER AND OTHER EMPLOYEES

An employer and employees are responsible for ensuring that care in an emergency is provided in a timely manner. Everyone on the work site should know how to access first aid assistance, including:

• The location of the first aid room

• How to contact the first aid attendant

• The location of first aid kits and other equipment (e.g., AED)

Figure 25–1 First aid attendants must document all first aid-related actions.

Return-to-Work Protocol

Each person has the right to choose to either return to work immediately after an illness or injury or to seek further medical attention. (This is a decision to be made by the ill or injured person based on recommendations by the first aid attendant.) Supervisors cannot override the decision of the first aid attendant with respect to treatment of an ill or injured person.

Regardless of the incident and whether or not the employee returns to work or seeks advanced medical care, documentation must be thorough and in accordance with legislative requirements. Across the country, different jurisdictions may have specific forms. First aid attendants must be familiar with legislative and employer requirements regarding documentation.

WORKPLACE EQUIPMENT

Workplace first aid attendants will likely have access to most of the equipment described throughout *Emergency Care*, however, here are exceptions. Workplace first aid attendants may not be required to assess blood pressure or may not have access to certain commercial products, such as a K.E.D.® or head immobilization devices for spinal precautions. As a workplace first aid attendant, it is important to be familiar with the equipment at each workplace and to consider alternative means of applying skills such as using a blanket roll instead of a commercial head immobilization device.

Some workplaces, depending on their size, the location, and the industry, may be required to have an emergency transport vehicle (ETV) to transport ill or injured people. An ETV is a dedicated vehicle that is available during emergencies and can arrive on site in three to five minutes.

There should be employees who can drive the ETV in the event that the first aid attendant is providing care. It is recommended that each ETV:

- Be capable of traversing the area it is intended to serve

- Has headspace of at least one metre (three feet)

- Provide protection from the elements (e.g., dust, sun, extreme temperatures, etc.)

- Has effective communication between driver and first aid attendant, as well as the vehicle and the hospital/medical direction

- Conform to any legislative requirements where it is operating

REGULATIONS AND DOCUMENTATION

Workplace Occupational Health and Safety Regulations

The Canadian Centre for Occupational Health and Safety (CCOHS) states that all Canadians have a fundamental right to a healthy and safe working environment.[39] It explains that a health and safety program is a plan of action designed to prevent injuries and illness at work, and that it is required under Occupational Health & Safety (OH&S) legislation in most Canadian jurisdictions.[40]

Part of such programs are regulations that outline the first aid requirements on a work site. Each province and territory of Canada interprets workplace health and safety regulations differently. In addition, there are regulations that apply to the federal government and other national organizations.

Employers are required to have a minimum number of first aid attendants on the work site at all times. The level of first aid training and the number of first aid attendants required are determined by the size and type of workplace. Workplace first aid attendants must be familiar with the legislation governing the jurisdiction in which they are employed.

> **NOTE:**
>
> *To better understand the regulations governing training levels and mandatory first aid equipment, contact or refer to the website of your legislative workers' compensation body (e.g., WorkSafe BC) or visit the Canadian Red Cross website at www.redcross.ca for more information.*

Workplace Hazardous Materials Information System

The Workplace Hazardous Materials Information System (WHMIS) is Canada's national hazard communication standard. The key elements of the system are cautionary labelling of hazardous materials, the provision of Material Safety Data Sheets (MSDSs), and worker education and training programs.

The federal *Hazardous Products Act* established the national standard for chemical classification and hazard communication in Canada and is the foundation for the workers' "right-to-know" legislation enacted in every province and territory. This single national system for mobile labour forces also minimized confusion and facilitated implementation of the system.[41]

WHMIS will be changing to the Globally Harmonized System (GHS) of Classification and Labelling of Chemicals. GHS is an international (as opposed to national) class identification system that provides employers and workers with information about the hazardous materials they work with. The GHS was initiated at the Rio Earth Summit in 1992, when the United Nations Conference on Environment and Development agreed to develop "a globally harmonized hazard classification and compatible labelling system, including Material Safety Data Sheets and easily understandable symbols." This harmonization is intended to better protect both people and the environment.

The GHS will introduce some new terminology, including Safety Data Sheets (SDSs) instead of Material Safety Data Sheets (MSDSs), and pictograms, which are the hazard symbols on labels. Health Canada is working on implementing the GHS in Canada.[42]

Prevention of Injuries Due to Hazardous Materials in the Workplace

About one-quarter of all workers are exposed to chemical hazards in their workplace. According to WHMIS regulations, employers must:

- Clearly label hazardous materials, including all toxic substances.

- Tell employees about risks and precautions.

- Have a detailed MSDS available for every hazardous substance in the workplace.

- Give workers who may be exposed to hazardous materials the proper training in safety measures and emergency procedures (Figure 25–2).

Employees should:

- Check all warning labels, tags, and posters in the workplace and follow the instructions carefully.

- Read labels and MSDSs to find out the risks of each hazardous material, the safety measures to prevent poisoning, and first aid for poisoning.

- Never use a product that is in an unidentified container.

Note that many everyday substances can be hazardous in large enough quantities.

Documentation

It is important to document any actions taken when providing first aid for a workplace emergency. Whether an employee is returning to work or being referred for further

Figure 25–2 Workers who may be exposed to hazardous materials, such as chemicals, need training in safety measures.

medical attention, documentation must be completed. More than one type of form may be required. Regardless, good documentation will include the following:

- The name of the ill or injured person

- The date the report was filed

- The time that the report was received, the time the response was made, the time care was provided, and the time care was handed off to advanced medical personnel

- A description of how the illness or injury occurred

- A description of the illness or injury

- A detailed description of the care provided

- A description of any problems or shortcomings at the scene that may have contributed to the injury or illness

- A description of the outcome

- The signature of both the first aid attendant and the ill or injured person (if possible)

- A description of the follow-up with the ill or injured person (approximately three days after the person's return to work)

ACCESSING APPROPRIATE MEDICAL CARE

Canadian geography varies from east to west and north to south. Workplaces range from densely populated urban environments, where a call to EMS/9-1-1 sees paramedics arriving within a matter of minutes, to workplaces in remote locations requiring air transport to the nearest hospital or nursing station. In some cases, transportation may be delayed due to weather or other factors.

Workplace first aid attendants need to be prepared to provide care until such a time as the ill or injured person is handed over to personnel with more advanced training, be that at the hospital or in the area of EMS/9-1-1 service.

WORKPLACE EMERGENCIES

Because of the nature of the work performed, some of the most serious injuries occur at industrial and agricultural sites. You should be prepared to encounter crush injuries, avulsions, amputations, and other major open and closed soft tissue and musculoskeletal injuries.

Scene Survey

As always, size up the scene of an emergency before entering. Never enter if there is any risk to your safety. Look for hazards such as toxic chemicals, fires or fire hazards, unstable structures, running machinery, or unsecured livestock/animals. If necessary, call specialized personnel, such as the fire department, the Emergency Response Team (ERT), or a hazardous materials (haz-mat) removal team, to stabilize the scene before entering (Figure 25–3).

Be sure to observe lockout/tagout procedures. Lockout/ tagout refers to a set of procedures and practices that safeguard against the unexpected startup of machinery and equipment or the possible release of hazardous energy when machinery is being maintained. The individual using the machinery turns off and disconnects it from its energy source before performing maintenance, and an authorized employee either locks or tags the energy-isolating device to prevent unwanted release of energy.

Machinery that is on and/or that might be leaking fuel or hydraulic fluid should not be approached. An agricultural storage area or similar storage facilities should not be entered alone.

Figure 25–3 Call specialized personnel, such as a haz-mat removal team, to safely remove toxic chemicals.

Specific Hazards

Confined Spaces

Working in confined spaces is another safety concern. A confined space is one with restricted openings for entry and exit; poor ventilation with possible air contaminants; and physical hazards related to engulfment (being surrounded and overwhelmed by a substance such as soil or grain), or collapse (Figure 25–4). Such scenes might include pits, tunnels, storage tanks, sewers, ventilation and exhaust ducts, underground utility vaults, and pipelines.

It is important that responders who are required to enter a confined space follow certain guidelines. An emergency rescue involving entry into a confined space must never be attempted without training in safe confined space entry and rescue procedures. Assume a confined space is hazardous. A person qualified to enter a confined space must ensure that structures are safe from collapse prior to anyone entering the confined space.

A first aid attendant must be present immediately outside the space to provide help to the responder inside, and there must be a plan for emergency rescue. There must be a safe method of communication between the responder inside the space and the first aid attendant.

Appropriate PPE must be worn by the responder entering the confined space. Exact equipment is determined by the specific hazards encountered in the confined space (e.g., eye/face and head and foot protection, respiratory protection, safety belts, lifelines, and harnesses).

Once a confined space has been identified, warning signs should be posted and, when possible, the entry physically blocked. The conditions must be tested prior to the responder entering and continuously monitored during entry. Testing must be performed by someone who is properly trained and has the appropriate equipment; one's senses should never be trusted to determine if the air in a confined space is safe. Many toxic gases and vapours cannot be seen or smelled. This is also not a reliable way to determine if sufficient oxygen is present.

Adequate air conditions must be maintained in the confined space, through proper ventilation. If safe atmospheric conditions cannot be maintained, the absolute necessity of entering should be evaluated. If it is necessary to enter, an appropriate respirator must be worn, and this equipment must be evaluated by someone with the proper training to do so.

Properly trained workers must control utilities prior to entry into confined spaces, including, for example, electrical services, gas, propane, water, sanitary systems, communications, and any secondary service systems. If an unsafe condition develops, the space should be exited immediately.

Roadside Construction

Working in traffic control zones is high risk. Traffic control personnel (TCP) may be struck by motor vehicles that do not slow down in traffic control zones, leading to injury or even death.

Use TCP only when signs and other traffic control devices and procedures cannot provide effective traffic control or when emergency or brief work makes it impractical to control traffic with signs and other

Figure 25–4 A confined space has restricted openings for entry and exit.

devices and procedures. Assess the level of risk faced by the TCP in each situation. Consider traffic speed, direction, and volume as well as weather conditions and the time of day or night.

Plan and assess escape routes based on the traffic control layout but also on the time needed to jump safely out of the way if a vehicle does not stop as directed. Ensure that TCP stand in a safe position, are clearly visible, and have an unobstructed view of approaching traffic. A safe position is usually on the side of the shoulder of the road, out of the way of vehicles.

Ensure that TCP are trained to the required standard and have current qualifications.[43]

Remote Locations

Working in remote locations, for example, in mining or forestry, exposes workers to a variety of hazards. This "workplace" may include vast areas of terrain that may vary from mountainous to swampy conditions. Safety concerns encompass a wide range of considerations.

Workers need to consider rising water or flooding at times of high runoff; vulnerability to potential forest fires; avalanche, rockfall, or slide dangers; and tall or dead trees, especially dead branches that could fall into a campsite with strong winds or lightning strikes.

They must also think about safe drinking water, animal habits (e.g., bear encounters may be increased near old garbage dumps or camps, bear trails, spawning creeks, or berry patches) and camp size (i.e., whether the area is sufficient to carry out operations safely).[44]

Hazardous Materials Incidents

When approaching any scene, you should be aware of dangers involving chemicals. Whether a motor vehicle collision or an industrial emergency is involved, you should be able to recognize clues that indicate the presence of hazardous materials. These include:

- Signs (placards) on vehicles or storage facilities identifying the presence of hazardous materials
- Spilled liquids or solids
- Unusual odours

NOTE:

Transport Canada's 2012 Emergency Response Guidebook *helps first responders to quickly identify the hazardous materials in a transportation incident and protect themselves and the general public during the initial response phase of the incident.*

- Clouds of vapour
- Leaking containers

Placards, or signs, are required by law to be placed on any vehicles that contain specific quantities of hazardous materials (Figure 25–5). In addition, manufacturers and others associated with the production and distribution of these materials are required by law to display the appropriate placard. Placards often clearly identify the danger of the substance. Terms such as "explosive," "flammable," "corrosive," and "radioactive" are frequently used. Universally recognized symbols are also used.

Unless you have received special training in handling hazardous materials and have the necessary equipment, clothing, and PPE to deal with it without danger, you should stay well away from the area. Stay out of low areas where vapours and liquids may

Figure 25–5 A hazardous material placard.

collect. Stay upwind and uphill from the scene. Be alert for wind changes that could cause vapours to blow toward you. Do not attempt to enter a scene for which you are not trained or prepared for. It is not uncommon for even responding paramedics approaching the scene to recognize a hazardous materials placard and immediately move to a safe area and summon more advanced help.

Many fire departments have specially trained teams to handle incidents involving hazardous materials. While awaiting help, keep people away from the danger zone.

Hazardous materials are not found only in industrial sites. They are often transported by rail or truck and may be exposed when a vehicle turns over or is in a collision. Homes contain many hazardous materials, such as natural gas, gasoline, kerosene, and pesticides.

Some hazardous materials, such as natural gas, are flammable and can cause an explosion. Even turning on a light switch or using a telephone or radio may create a spark that sets off an explosion. When you call for help at a scene with suspected hazardous material, use a telephone or radio well clear of the scene.

Working with Equipment

Various injuries are associated with different types of machinery, and care for each involves a different approach. It is important to have a basic understanding of how each piece of equipment works and how it can harm a person in order to avoid injuries to yourself or further harm to the injured person.

Before trying to extricate a person from industrial/agricultural equipment, the equipment must be stabilized and shut down. If necessary, call a specialized crew to do this (Figure 25–6).

As a general principle, equipment can be stabilized by blocking or chocking the wheels, putting on the parking brake, or tying the equipment to another vehicle. The equipment should be shut down by entering the cab to access the main controls. The engine should be slowed down with the throttle and then the machine switched off using the ignition key. Some diesel-powered machines are shut down via an air shut-off lever rather than an ignition key.

The engine can also be shut off by shutting the fuel line. This is done using the shut-off valve at the bottom of the fuel tank or using vice-grip pliers. If a diesel engine cannot be shut down and the person is in a life-threatening situation, a 9-kilogram (20-pound) CO_2 fire extinguisher can be emptied into the air intake. This will shut down the engine but will also cause considerable damage to the engine.

Never touch a control on a piece of machinery unless you are sure you know what it does.

Chainsaws

Anyone working with chainsaws needs to understand how to control major bleeding and to deal with crush injuries, so it is recommended that operators hold an emergency first aid certificate. In remote sites, people who have been injured may also be at risk of hypothermia. Make sure operators always carry a personal first aid kit (that includes a large-wound dressing) with them and have reasonable access to a more comprehensive kit.

It is also important to consider the health risks chainsaws pose to operators due to high levels of noise and

Figure 25–6 If necessary, call specialized personnel, such as the fire department, to stabilize and shut down heavy equipment.

hand-arm vibration. These risks can be controlled by using low-noise/low-vibration chainsaws, providing suitable hearing protection, maintaining chainsaws and protective equipment, and providing operators with training on the health risks associated with operating chainsaws.[45]

Ride-on Rollers/Compactors

Those who work around or operate rollers/compactors face risks of injury related to a machine rollover or being struck by the machine or its components. Measures must be taken to prevent injury or death.

Develop site-specific safety plans for all aspects and stages of the job. Have plans analyzed by a qualified person to determine the safest possible methods to perform the work. Provide all workers on site with training in site-specific safety procedures and in hazards they may encounter at the site. Continually evaluate safety plans to address changing conditions at the work site.

Minimize the presence of workers on foot near machinery. Use barriers to separate workers, pedestrians, and vehicles from moving equipment. Provide appropriate protective equipment, such as high-visibility reflective vests and hard hats, and ensure that workers use and maintain them.

Ensure that machines are not operated on grades steeper than those specified by the manufacturer. Make sure that all the manufacturers' safety features are operational.[46]

Tractors/Forklifts

Be aware that tractors can be fuelled by diesel, gasoline, or propane, and that fuel leaks, fires, and explosions are a real possibility. Tractors often injure people by rolling over onto the rider. Do not approach the site until the tractor has been stabilized.

An injured person trapped by a tractor can be freed by digging a trench underneath the person's body or by cutting off a piece of the machine, such as the steering wheel. In some cases, however, the tractor may need to be lifted off the person by a specialized team.

Combines

Some common trouble spots on a combine include the auger, which is the rotating part of the screw conveyor; the heads, with their oscillating cutting bars; the reels, steel tines that can impale someone; and the snapping rollers, which can cause crush injuries (Figure 25–7).

The reverse feature should never be used in an attempt to extricate a person from a combine. The safest approach is to keep the machinery from moving, so pry bars and other tools should be used to jam the moving parts into place before beginning extrication. The hydraulic system must be locked. Usually a bar near the hydraulic cylinder will lock the header. If possible, the combine header should be divided from the drive mechanism. An acetylene torch can be used to cut pieces of the combine to free a person, but the combine and surrounding soil should first be washed down and the inside of the combine flushed, to reduce the risk of fire.

If a person is trapped in the auger, the auger may need to be first cut free, in which case it should be transported with the person. First, a large pipe wrench should be wedged on the shaft to prevent it from reversing, and then the auger drive should be disconnected. No attempt should be made to extricate a person in the field if the auger has caused an avulsion.

Figure 25–7 Combine parts, such as the auger, heads, reels, and snapping rollers can cause serious injuries.

On older equipment, rescue tools can be used to spread snapping rollers, but this approach will not work on newer equipment.

Hay Balers

To free a person caught in a hay baler, the tines may need to be disassembled by unscrewing the bolts holding it together. The drive belts that drive the cross auger or raise the auger may need to be disassembled with rescue tools. To prevent reverse motion, a pipe wrench can be used to hold on to the input shaft as the auger is cut free. To release a person from the smooth rollers, the mounting bolts at each end should be removed, to remove the bearings.

An acetylene torch should never be used to take apart a hay baler, as the combustible dust inside the baler may ignite.

Silos

The major hazard in a silo is the gas formed during fermentation of stored crops, which, when inhaled, can kill within minutes (Figure 25–8). Keep in mind that "silo gas" can leak out to the surrounding area. Signs of this gas include a bleach-like smell, the presence of dead birds and insects, a yellowish or reddish vapour, and sick livestock nearby. A self-contained breathing apparatus (SCBA) must be worn to rescue a person in the presence of silo gas. Administer emergency oxygen to the person if it is available, and transport as soon as possible.

Manure Storage

Manure is often flushed from livestock facilities into a holding pond or a closed structure. The hazards include toxic fumes and risk of drowning. To rescue a person in a manure storage area, you must wear an SCBA and lifeline. Treat an immersed person as you would a person who has survived a drowning incident. If the person is breathing, connect the person to an SCBA. Also administer emergency oxygen if it is available. Before transporting the person, remove any contaminated clothing and flush the person's body with water. Do not bring any contaminated materials into the transport vehicle. Anyone and everything that came into contact with manure will require decontamination.

Livestock

Never enter an area with unsecured livestock. Treat injuries inflicted by livestock as you would any similar injury but be sure to flush animal feces from any wound.

Chemicals

Various industrial chemicals are used across many industries, and they may be found in a gas, aerosol, liquid, or solid state. These chemicals can be hazardous either because of the chemicals they contain (e.g., carcinogens, reproductive hazards, corrosives, or agents that affect the lungs or blood) or because of their physical properties (e.g., flammable, combustible, explosive, or reactive). Large quantities of these chemicals may pose a risk because of exposure through routine use. If these hazardous chemicals are released, they could have extremely serious effects on exposed individuals.

Many types of chemicals, particularly pesticides and fertilizers, are used in agriculture. Use protective clothing before entering a scene that may contain pesticides or other chemicals. If necessary, call a haz-mat removal team. If you know which pesticide was involved in a particular emergency, check the label for instructions and precautions, and take the label with you to the hospital. Before transporting a person, remove all clothing and flush the person's body with water.

Figure 25–8 The gas formed during fermentation of crops stored in a silo can kill within minutes when inhaled.

In any of their states (gas, aerosol, liquid, or solid), these toxic industrial chemicals could enter the body by being inhaled, absorbed through the skin, or ingested. The time it takes for these substances to have an effect depends mainly on the route they use to enter the body. Generally, poisoning occurs more quickly if the chemical is inhaled. MSDSs or chemical information cards will provide information on the effects of each chemical and the symptoms of exposure.

If you or someone you are helping is exposed to a toxic industrial chemical, get yourself and the person away from the area as quickly as you can. Avoid passing through the contaminated area, if possible.

Employers should have an effective plan in place to assist employees in reaching shelter safely. They may be required to "shelter-in-place" if they cannot get out of a building or if the only place with clean air is indoors. Health and safety plans should take into account the possible impact of a release of toxic industrial chemicals. Plans should include guidelines such as monitoring, detection, awareness training, PPE, decontamination, and medical surveillance of acutely exposed workers.

Health Canada provides guidelines on the PPE to be used during or after a toxic chemical release and when the duration of the chemical release or airborne concentration of chemicals is unknown. Details are available on the Health Canada website.[47]

Typical Injuries

At a workplace, injuries most often involve the hands and arms, which can get caught in machinery (Figure 25–9). The most common injuries include:

- Soft tissue injuries (see Chapter 12):
  - Abrasions
  - Amputations
  - Avulsions
  - Burns
  - Contusions
  - Impaled fish hooks

Figure 25–9 In the workplace, injuries often involve the hands and arms.

  - Lacerations
  - Punctures
  - Subungual hematomas
- Employees can also develop various skin conditions, such as abscesses, dermatitis, and gangrene (see Chapter 12)
- Musculoskeletal injuries (see Chapter 13):
  - Fractures
  - Sprains
  - Strains
- Head and/or spine Injuries (see Chapter 14):
  - Concussions
  - Eye injuries
- Poisoning (see Chapter 17):
  - Animal bites

SUMMARY

All Canadians have a right to a safe and healthy work environment. As a first aid attendant, your role is to contribute to that environment by responding to situations requiring first aid and applying your knowledge and skills to the best of your ability.

The rules and regulations around health and safety differ in each province and territory. You will need to be familiar with the ones that apply to your place of work. As well, there will be particular health and safety concerns that relate specifically to your type of workplace, whether in an office, factory, agricultural setting, construction site, or other. Being familiar with programs such as WHMIS, Canada's national hazard communication standard, will help reduce dangers in your workplace that could result in injury or illness.

When you arrive on the scene, you realize your co-worker has suffered a crush injury and is unconscious. What do you do?

Common Abbreviations for Documentation

♀	Female		CIS	Critical incident stress
♂	Male		CO_2	Carbon dioxide
↓	Diminished, decreased, lower		COPD	Chronic obstructive pulmonary disease
↑	Elevated, increased, upper		CP	Chest pain
>	Greater than		CPR	Cardiopulmonary resuscitation
<	Less than		CSF	Cerebrospinal fluid
=	Equals		CT (CAT)	Computed tomography
≠	Not equal		CVA	Cerebrovascular accident
i, ii, iii	One, two, three			
Ø	None, not present, not found		D_5W	Dextrose 5% in water
			$D_{10}W$	Dextrose 10% in water
abd	Abdomen		DNR	Do not resuscitate
ac	Before meals		DOA	Dead on arrival
AED	Automated external defibrillator		DPU	Discharge planning unit
AE, A/E	Air entry		Dx	Diagnosis
am	Before noon			
ANU	Ambulance not used		ECG, EKG	Electrocardiogram
AOB	Alcohol on breath		ECU	Extended care unit
approx	Approximately		EEG	Electroencephalograph
ASA	Acetylsalicylic acid, Aspirin®		EP	Emergency physician
ASAP	As soon as possible		ER, ED	Emergency room, department
			ET	Endotracheal
bG	Blood glucose		ETA	Estimated time of arrival
bid	Twice a day			
BM	Bowel movement		°F	Degrees Fahrenheit
BP	Blood pressure		FR	First responder
			Fx, #	Fracture
c̄	With			
°C	Degrees Celsius		GI	Gastrointestinal
C-section	Caesarean section		GOA	Gone on arrival
C/C	Chief complaint		gtt	Drop
c/o	Complains of			
Ca	Cancer		Hb	Hemoglobin
CABG	Coronary artery bypass graft		Hct	Hematocrit
CAD	Coronary artery disease		Hg	Chemical symbol for mercury
cath	Catheter		H_2O	Water
CBC	Complete blood count		hr	Hour
cc	Cubic centimetre		Hs	Evening, at bedtime
CCU	Cardiac care unit		Hx	History
CHF	Congestive heart failure			

ICN	Intensive care nursery	PEARL	Pupils equal and react to light
IDDM	Insulin-dependent diabetes mellitus	PERLA	Pupils equal, round, react to light and accommodation
IM	Intramuscular	pm	After noon
IV	Intravenous	PO	By mouth, oral
		post-op	Postoperative
kg	Kilogram	pre-op	Preoperative
		prn	As needed, as required
L1	First lumbar vertebrae	pt	Patient
l, L	Litre		
lg	Large	q am	Every morning
LLQ	Left lower quadrant	QID/qid	Four times per day
LOC	Level of consciousness	q1h, q2h	Every hour, every two hours
LUQ	Left upper quadrant		
		R, resp	Respirations
MCG, mcg	Microgram	RBC	Red blood cells
MCI	Multiple casualty incident	RLQ	Right lower quadrant
mEq/L	Milliequivalents per litre	RUQ	Right upper quadrant
mg	Milligram	Rx	Medications
MI	Myocardial infarction	R/O	Rule out
ml, mL	Millilitre		
mmHg	Millimetres of mercury	s, w/o	Without
MO	Mental observation point	SA	Sinoatrial node
MRI	Magnetic resonance imaging	SC, sc	Subcutaneous
MVC	Motor vehicle collision	SCN	Special care nursery
		SIDS	Sudden infant death syndrome
N/A	Not applicable/Not available	SL, sl	Sublingual
NIDDM	Non-insulin-dependent diabetes mellitus	SOB	Shortness of breath
nitro	Nitroglycerin	stat	Immediately
NKA	No known allergies	SV	Stroke volume
N_2O	Nitrous oxide (Entonox®)		
NPO	Nothing by mouth, oral	T2	Second thoracic vertebrae
NS	Normal saline	tab	Tablet
NYD	Not yet diagnosed	TIA	Transient ischemic attack
		tid	Three times per day
O_2	Oxygen	TKO, TKVO	To keep vein open
OB, OBS	Obstetrics	TPR	Temperature, pulse, respiration
od	Once per day	TPN	Total parenteral nutrition
OD	Overdose	Tx	Treatment
OR	Operating room	tx	Transmit
OTC	Over the counter		
		U/K	Unknown
P	Pulse		
palp	Palpation	vag	Vaginal
PAU	Psychiatric assessment unit		
pc	After meals, after food	yr	Year
per	Through, by		

Appendix *B*

SAMPLE AMBULANCE EQUIPMENT LIST

Quantity	Size	Description
1		Multi-level (with a minimum of 3 height-adjustment levels) ambulance cot with waterproof covered mattress and minimum of 2 restraint belts (preferably equipped with 5-point harness system)
1		Pediatric transport device
1		Folding stretcher with a minimum of 2 restraint belts (Ferno model 9 or equivalent with/without wheels)
1	3 (or D)	Oxygen tank with oxygen and regulator/flowmeter assembly, complete with cylinder wrench; the tank's oxygen level must not be less than 700 psi (must not be equipped with a pressure compensated flowmeter)
2	5 (or E)	Oxygen tanks, with a minimum of 1 oxygen and regulator/flowmeter assembly; the in-use tank must be equipped with a cylinder wrench. The spare tank's oxygen level must not be less than 2,000 psi and the in-use tank's oxygen level must not be less than 500 psi
3	Adult	Oxygen face masks—3-in-1 type (non-rebreather)
2	Adult	Oxygen face masks—Venturi type with 6 diluters or dials between 24 and 50% oxygen
2	Adult	Nasal cannulas, complete with tubing
1	Pediatric	Oxygen face mask—Venturi type with 6 diluters or dials between 24 and 50% oxygen
2	Pediatric	Oxygen face masks—3-in-1 type (non-rebreather)
1	Adult (1,500–1,600 mL)	Resuscitator (bag-valve-mask), complete with mask, bag, and reservoir/accumulator
1	Child (450–500 mL)	Resuscitator (bag-valve-mask), complete with mask, bag, and reservoir/accumulator
1	Baby (150–300 mL)	Resuscitator (bag-valve-mask), complete with mask, bag, and reservoir/accumulator

1	Adult	CPR pocket mask in protective case with one-way valve, filter, oxygen outlet, and head strap
1	50 mm (or 55 mm)	Oropharyngeal airway
1	60 mm	Oropharyngeal airway
1	70 mm	Oropharyngeal airway
1	80 mm	Oropharyngeal airway
1	90 mm	Oropharyngeal airway
1	100 mm	Oropharyngeal airway
1	110 mm	Oropharyngeal airway
1		Fixed electric suction apparatus with suction catheters in sizes 8, 10, 12 and 14, complete with tubing (intake manifold powered not permitted)
3		Yanker suction catheters, complete with tubing
1		Portable suction apparatus (Res-, Q-Vac, V-Vac, Vac-Pac, or equivalent), rubber bulb-type not equivalent, complete with pump, 2 canisters, catheter set, adapters, etc.
1	Approximately 180 cm (71 in.) × 40 cm (16 in.)	Long backboard with a minimum of 3 straps and shoulder harness (Fastrap, V-8, Spider Straps, or equivalent); if backboard is wooden, it must be 2 cm (¾ in.) plywood, sanded and coated/sealed on all sides and of an appropriate design (approved backboard restraints only)
1		Head immobilizer set (Ferno model 445, Ferno Red Head, Ambu disposable, Headgrip II, or equivalent)
1	Approximately 85 cm (33 in.) × 40 cm (16 in.)	Short spinal motion restriction device, (K.E.D.® board or equivalent); a short wooden backboard of an appropriate design and construction is minimally acceptable, but only if equipped with a head pad, two 3 m (9 ft.) belts or three 2 m (7 ft.) belts as well as head and chinstraps
1	Baby	Cervical immobilization device (CID)/rigid collar
1	Pediatric	CID/rigid collar
1	Adult short	CID/rigid collar
1	Adult regular	CID/rigid collar
1	Adult tall	CID/rigid collar

2		CSA class 2 traffic safety vests
2		Fluid-impervious thigh splints
2		Fluid-impervious lower leg splints
2		Fluid-impervious arm splints
1	Adult size	Femoral traction apparatus (Fernotrac, Sager, Hare, Klipple, Speed-splint or equivalent)
1		Bed pan
1		Urinal
1	Large	Emesis basin
3	Large	Biohazard bags
3		Urine and vomit convenience bags of a commercial design
1		Blood pressure apparatus with 1 gauge and at least 5 different cuff sizes, including baby, child, adult, large-size adult, and thigh-sized
1		Stethoscope (dual head)
1	14 cm (6 in.)	Lister bandage scissors
1	19 cm (7 in.)	Super shears/paramedic shears
1	14 cm (6 in.)	Kelly forceps
1	Standard size (10 cm/4 in.)	Dressing tweezers
1		Penlight
1		Commercially designed medical sharps container
2	2.3 kg (5 lb.)	Dry chemical fire extinguishers (ABC, ULC rated), inspected as per fire code requirements
1	Standard hatchet size	Axe
2	Sized-to-fit tires	Tire chains (optional)
2	7.5 cm (3 in.) diameter lense	Battery operated hand lanterns
3		Roadside reflectors (or 2 red traffic triangles)
1	Standard short handle	Steel shovel

1	90 cm (35 in.) and minimum 1.27 cm (0.5 in.) in diameter	Straight pry bar of a commercial design (to be stored under the squad bench)
1	roll	Duct tape
2		Level C haz-mat suit with hood (Tyvek®)
1	1 cm (0.4 in.) × 10 m (33 ft.) or 21 cm (8 in.) × 5 m (16 ft.)	Rope
2		Helmets

PHONETIC ALPHABET

Use plain language whenever possible. However, due to differences in accents and pronunciations throughout the world, or when conditions for reception are not completely clear, it is standard procedure to use the phonetic alphabet for your call sign and for completing your communication.

Letter	Word	Pronounced as	Letter	Word	Pronounced as
A	Alpha	AL FAH	N	November	NO VEM BER
B	Bravo	BRAH VOH	O	Oscar	OSS CAR
C	Charlie	CHAR LEE or SHAR LEE	P	Papa	PAH PAH
D	Delta	DELL TAH	Q	Quebec	KEH BECK
E	Echo	ECK OH	R	Romeo	ROW ME OH
F	Foxtrot	FOKS TROT	S	Sierra	SEE AIR RAH
G	Golf	GOLF	T	Tango	TANG GO
H	Hotel	HOH TELL	U	Uniform	YOU NEE FORM or OO NEE FORM
I	India	IN DEE AH	V	Victor	VIK TAH
J	Juliette	JEW LEE ETT	W	Whiskey	WISS KEY
K	Kilo	KEE LOH	X	X-ray	ECKS RAY
L	Lima	LEE MAH	Y	Yankee	YANG KEY
M	Mike	MIKE	Z	Zulu	ZOO LOO

Example of Urgency Call and Message

PAN PAN, PAN PAN, PAN PAN

HALIFAX COAST GUARD RADIO, HALIFAX COAST GUARD RADIO, HALIFAX COAST GUARD RADIO

THIS IS CANCROSS VY1896, CANCROSS VY1896, CANCROSS VY1896

ONE OF THE RESCUED PERSONS HAS GONE INTO DEEP SHOCK REQUEST HELICOPTER AIR LIFT

MY POSITION IS 30 MILES SOUTH OF HALIFAX

CANCROSS VY1896 OVER

Example of Reply

PAN PAN

CANCROSS VY1896, CANCROSS VY1896, CANCROSS VY1896

THIS IS HALIFAX COAST GUARD RADIO, HALIFAX COAST GUARD RADIO, HALIFAX COAST GUARD RADIO

HELICOPTER HAS BEEN DISPATCHED

ESTIMATED TIME OF ARRIVAL IS 1215z
(say "zulu" for "z")

HALIFAX COAST GUARD RADIO OVER

If the vessel Cancross VY1896 had been asked to spell its name and call sign phonetically it would do so as follows: "CHARLIE, ALPHA, NOVEMBER, CHARLIE, ROMEO, OSCAR, SIERRA, SIERRA, VICTOR, YANKEE, one, eight, niner, six."

Glossary

A

Abandonment: Ending care of a patient without that patient's consent or without ensuring that someone with equal or greater training will continue that care.

ABCs: Airway, breathing, and circulation.

Abdomen: The part of the trunk below the ribs and above the pelvis.

Abdominal aortic aneurysm: A rupturing of the abdominal aorta.

Abdominal cavity: An area located in the trunk that contains the liver, pancreas, intestine, stomach, and spleen.

Abdominal thrusts: A technique for unblocking an obstructed airway by forcefully squeezing the abdomen.

Abrasion: A wound characterized by skin that has been scraped or rubbed away.

Abruptio placentae: A partial or complete detachment of a normally implanted placenta at more than 20 weeks gestation.

Absorbed poison: A poison that enters the body through the skin or mucous membranes.

Acid: A substance with a pH less than seven; usually corrosive and can cause chemical burns on the skin.

Acquired immune deficiency syndrome (AIDS): A condition caused by the human immunodeficiency virus (HIV).

Active listening: A process that helps you more fully communicate with a patient by focusing on what the patient is saying.

Acute: Having a rapid and severe onset and then quickly subsiding.

Acute coronary syndrome (ACS): A range of clinical conditions, including unstable angina, that are due to insufficient blood supply to the heart muscle, resulting from coronary heart disease.

Acute mountain sickness (AMS): One of three forms of high-altitude illness; not a specific disease but a group of varied symptoms caused by altitude.

Acute myocardial ischemia: An episode of chest pain due to reduced blood flow to the heart muscle.

Acute pulmonary edema: Fluid buildup in the lungs.

Acute respiratory distress syndrome (ARDS): Serious lung disease caused by a variety of conditions that lead to an increase in the quantity of fluid between the alveolar membrane and the surrounding pulmonary capillaries, which decreases the amount of oxygen the red blood cells can absorb.

Adolescent: A person between 13 and 18 years of age.

Adverse effects: Side effects that cause problems in a patient. These are the effects you must watch for when administering medications such as nitroglycerin.

Agonal respiration: Isolated or infrequent gasping in the absence of other breathing in an unconscious person; can occur after the heart has stopped beating; not considered breathing.

Airborne transmission: The transmission of a disease by inhaling infected droplets that become airborne when an infected person coughs or sneezes.

Airway: The pathway for air from the mouth and nose to the lungs.

Airway obstruction: A blockage of the airway that prevents air from reaching a person's lungs.

Alkali: A substance with a pH greater than seven that neutralizes an acid; can cause chemical burns on the skin.

Altered mental status: A disturbance in a person's level of consciousness, including confusion and delirium; causes include injury, infection, poison, drug abuse, and fluid/electrolyte imbalance.

Altitude sickness: Illness due to a change in altitude.

Alveoli: Small air sacs in the lungs where gases and waste are exchanged between the lungs and the blood.

Alzheimer's disease: A progressive, degenerative disease that affects the brain, resulting in impaired memory, thinking, and behaviour.

Amniotic sac: A fluid-filled sac that encloses, bathes, and protects the developing baby.

Amputation: The complete removal or severing of a body part.

Anal fissure: A small tear in the skin that lines the anus.

Anaphylaxis: A severe allergic reaction in which the air passages constrict and restrict the person's breathing.

Anatomical splint: A splint that uses an uninjured body part to immobilize an injured body part.

Anatomical obstruction: The blockage of the airway by an anatomical structure, such as the tongue.

Anatomical position: A position in which a person is standing erect with arms down at the sides, and palms facing forward.

Anatomy: The study of structures, including gross anatomy (structures that can be seen with the naked eye) and microscopic anatomy (structures seen under the microscope).

Aneurysm: A condition in which the wall of an artery or vein weakens, balloons out, and ruptures.

Angina: Chest pain or pressure resulting when the heart needs more oxygen-rich blood than it is getting; pain or pressure usually lasts less than 10 minutes; can be stable (occurring under exertion or stress) or unstable (occurring at rest, without reason); also called angina pectoris.

Anterior: Toward the front of the body.

Antibodies: A type of protein found in blood or other bodily fluids; used by the immune system to identify and neutralize pathogens, such as bacteria and viruses.

Appendicitis: Acute inflammation of the appendix.

Arrhythmia: A disturbance in the conduction of electrical impulses within the heart; also called dysrhythmia.

Arteries: Large blood vessels that carry oxygen-rich blood from the heart to all parts of the body.

Arthritis: An inflamed condition of the joints, causing pain and swelling and sometimes limiting motion.

Aseptic technique: The use of sterile procedures to prevent bacteria from entering the body, thus limiting the risk of infection.

Aspiration: Taking blood, vomit, saliva, or other foreign material into the lungs.

Assault: Abuse, either physical or sexual, resulting in injury and often emotional crisis.

Asthma: A condition that narrows the air passages and makes breathing difficult.

Asystole: The stopping of all electrical activity in the heart.

Atherosclerosis: A form of cardiovascular disease marked by a narrowing of the arteries in the heart and other parts of the body.

Atria: The upper chambers of the heart.

Aura: An unusual sensation or feeling a person may experience before an epileptic seizure; may be a visual hallucination; a strange sound, taste, or smell; or an urgent need to get to safety.

Auscultation: Listening to the internal sounds of the body; usually with a stethoscope.

Automated external defibrillator (AED): An electronic device that shocks a patient's heart to stop certain arrhythmias.

Avulsion: A wound in which a portion of the skin, and sometimes other soft tissue, is partially or completely torn away.

B

Baby: A child up to one year of age.

Bacteria: One-celled micro-organisms that may cause infections.

Bag-valve-mask (BVM) resuscitator: A hand-held ventilation device consisting of a self-inflating bag, a one-way valve, and a face mask; can be used with or without supplemental oxygen.

Bandage: Material used to wrap or cover a part of the body; commonly used to hold a dressing or splint in place.

Behavioural disorder: Any of various forms of behaviour, resulting from situational, organic, or psychiatric causes, that are dangerous or disturbing to the person or those around him.

Biological death: The irreversible damage caused by the death of brain cells.

Birth canal: The passageway from the uterus to the vaginal opening through which a baby passes during birth.

Bladder: An organ in the pelvis in which urine is stored until released from the body.

Blast injury: An injury resulting from an explosion; caused by pressure waves, flying debris, or being thrown.

Blood-borne pathogens: Bacteria and viruses present in human blood and body fluids that can cause disease in humans.

Blood glucose level (BGL): The amount of sugar (glucose) in the blood.

Blood pressure (BP): The force exerted by blood against the blood vessel walls as it travels throughout the body.

Blood pressure cuff: A device used to measure a patient's blood pressure.

Blood volume: The total amount of blood circulating within the body.

Body cavity: A hollow place in the body that contains organs, glands, blood vessels, and nerves.

Body mechanics: Using the body to gain mechanical advantage in the safest and most efficient way.

Body system: A group of organs and other structures working together to carry out specific functions.

Bone: A dense, hard tissue that forms the skeleton.

Bowel obstruction: An occlusion of the intestinal cavity resulting in blockage of normal flow of intestinal contents.

Brachial artery: A large artery located in the upper arm.

Brain: The centre of the nervous system that controls all body functions.

Breathing emergency: An emergency in which breathing is so impaired that life can be threatened.

Breech birth: The delivery of a baby, feet or buttocks first.

Bronchi: The air passages that lead from the trachea to the lungs.

Bronchitis: A disease causing excessive mucous secretions and inflammatory changes to the bronchi.

Burn: An injury to the skin or other body tissues caused by heat, chemicals, electricity, or radiation.

C

Capillaries: Tiny blood vessels linking arteries and veins that transfer oxygen and other nutrients from the blood to all body cells and remove waste products.

Capillary refill: An estimate of the amount of blood flowing through the capillary beds, such as those in the fingertips.

Carbon dioxide: A colourless, odourless gas; a waste product of respiration.

Cardiac arrest: A condition in which the heart has stopped functioning.

Cardiopulmonary resuscitation (CPR): A technique that combines rescue breathing and chest compressions for a patient whose breathing and heart have stopped.

Cardiovascular disease: A disease of the heart and blood vessels; commonly known as heart disease.

Carotid arteries: Arteries located in the neck that supply blood to the head and neck.

Cartilage: An elastic tissue that acts as a shock absorber when a person is walking, running, or jumping.

Cell: The basic unit of all living tissue.

Cervical collar: A rigid device positioned around the neck to limit movement of the head and neck.

Cervix: The upper part of the birth canal.

Chemical burns: Burns that are caused by caustic chemicals, such as strong acids or alkalis.

Chest thrusts: Forceful pushes on the chest; delivered to a patient with an obstructed airway in an attempt to expel any foreign object blocking the airway.

Chief complaint: A brief description, usually in the patient's own words, of why EMS personnel were called to the scene.

Child: For the purpose of providing emergency medical care, anyone who appears to be between the ages of about one year and puberty; when using an AED, anyone between the ages of one and eight.

Child abuse: The physical, psychological, or sexual assault of a child, resulting in injury and emotional trauma.

Chocking: The use of items, such as wooden blocks, placed against the wheels of a vehicle to help stabilize the vehicle.

Cholesterol: A fatty substance made by the body and found in certain foods.

Chronic: Persistent over a long period of time.

Chronic obstructive pulmonary disease (COPD): A disease characterized by a loss of lung function.

Circulatory emergencies: Sudden illnesses or injuries involving the heart or blood vessels.

Circulatory system: A group of organs and other structures that carry oxygen-rich blood and other nutrients throughout the body and remove waste.

Clavicle: See collarbone.

Clinical death: The condition in which the heart stops beating and breathing stops.

Closed fracture: A fracture in which the skin is left unbroken.

Closed wound: A wound in which soft tissue damage occurs beneath the skin and the skin is not broken.

Clotting: The process by which blood thickens at a wound site to seal an opening in a blood vessel and stop bleeding.

Collarbone: A horizontal bone that connects with the sternum and the shoulder; also called the clavicle.

Community-associated MRSA (CA-MRSA): Methicillin-resistant *Staphylococcus aureus* (MRSA) that occurs in groups of people who have not been recently hospitalized or have not had a medical procedure.

Compassion: An understanding of the emotional state of another person, combined with the desire to alleviate or reduce the suffering of that person.

Competence: The state or quality of being adequately qualified for, or the ability to perform, a particular role; the ability of a patient to understand a responder's questions and the implications of a decision.

Concussion: A temporary impairment of brain function, usually without permanent damage to the brain.

Confidence: The state of being certain that a chosen course of action is the best or most effective.

Confidentiality: Protecting a patient's privacy by not revealing any personal information you learn about the patient except to law enforcement personnel or more advanced medical care.

Conflict: An internal or external state of unrest due to the opposition of one's needs, values, and interests.

Congestive heart failure (CHF): A condition in which the heart loses its pumping ability, causing fluid buildup in the body; results in heart failure.

Consciousness: The state of being aware of one's self and one's surroundings.

Consent: Permission to provide care, given by a patient to a responder.

Contraction: The rhythmic tightening of muscles in the uterus during labour; or the pumping action of the heart.

Coronary arteries: Blood vessels that supply the heart muscle with oxygen-rich blood.

Coronary heart disease (CHD): A disease in which cholesterol and plaque build up on the inner walls of the arteries that supply blood to the heart; also called coronary artery disease (CAD).

Cranial cavity: An area in the body that contains the brain and is protected by the skull.

Crepitus: A grating, crackling, or popping sound under the skin that can be due to a number of causes, including two pieces of bone rubbing against each other.

Critical burn: Any burn that is potentially life-threatening, disabling, or disfiguring; a burn requiring more advanced emergency care.

Croup: A viral infection that causes swelling of the tissues below the vocal cords; a common childhood illness.

Crowning: The time in labour when the baby's head is at the opening of the vagina.

Crush injury: An injury caused when a crushing force is applied to any part of the body over a short or long period of time.

Cyanosis: A bluish coloration of the skin and mucous membranes due to the presence of deoxygenated blood in the vessels near the skin surface.

D

Decomposition: The breaking down of the body's chemical composition after death.

Defibrillation: An electric shock administered to correct a life-threatening heart rhythm.

Depressants: Substances that affect the central nervous system to slow physical and mental activity.

Dermis: The deeper of the two layers of skin.

Designer drug: A potent and illegal street drug formed from a medicinal substance whose chemical composition has been modified ("designed").

Developmental disability: Impaired mental function, resulting from injury or genetics.

Diabetes: A disease in which there are high levels of blood glucose due to defects in insulin production, insulin action, or both.

Diabetic emergency: A situation in which a person becomes ill because of an imbalance of insulin.

Diaphragm: A dome-shaped muscle that aids breathing and separates the chest from the abdomen.

Diastolic pressure: The pressure in the arteries when the heart is at rest.

Digestive system: A group of organs and other structures that digests food and eliminates wastes.

Dignity: The state of being worthy of honour and respect.

Diplomacy: Using tact and skill when dealing with people.

Direct contact transmission: The transmission of a disease by touching an infected person's body fluids.

Direct pressure: The pressure applied on a wound to control bleeding.

Discretion: The ability to make responsible decisions.

Dislocation: The displacement of a bone from its normal position at a joint.

Distal: Away from the trunk of the body.

Distal circulation: Blood flow below the site of an injury.

Downwind: In the direction in which the wind blows.

Dressing: A pad placed directly over a wound to absorb blood and other bodily fluids and to prevent infection.

Drowning: A form of suffocation caused by being immersed in water or other liquid.

Drug: Any substance other than food intended to affect the functions of the body.

Duty to act: A legal responsibility of some individuals to provide a reasonable standard of emergency care; may be required by case law, statute, or job description.

Dyspnea: Difficulty breathing; shortness of breath.

Dysrhythmia: A disturbance in the conduction of electrical impulses within the heart; also called arrhythmia.

E

Ectopic pregnancy: When a fertilized ovum implants anywhere other than in the uterus.

Elder abuse: Any of four types of abuse: the infliction of pain or injury (physical abuse); mental anguish or suffering (psychological abuse); financial or material abuse; or unnecessary confinement or willful deprivation (neglect) by an older adult's caretaker.

Electrical burn: A burn caused by an electrical source, such as an electrical appliance or lightning.

Embolism: A sudden blockage of a blood vessel by a travelling clot or other material, such as fat or air.

Emergency medical responder (EMR): a responder who has successfully completed a recognized training program in the care and transportation of a patient.

Emergency medical services (EMS) system: A network of community resources and medical personnel that provides emergency care to people who are injured or suddenly ill.

Emergency move: Moving a patient before completing care; done only in certain necessary circumstances.

Emotional crisis: A highly emotional state resulting from stress, often involving a significant event in a person's life, such as the death of a loved one.

Empathy: Feeling or expressing emotion for another.

Emphysema: A disease in which the alveoli lose their elasticity, become distended with trapped air, and stop working.

Endocrine system: A group of organs and other structures that regulate and coordinate the activities of other systems by producing chemicals that influence the activity of tissues.

Endotracheal: Pertaining to something within the trachea.

Enteral: Pertaining to the small intestine; within the small intestine; also called enteric.

Epidermis: The outer layer of skin.

Epidural hematoma: Arterial bleeding between the skull and dura mater.

Epiglottis: The flap of tissue that covers the trachea to keep food and liquid out of the lungs.

Epiglottitis: A bacterial infection that causes a severe inflammation of the epiglottis.

Epilepsy: A chronic condition characterized by seizures that vary in type and duration; can usually be controlled by medication.

Epinephrine: A naturally occurring hormone; can be used to counter the effects of anaphylaxis.

Epistaxis: A nosebleed.

Esophagus: The tube leading from the mouth to the stomach.

Ethical: Conforming to accepted standards of conduct.

Exhale: To breathe air out of the lungs.

External bleeding: Bleeding from an open wound in the skin.

Extremities: The limbs of the body.

Extrication: The freeing of someone or something from an entanglement or difficulty.

F

Fainting: A loss of consciousness resulting from a temporary reduction in blood flow to the brain; also called syncope.

Febrile seizure: A seizure caused by an elevated body temperature.

Femur: The thighbone.

Fibula: One of the bones in the lower leg.

Finger sweep: A technique used to remove foreign material from a patient's airway.

First aid attendant: A designated person who provides advanced first aid in the workplace.

First responder: A person trained in emergency care who may be called on to provide such care as a routine part of his job; often the first trained professional to respond to emergencies.

Flail chest: An injury involving fractured ribs that do not move normally with the rest of the chest during breathing.

Flowmeter: A device used to regulate in litres per minute (lpm) the amount of oxygen administered to a patient.

Fracture: A break or disruption in bone tissue.

Freeboard: The distance between the top of a watercraft, or the deck of a ship, and the waterline.

Frostbite: A serious condition in which body tissues freeze, most commonly in the fingers, toes, ears, and nose.

Full-thickness burn: A burn injury involving both layers of skin and underlying tissues; skin may be brown or charred, and underlying tissues may appear white.

G

Gastric distention: Air in the stomach, causing it to bloat.

Gastroenteritis: A condition often resulting from an infection of the gastrointestinal tract.

Genitalia: The external reproductive organs.

Genitourinary system: A group of organs and other structures that eliminate waste and enable reproduction.

Glands: Organs that release fluid and other substances into the blood or on the skin.

Glasgow Coma Scale (GCS): A standardized system used to determine a patient's level of consciousness; often performed on patients with suspected head injuries.

Glucometer: A device used to measure a patient's blood glucose level.

Glucometry: The process of measuring the level of glucose circulating in the blood.

Good Samaritan laws: Laws that protect people who willingly give emergency care while acting in good faith, without negligence, and within the scope of their training.

H

H.A.IN.E.S. recovery position: A recovery position for an unconscious patient that helps to keep the airway open and allows any blood or vomit to drain from the mouth; stands for High Arm in Endangered Spine.

Hallucinogens: Substances that affect mood, sensation, thought, emotion, and self-awareness; alter perceptions of time and space; and produce delusions.

Hazardous materials: Substances that are harmful or toxic to the body; can be liquids, solids, or gases.

Head-tilt/chin-lift: A method of opening the airway when there is no suspected head and/or spine injury.

Hearing impairment: Partial or complete deafness.

Heart: A fist-sized muscular organ that pumps blood throughout the body.

Heart attack: A sudden illness involving the death of heart muscle tissue when it does not receive enough oxygen-rich blood; also called myocardial infarction (MI).

Heat cramps: Painful spasms of skeletal muscles following exercise or work in warm or moderate temperatures; usually involve the calf and abdominal muscles.

Heat exhaustion: A form of shock, often resulting from strenuous work or exercise in a hot environment.

Heat stroke: A life-threatening condition that develops when the body's cooling mechanisms are overwhelmed and body systems begin to fail.

Hemorrhage: A loss of a large amount of blood in a short time.

Hemorrhoids: Clumps of tissue within the anal canal that contain blood vessels and the surrounding, supporting tissue made up of muscle and elastic fibres.

Hemothorax: A condition in which blood enters the pleural space as a result of a blunt or penetrating trauma.

Hepatitis: A viral infection of the liver.

Herpes: A viral infection that causes eruptions of the skin and mucous membranes.

High-altitude cerebral edema (HACE): An accumulation of fluid between the brain and skull; a progressive stage of acute mountain illness that occurs two to three days after arrival at altitude; a serious condition that is difficult to diagnose.

High-altitude pulmonary edema (HAPE): A serious, life-threatening condition in which fluid pools in the lungs, resulting in a breathing emergency; a progressive stage of acute mountain illness that usually occurs one to four days after arrival at altitude.

Homeostasis: A constant state of balance or well-being of the body's internal systems that is continually and automatically adjusted.

Human immunodeficiency virus (HIV): The virus that destroys the body's ability to fight infection. The resultant state is referred to as AIDS.

Humerus: The bone of the upper arm.

Hyperglycemia: A condition in which too much sugar is in the bloodstream.

Hypertension: High blood pressure.

Hyperventilation: Rapid breathing that upsets the body's balance of oxygen and carbon dioxide.

Hypoglycemia: A condition in which too little sugar is in the bloodstream.

Hypothermia: A life-threatening condition in which the body's warming mechanisms fail to maintain normal body temperature and the entire body cools.

Hypoxia: A decrease in oxygen in the blood.

I

Immobilize: To use a splint or other method to keep an injured body part from moving.

Immune system: The body's group of responses for fighting disease.

Immunization: A specific substance containing weakened or killed pathogens that is introduced into the body to build resistance to specific infection.

Impaled object: An object remaining in a wound.

Implied consent: A legal concept assuming that patients who are unconscious, or so severely injured or ill that they cannot respond, would consent to receive emergency care.

Incident command system (ICS): A system used to manage resources, such as personnel, equipment, and supplies, at the scene of an emergency.

Indication: A condition that makes administration of a drug appropriate.

Indirect contact transmission: The transmission of a disease by touching a contaminated object.

Infection: A condition caused by disease-producing micro-organisms, also called pathogens or germs, in the body.

Infectious disease: Disease capable of being transmitted from people, objects, animals, or insects.

Inferior: Toward the feet.

Influenza: Respiratory illness caused by influenza viruses and transmitted from person to person via large virus-laden droplets from coughing or sneezing.

Informed (actual) consent: Permission the patient, parent, or guardian gives the responder to provide care. This consent requires the responder to explain his level of training, what the responder thinks is wrong, and the care the responder intends to give.

Ingested poison: A poison that is swallowed.

Inhalants: Substances inhaled to produce an effect.

Inhale: To breathe in.

Inhaled poison: A poison breathed into the lungs.

Injected poison: A poison that enters the body through a bite, sting, or syringe.

In-line stabilization: A technique used to minimize movement of a patient's head and neck.

Insulin: A hormone that enables the body to use sugar for energy; frequently used to treat diabetes.

Integumentary system: A group of organs and other structures that protect the body, retain fluids, and help prevent infection.

Interaction: The beneficial or detrimental modification of the effects of one drug by the prior or concurrent administration of another drug, thereby increasing or decreasing the pharmacological or physiological action of one or both drugs.

Internal bleeding: Bleeding that occurs inside the body.

Interpersonal communication: The process of speaking and listening to other people at an emergency scene; can be verbal or nonverbal.

Intervention: A medication, device, therapy, or action that produces an effect or that is intended to alter the course of an illness or injury.

Intramuscular: Within the muscle; a route for administering a drug.

J

Jaw thrust: A method of opening the airway when there is a suspected head and/or spine injury.

Joint: A structure in which two or more bones are joined.

K

Kidney: An organ that filters waste from the blood to form urine.

Kidney stones: Solid concentrations of dissolved minerals found in the kidneys or ureters.

L

Labour: The birth process; beginning with the contraction of the uterus and dilation of the cervix and ending with the stabilization and recovery of the mother.

Laceration: A cut, usually from a sharp object; may have jagged or smooth edges.

Landing zone: The area where aircraft land.

Larynx: A part of the airway connecting the pharynx with the trachea; commonly called the "voice box."

Lateral: Away from the midline.

Level of consciousness (LOC): A patient's state of awareness, ranging from being fully alert to unconscious.

Ligament: A fibrous band that holds bones together at a joint.

Lividity: Following death, a large pooling of blood in the trunk resulting in discoloration.

Lungs: A pair of organs in the chest that provides the mechanism for taking oxygen in and removing carbon dioxide during breathing.

Lyme disease: An illness transmitted by a certain kind of infected tick.

M

Mechanism of injury (MOI): The event or forces that caused a patient's injury.

Medial: Toward the midline.

Medical control: The process that allows a physician to direct care given to a patient by pre-hospital professionals (may also be known as transfer of function, or medical delegation).

Medication: A drug given to prevent or correct the effects of a disease or condition or otherwise enhance mental or physical well-being.

Membranes: A thin sheet of tissue that covers a structure or lines a cavity, such as the mouth or nose.

Meningitis: An inflammation of the brain or spinal cord caused by a viral or bacterial infection.

Mental disability: Impaired mental function that interferes with normal activity.

Metered-dose inhaler (MDI): A device prescribed to many people with asthma, containing a medication that counters the effects of an asthma attack.

Methicillin-resistant *Staphylococcus aureus* (MRSA): A staph bacterium that can cause infection by being spread from one person to another through casual contact or contaminated objects and is resistant to many types of antibiotics.

Miscarriage: The spontaneous termination of pregnancy before 20 weeks of gestation.

Multiple casualty incident (MCI): An emergency situation involving two or more patients.

Muscle: A tissue that lengthens and shortens to create movement.

Musculoskeletal system: A group of tissues and other structures that supports the body, protects internal organs, allows movement, stores minerals, manufactures blood cells, and creates heat.

Myocardial infarction (MI): The death of cardiac muscle tissue due to a sudden deprivation of circulating blood; heart attack.

N

Narcotics: Powerful depressant substances used to relieve anxiety and pain.

Nasal cannula: A device used to administer oxygen through the nostrils to a breathing patient.

Nasopharyngeal airway (NPA): A curved tube inserted into the nose to assist in maintaining an open airway.

Nebulization: The use of a small-volume nebulizer to administer aerosolized medication (mist) over a few minutes, ensuring efficient drug delivery.

Negligence: The failure to provide the level of care a person of similar training would provide, thereby causing injury or damage to another.

Nervous system: A group of organs and other structures that regulates all body functions.

Nitroglycerin: A medication often prescribed to people diagnosed with angina.

Non-rebreather mask: A special mask combined with a reservoir bag, used to administer high-concentration oxygen to a breathing patient through a mask covering both the nose and the mouth.

Nonverbal communication: Communication through body actions, such as assuming a nonthreatening posture or the use of hand gestures.

O

Occlusive dressing: A dressing or bandage that seals a wound and protects it from the air.

Older adult: An individual who is 65 years of age or older.

Open fracture: A fracture that results when bone ends tear the skin and surrounding tissue or when an object penetrates the skin and breaks a bone.

Open wound: A wound resulting in a break in the skin surface.

Organ: A collection of similar tissues acting together to perform specific body functions.

Oropharyngeal airway (OPA): A curved plastic tube inserted into the mouth and positioned at the back of the throat to keep the tongue from blocking the airway.

Osteoporosis: A disease characterized by low bone mass and bone tissue deterioration.

Overdose: A situation in which a person takes enough of a substance that it has poisonous or fatal effects.

Oxygen: A tasteless, colourless, odourless gas necessary to sustain life.

Oxygen cylinder: A steel or alloy cylinder that contains 100% oxygen under high pressure.

Oxygen delivery device: A device used to administer oxygen from an oxygen cylinder to a patient.

P

Palpation: The method of feeling with the hands by a responder during a physical examination of a patient.

Pandemic influenza: A respiratory illness caused by virulent human influenza A virus; spreads easily and sustainably and can cause global outbreaks of serious illness in humans.

Paradoxical movement: The movement of one part of the chest wall in the opposite direction from the rest of the chest wall.

Paralysis: A loss of muscle control; a permanent loss of feeling and movement.

Parenteral: Introduction of a substance into the body through a route other than the digestive system (e.g., subcutaneous, intramuscular, or intravenous).

Partial-thickness burn: A burn injury involving both layers of skin; characterized by red, wet skin and blisters.

Patella: The kneecap.

Pathogen: A disease-causing agent; also called a micro-organism or germ.

Pathophysiology: The study of the abnormal changes in mechanical, physical, and biochemical functions that are caused by injury or illness.

Pelvic cavity: The lowest part of the trunk that contains the bladder, rectum, and the reproductive organs in females.

Pelvis: The lower part of the trunk that includes a group of large bones that form a protective girdle around the organs in the pelvic cavity.

Peptic ulcer: A small erosion in the gastrointestinal tract caused by the destruction of the gastric or intestinal mucosal lining by hydrochloric acid.

Perfusion: The circulation of blood throughout the body.

Peritonitis: An inflammation of the peritoneum.

Personal flotation device (PFD): A buoyant device designed to be worn to keep a person afloat.

Personal protective equipment (PPE): Specialized clothing or equipment worn for protection from a hazard.

Pharmacology: The study of drugs and how they interact with the body.

Pharynx: A part of the airway formed by the back of the nose and throat.

Physical assault: Abuse that may result in injury to the body.

Physical disability: A serious injury that results in the loss of limb function or a condition with which there is an impairment that interferes with activity or movement.

Physiology: How living organisms function (e.g., movement and reproduction).

Placard: A sign or notice; a poster.

Placenta: An organ attached to the uterus and unborn child through which nutrients are delivered to the baby; expelled after the baby is delivered.

Placenta previa: A condition in which the placenta is attached in the lower uterus.

Plasma: The liquid part of blood.

Platelets: Disc-shaped structures in the blood that are made of cell fragments; help stop bleeding by forming blood clots at wound sites.

Pneumonia: A group of illnesses characterized by lung infection and fluid of pus-filled alveoli, resulting in inadequate oxygen in the blood.

Pneumothorax: A condition in which air enters the pleural space usually as a result of a blunt or penetrating trauma.

Poison: Any substance that causes injury, illness, or death when introduced into the body.

Poison Control Centre: A specialized health centre that provides information in cases of poisoning or suspected poisoning emergencies.

Posterior: Toward the back.

Postpartum bleeding: Bleeding after the birth of a newborn; characterized by more than 500 mL (17 oz.) of blood loss.

Pregnancy: A condition in which the egg (ovum) of the female is fertilized by the sperm of the male, forming an embryo.

Preschooler: A child three to five years of age.

Pressure bandage: A bandage applied snugly to create pressure on a wound to aid in controlling bleeding.

Pressure regulator: A device attached to an oxygen cylinder that reduces the delivery pressure of oxygen to a safe level.

Primary survey: A check for conditions that are an immediate threat to a patient's life.

Prolapsed cord: A complication of childbirth in which a loop of umbilical cord protrudes through the vagina prior to delivery of the baby.

Prone: A position in which a person is lying face down on her stomach.

Protocols: Standardized methods.

Proximal: Closer to the trunk of the body.

Pulmonary embolism: A blockage of a pulmonary artery by a clot or other foreign material.

Pulse: The beat felt in arteries with each contraction of the heart.

Pulse oximeter: A device used to measure the percentage of red blood cells that are saturated with oxygen.

Puncture: A wound that results when the skin is pierced with a pointed object, such as a nail, a piece of glass, or a knife.

Q

Quality assurance: Providing evidence needed to establish quality in work.

R

Rabies: A disease caused by a virus transmitted through the saliva of an infected animal.

Radial pulse: The pulse felt in the wrist.

Radiation burn: A burn caused by rays, energy, or electromagnetic waves.

Rapid body survey: A hands-on check that is completed quickly, unless intervention is required; used to look for life-threatening injuries and conditions.

Rapid transport category: The category that describes patients who require immediate transport to medical care; associated with "load-and-go" emergencies.

Refusal of care: The declining of care by a person.

Reproductive system: A group of organs and other structures that enable sexual reproduction.

Rescue breathing: A technique of breathing for a non-breathing patient.

Respiration: The breathing process of the body that takes in oxygen and eliminates carbon dioxide.

Respiratory arrest: A condition in which breathing has stopped.

Respiratory distress: A condition in which breathing is difficult.

Respiratory rate: The number of times a person breathes per minute.

Respiratory system: A group of organs and other structures that bring air into the body and remove wastes through a process called breathing, or respiration.

Resuscitation mask: A pliable, dome-shaped device that fits over the nose and mouth; used to administer oxygen and assist with rescue breathing.

Rib cage: The cage of bones formed by the 12 pairs of ribs, the sternum, and the spine.

Ribs: Bones that attach to the spine and sternum and protect the heart and lungs.

Right-of-way: The right of a vessel or vehicle to cross in front of other vessels or vehicles.

Rigid splint: A splint made of boards, metal strips, and folded magazines or newspaper.

Rigor mortis: The rigid stiffening of heart and skeletal muscle after death.

Risk factors: Conditions or behaviours that increase the chance that a person will develop a disease.

Roller bandage: A bandage made of gauze or gauzelike material used to wrap around a dressing.

Routine maintenance: Maintenance work that is planned and performed on a regular basis to ensure proper working order of equipment and/or vehicles.

Rule of Nines: A method in which to estimate the percent of body surface area burned.

Rule of Palms: A method in which to estimate the percent of body surface area burned.

Rule of Thirds: A method of determining if an injury is a joint or mid-shaft injury; works by dividing the long bones into thirds.

S

SAMPLE: An acronym for remembering the questions to ask when gathering important information about a patient; stands for Signs and symptoms, Allergies, Medications, Past medical history, Last meal, and Events before the incident.

Scapula: See shoulder blade.

School age: A child between 5 and 12 years of age.

Secondary survey: A check for injuries or conditions that could become life-threatening if not cared for.

Seizure: A disorder in the brain's electrical activity, marked by loss of consciousness and often uncontrollable muscle movement.

Sepsis: A life-threatening illness in which the body is overwhelmed by its response to infection; commonly referred to as blood poisoning.

Severe acute respiratory syndrome (SARS): A viral respiratory illness caused by the SARS-associated Coronavirus (SARS-CoV).

Sexual assault: Forcing another person to take part in a sexual act.

Shock: A life-threatening condition that occurs when the circulatory system fails to provide adequate oxygen-rich blood to all parts of the body.

Shoulder blade: A large, flat, triangular bone at the back of the shoulder in the upper part of the back; also called the scapula.

Shoulder dystocia: When, during childbirth, the baby's head emerges, but one or both of the baby's shoulders unexpectedly get stuck behind the mother's pelvic bone, preventing the baby's body from emerging.

Side effect: An often unavoidable effect of using a drug; an action or effect other than those for which the drug was originally given.

Signs: Any observable evidence of injury or illness, such as bleeding or an unusually pale skin colour.

Skeletal muscles: Muscles that attach to bones.

Skeleton: The 206 bones of the body that protect vital organs and other soft tissue.

Skin: A tough, supple membrane that covers the entire surface of the body.

Sling: A bandage used to hold and support an injured part of the body; often used to support an injured arm.

Soft tissues: Body structures that include the layers of skin, fat, and muscles.

Spinal cavity: An area in the body that contains the spinal cord and is protected by the bones of the spine.

Spinal column: The series of vertebrae extending from the base of the skull to the tip of the tailbone (coccyx).

Spinal cord: A bundle of nerves extending from the base of the skull to the lower back, protected by the spinal column.

Spine: A series of bones (vertebrae) that surrounds and protects the spinal cord; also called the backbone.

Splint: A device used to immobilize body parts.

Sprain: The excessive stretching and tearing of ligaments and other soft tissue structures at a joint.

Standard of care: The minimal standard and quality of care expected of an emergency care provider.

START system: A simple system used at the scene of multiple casualty incidents to quickly assess and prioritize care according to three conditions: breathing, circulation, and level of consciousness.

Status epilepticus: A continuous seizure or two or more seizures without a period of consciousness.

Sternum: The long, flat bone in the middle of the front of the rib cage; also called the breastbone.

Stimulants: Substances that affect the central nervous system to speed up physical and mental activity.

Stimuli: Anything that rouses or excites an organism or body part to respond.

Stoma: An opening connecting a part of a body cavity to the outside environment.

Stomach: One of the main organs of digestion, located in the abdomen.

Strain: The excessive stretching and tearing of muscles and tendons.

Stress management: Techniques or interventions designed to help an individual cope with psychological stress.

Stroke: A disruption of blood flow to a part of the brain that causes permanent damage; also called a cerebrovascular accident (CVA).

Subcutaneous: Under the skin.

Subdural hematoma: Venous bleeding in the subdural space.

Substance abuse: The deliberate, persistent, excessive use of a substance without regard to health concerns or accepted medical practices.

Substance misuse: The use of a substance for unintended purposes or for intended purposes but in improper amounts or doses.

Sucking chest wound: A type of penetrating chest injury in which a sucking sound is heard with each breath a person takes due to air freely passing in and out of the chest cavity.

Suctioning: The process of removing matter such as saliva, vomitus, or blood from a patient's mouth and throat by means of a mechanical or manual device.

Suction tip: A rigid or flexible tubing attached to the end of a suction device and placed in the mouth or throat of a patient to remove foreign matter.

Sudden infant death syndrome (SIDS): The sudden death of a seemingly normal, healthy baby that occurs during the baby's sleep without evidence of disease.

Suicide: Self-inflicted death.

Superficial burn: A burn injury involving only the top layer of skin, characterized by red, dry skin.

Superior: Toward the head.

Supine: A position in which a person is lying face up on his back.

Sympathy: Understanding another's emotions, and feeling concern for that person.

Symptoms: Something the patient tells you about her condition, such as "my chest hurts," or "I feel sick to my stomach."

Syncope: Temporary loss of consciousness; usually related to temporary insufficient blood flow to the brain; also known as fainting, "blacking out," or "passing out."

Systolic pressure: The pressure in the arteries when the heart is contracting.

T

Tachypnea: Rapid breathing.

Tact: Acting appropriately according to one's situation and environment; the ability to communicate without offending others.

Tendon: A fibrous band that attaches muscle to bone.

Tension pneumothorax: The continual flow of air into the pleural space, which cannot escape.

Third trimester bleeding: Bleeding during the last three months of pregnancy. Usually caused by abruptio placentae, placenta previa, or uterine rupture.

Thoracic cavity: An area in the body that contains the heart and lungs and is protected by the rib cage and upper portion of the spine.

Tibia: One of the bones in the lower leg.

Tissue: A collection of similar cells acting together to perform specific body functions.

Toddler: A child one to three years of age.

Tourniquet: A constricting band used over an artery above the site of an open wound with severe bleeding to decrease blood flow to the injured area for a short period of time.

Trachea: A tube leading from the upper airway to the lungs.

Traction: A pulling force applied to a body part to care for specific musculoskeletal injuries.

Transient ischemic attack: A temporary disruption of blood flow to the brain; sometimes called a ministroke or TIA.

Trauma: Physical injury caused by an outside force.

Triage: The process of sorting and providing care to multiple patients according to the severity of their injuries or illnesses.

Triangular bandage: A bandage that can be used as a sling or to hold a dressing or splint in place.

Tripod position: A position in which a person is sitting upright, leaning forward, struggling to breathe.

Trunk: The part of the body containing the chest, abdomen, and pelvis.

Tuberculosis (TB): A respiratory disease caused by a bacterium.

U

Umbilical cord: A flexible structure that attaches the placenta to the unborn child, allowing for the passage of blood, nutrients, and waste.

Unconsciousness: The state of a person who is unaware of the surrounding environment and is unresponsive to stimuli.

Universal precautions: Safety measures taken to prevent occupational-risk exposure to blood or other body fluids.

Upwind: In the direction from which the wind blows.

Urinary system: A group of organs and other structures that eliminates waste products from the blood.

Urinary tract infection: An infection, usually bacterial, at any site within the urinary tract.

Uterine rupture: A spontaneous or traumatic rupture of the uterine wall.

Uterus: A pear-shaped organ in a woman's pelvis in which an embryo is formed and develops into a baby.

V

Vaccine: A medical substance containing killed or weakened micro-organisms that is introduced into the body to prevent, kill, or treat a disease.

Vagina: The lower part of the birth canal through which the baby passes during birth.

Vector-borne transmission: The transmission of a disease by an animal or insect bite through exposure to blood or other body fluids.

Veins: Blood vessels that carry oxygen-poor blood from all parts of the body to the heart.

Ventilation: The process of providing oxygen to the lungs through rescue breathing or by other means.

Ventilation devices: Devices used to help with ventilation.

Ventricles: The two lower chambers of the heart.

Ventricular fibrillation: A life-threatening arrhythmia in which the heart muscle quivers rather than pumping blood.

Ventricular tachycardia: A life-threatening arrhythmia in which the heart muscle contracts too quickly for an adequate pumping of blood to the body.

Vertebrae: The 33 bones of the spinal column.

Virus: A disease-causing agent, or pathogen, that requires another organism to live and reproduce.

Visual impairment: Inability to see adequately, or at all; also referred to as blindness or partial blindness.

Vital organs: Organs whose functions are essential to life, including the brain, heart, and lungs.

Vital signs: Important information about the patient's condition, obtained by checking level of consciousness, breathing, pulse, skin characteristics, blood pressure, and pupils.

W

Wound: An injury to the soft tissues.

References

Chapter 1

[1] Adapted from the Paramedic Association of Canada. *National Occupational Competency Profile*. 2011. Available at www.paramedic.ca/nocp/ (accessed February 2012).

[2] Adapted from the Canadian Organization of Paramedic Regulators. *History*. Available at www.copr.ca/Content.aspx?ContentID=2 (accessed February 2012).

[3] Adapted from the Paramedic Association of Canada. *National Occupational Competency Profile*. 2011. Available at www.paramedic.ca/nocp/ (accessed February 2012).

[4] Adapted from Human Resources and Skills Development Canada. *Labour Mobility.* 2011. Available at www.hrsdc.gc.ca/eng/workplaceskills/labour_mobility/index.shtml (accessed February 2012).

[5] Adapted from the Paramedic Association of Canada. *National Occupational Competency Profile*. 2011. Available at www.paramedic.ca/nocp/ (accessed February 2012).

[6] Ibid.

[7] Adapted from the Paramedic Association of Canada. *NOCP Area 2: Communication*. 2011. Available at www.paramedic.ca/nocp/nocp_communication/ (accessed February 2012).

[8] Canadian Criminal Code, Articles 45, 215, 216, and 217.

[9] Paramedic Association of Canada. *NOCP Area 2: Communication*. 2011. Available at www.paramedic.ca/nocp/nocp_professionalresponsibilities/ (accessed February 2012).

[10] Paramedic Association of Canada. *NOCP Area 1: Professional Responsibilities*. 2011. Available at www.paramedic.ca/nocp/nocp_professionalresponsibilities/ (accessed February 2012).

Chapter 3

[11] Adapted from the Public Health Agency of *Canada. Hepatitis C.* 2011. Available at www.phac-aspc.gc.ca/hepc/index-eng.php (accessed March 2012).

[12] Adapted from the Public Health Agency of Canada. *Hepatitis D Fact Sheet.* 2004. Available at www.phac-aspc.gc.ca/hcai-iamss/bbp-pts/hepatitis/hep_d-eng.php (accessed March 2012).

[13] Adapted from the Public Health Agency of Canada. *Hepatitis E Fact Sheet.* 2004. Available at www.phac-aspc.gc.ca/hcai-iamss/bbp-pts/hepatitis/hep_e-eng.php (accessed March 2012).

[14] Adapted from the Emergency Health Services Branch of the Ministry of Health and Long-Term Care (Ontario Government). *Infection Prevention and Control—Best Practices Manual for Land Ambulance Paramedics.* March 2007.

Chapter 6

[15] Adapted from The Lung Association. *Get Help: How to Use Puffers, Inhalers, and Other Devices.* 2012. Available at www.lung.ca/diseases-maladies/help aide/devices-dispositifs/index_e.php (accessed February 2012).

Chapter 12

[16] Gookin, John. *NOLS Backcountry Lightning Safety Guidelines.* Available at www.rendezvous.nols.edu//content/view/1718/739/ (accessed March 2012).

Chapter 14

[17] Summary and Agreement Statement of the 2nd International Conference on Concussion in Sport, Prague, 2004, *Clinical Journal of Sport Medicine*, Vol 15, Number 2, March 2005.

Chapter 16

[18] Adapted from the Canadian *Diabetes Association. Diabetes in Special Populations.* 2012. Available at www.diabetes.ca/research/specialpopulations/ (accessed February 2012).

[19] Ibid.

[20] Ibid.

[21] Adapted from Livestrong.com. *Use and Dosage for Oral Glucose Gel.* 2012. Available at www.livestrong.com/article/459422-use-dosage-for-oral-glucose-gel/ (accessed February 2012).

[22] Adapted from Epilepsy Canada. *Epidemiology.* Available at www.epilepsy.ca/en-CA/Facts/Epidemiology.html (accessed March 2012).

[23] Ibid.

[24] Adapted from The Kidney Foundation of Canada. *Urinary Tract Infections.* 2007. Available at www.kidney.ca/document.doc?id=316 (accessed March 2012).

Chapter 19

[25] Adapted from Keith J. Karren, PhD, et al. *Emergency Medical Responder: A Skills Approach.* Toronto: Prentice Hall, 1998: 447.

[26] Mount Sinai Hospital Department of Microbiology. *FAQ: Chickenpox (Varicella).* 2007. Available at www.microbiology.mtsinai.on.ca/faq/chickenpox.shtml (accessed April 2012).

[27] Kids Health. Infections: *Impetigo.* 2011. Available at www.kidshealth.org/parent/infections/bacterial_viral/impetigo.html# (accessed April 2012).

[28] Adapted from Livestrong.com. *How long is ringworm contagious during treatment?* 2011. Available at www.livestrong.com/article/35018-long-ringworm contagious-during-treatment/ (accessed April 2012).

[29] Adapted from Centers for Disease Control and Prevention. *Scabies Frequently Asked Questions.* 2010. Available at www.cdc.gov/parasites/scabies/gen_info/faqs.html (accessed April 2012).

[30] Adapted from Kids Health. *Pinkeye (Conjunctivitis).* 2009. Available at www.kidshealth.org/teen/infections/common/conjunctivitis.html# (accessed April 2012).

Chapter 24

[31] Adapted with permission from World Health Organization, *International Medical Guide for Ships, 3rd Edition.* Geneva: World Health Organization, 2007.

[32] Adapted with permission from Marine Occupational Health and Safety Regulations, Canada Labor Code, Subsection 13.6(1).

[33] Adapted with permission from Transport Canada. For full regulations, go to laws-lois.justice.gc.ca/eng/regulations/C.R.C.,_c._1436/page-52.html.

[34] Adapted from Health Canada. *The GHS: The Globally Harmonized System for Hazard Classification and Labelling.* 2009. Available at www.hc-sc.gc.ca/ahc-asc/intactiv/ghs-sgh/implement/ghs1-eng.php (accessed February 2012).

[35] Ibid.

[36] Adapted with permission from World Health Organization, *International Medical Guide for Ships, 3rd Edition.* Geneva: World Health Organization, 2007.

[37] Ibid.

[38] Ibid.

Chapter 25

[39] Adapted from the Canadian Centre for Occupational Health and Safety. *About CCOHS.* 2012. Available at www.ccohs.ca/ccohs.html (accessed February 2012).

[40] Adapted from the Canadian Centre for Occupational Health and Safety. *Occupational Health & Safety (OH&S Programs and Management Systems).* 2012. Available at www.ccohs.ca/keytopics/oshprograms.html (accessed February 2012).

[41] Adapted from Health Canada. *Workplace Hazardous Materials Information System (WHMIS).* 2010. Available at www.hc-sc.gc.ca/ewh-semt/occup-travail/whmis-simdut/index-eng.php (accessed February 2012).

42 Adapted from Health Canada. *The GHS: The Globally Harmonized System for Hazard Classification and Labelling.* 2009. Available at www.hc-sc.gc.ca/ahcasc/intactiv/ghs-sgh/implement/ghs1-eng.php (accessed February 2012).

43 Adapted from the Workers' Compensation Board of British Columbia. *Working in Traffic Control Zones—Be Prepared For High Risk!* Available at www2.worksafebc.com/i/posters/2009/2009-01/ha2009-01_traffic.html (accessed April 2012).

44 Adapted from the Yukon Mine Training Association. *Safety Guidelines for Mineral Exploration in Yukon.* 2009. Available at www.yukonminetraining.com/uploads/documents/YMTA-ExplorationSafetyGuidelines-Final.pdf (accessed April 2012).

45 Adapted from Health and Safety Executive. *Chainsaws at Work.* 2006. Available at www.hse.gov.uk/pubns/indg317.pdf (accessed April 2012).

46 Adapted from the Centers for Disease Control and Prevention: National Institute for Occupational Safety and Health. *Preventing Injuries When Working on Ride-On Roller/Compactors.* 2004. Available at www.cdc.gov/niosh/docs/wp-solutions/2005-101/pdfs/2005-101.pdf (accessed April 2012).

47 Adapted from Health Canada. *Personal Protective Equipment (PPE).* 2009. Available at www.hc-sc.gc.ca/ewh-semt/pubs/occup-travail/personal-individuelle/index-eng.php (accessed April 2012).

We would like to thank the American Red Cross for permission to use the following illustrations and photographs (copyright © The American National Red Cross).

Chapter 4
Figures 4–3, 4–4, 4–7, 4–11, 4–15, 4–16 b, 4–17, 4–22, 4–27, 4–28, 4–29, 4–30, 4–31, 4–32 a-b

Chapter 5
Figure 5–11

Chapter 7
Figures 7–5, 7–9

Chapter 8
Figures 8–1, 8–4 a-b, 8–12, 8–17

Chapter 9
Figure 9–1

Chapter 10
Figure 10–3

Chapter 12
Figures 12–2 b, 12–3 b, 12–4 b, 12–6 b, 12–7 b

Chapter 13
Figures 13–1, 13–2, 13–3, 13–5, 13–7, 13–17, inset illustration page 218, 13–21, 13–25, 13–26

Chapter 15
Figures 15–2, 15–3, 15–4, 15–5, 15–6, 15–9 a-d

Chapter 16
Figure 16–1

Chapter 17
Figures 17–1 (top left), 17–5

Chapter 18
Figures 18–1 a-b, 18–2, 18–6 a-b

Chapter 20
Figures 20–1, 20–2, 20–3, 20–6, 20–7, 20–8, 20–9, 20–10

Chapter 21
Figure 21–9

Chapter 25
Figures 25–6, 25–7, 25–8

Index